Mesothelioma

Mesothelioma

Edited by

Bruce W. S. Robinson MD
*Professor of Medicine, University of Western Australia,
Perth, WA, Australia*

and

A. Philippe Chahinian MD
*Professor, Division of Neoplastic Diseases,
Mount Sinai Hospital, New York, NY, USA*

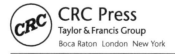

CRC Press
Taylor & Francis Group
Boca Raton London New York

CRC Press is an imprint of the
Taylor & Francis Group, an **informa** business

CRC Press
Taylor & Francis Group
6000 Broken Sound Parkway NW , Suite 300
Boca Raton, FL 33487-2742

First issued in paperback 2019

ISBN-13: 978-90-5823-180-2 (hbk)
ISBN-13: 978-0-367-39637-4 (pbk)

A CIP record for this book is available from the British Library.

Visit the Taylor & Francis Web site at
http://www.taylorandfrancis.com

and the CRC Press Web site at
http://www.crcpress.com

Contents

Contributors

Steven M. Albelda, MD
William Maul Measey Associate Professor of Medicine, Associate Chief, Pulmonary and Critical Care Division, Department of Medicine; and Thoracic Oncology Research Laboratories, University of Pennsylvania Health System, Philadelphia, PA, USA.

Philippe Astoul, MD
Department of Pulmonary Diseases, Hôpital Sainte Marguerite, University of the Mediterranean, Marseille, France.

Eric Bateman, MD(UCT), FRCP
Professor of Respiratory Medicine, Respiratory Clinic, University of Cape Town / Groote Schuur Hospital, Cape Town, South Africa.

Jean Bignon, MD
Service de Pneumologie, Hôpital Intercommunal de Creteil, 40 Avenue de Verdun, 94010 Creteil Cedex, France.

Christian Boutin, MD
UPRES 2050, University of the Mediterranean, Marseille, France.

Robert Bright, MD
Karmanos Cancer Institute, Wayne State University, Detroit, MI 48201, USA.

V. Courtney Broaddus, MD
Associate Professor of Medicine, Lung Biology Center, San Francisco General Hospital, 1001 Potrero Avenue, San Francisco, CA 94110, USA.

Michele Carbone, MD
Cancer Immunology Program, Cardinal Bernardin Cancer Center, Department of Pathology, Loyola Medical School, Maywood, IL 60153, USA.

A. Philippe Chahinian, MD
Professor, Division of Medical Oncology, Mount Sinai School of Medicine, One Gustave L. Levy Place, New York, New York 10029, USA.

Nicholas H. de Klerk, PhD
Child Health Research Institute and Department of Public Health, University of Western Australia, Nedlands, WA 6009, Australia.

Andrew Dean, MD
Palliative Care Physician, Sir Charles Gairdner Hospital, Monash Avenue, Nedlands, WA 6009, Australia.

Susan Fisher
Cancer Immunology Program, Cardinal Bernardin Cancer Center, Department of Pathology, Loyola Medical School, Maywood, IL 60153, USA.

Francoise Galateau-Salle
Department of Pathology, 'MesoPath Group', University of Caen, 140. 033 Caen, Cedex, France

John Gordon
Barrister, c/o Clerk Hyland, Ground Floor, Owen Dixon Chambers, 205 William St, Melbourne, Victoria 3000, Australia.

Alissa K. Greenberg, MD
Division of Pulmonary & Critical Care Medicine and Bellevue Chest Service, New York University School of Medicine, New York, NY 10016, USA.

Douglas Henderson, MBBS, FRCPA, FRCPath
Professor of Pathology, Flinders University of South Australia, and Head of the Department of Anatomical Pathology, Flinders Medical Centre, SA, Australia.

Yunico Iwatsubo
INSERM, U.139 University of Paris, 12 Cetreil 94010, France.

Marie-Claude Jaurand, PhD
Director of Research, Head, INSERM EMI 99.09, Respiratory and Urogenital Oncogenesis, University of Paris XII, France.

Larry Kaiser, MD
John Rhea Barton Professor and Chairman, Department of Surgery, University of Pennsylvania School of Medicine, Philadelphia, PA, USA

Theodore C. Lee, MD
Division of Pulmonary & Critical Care Medicine, and Bellevue Chest Service New York University School of Medicine, New York, NY 10016, USA

Y. C. (Gary) Lee, MD
Senior Registrar, Department of Respiratory Medicine, Sir Charles Gairdner Hospital, Monash Avenue, Nedlands, WA 6009, Australia.

James Leigh, MD, PhD
Head, Research Unit, National Occupational Health and Safety Commission, Coordinator, Australian Mesothelioma Register and Senior Lecturer, Department of Public Health and Community Medicine, University of Sydney, Sydney, NSW 2006, Australia.

Blair R. Mclaren, MD
The Tumor Immunology Group, University Department of Medicine, QEII Medical Centre, Nedlands, WA 6009, Australia.

Sutapa Mukherjee, MD
Research Fellow, Tumour Immunology Group, University Department Medicine, University of Western Australia, Verdun Street, Nedlands, WA 6009, Australia.

A. William Musk, MD
Departments of Respiratory Medicine, Sir Charles Gairdner Hospital, Nedlands, WA 6009, Australia.

Takashi Nakano, MD
Division of Geriatrics and Medical Oncology, Depatment of Internal Medicine, Hyogo College of Medicine, 1-1, Mukogawacho, Nishinomiya, Hyogo 663-8501, Japan.

Harvey I. Pass, MD
Professor of Surgery and Oncology, Wayne State University, and Chief, Thoracic Oncology, Karmanos Cancer Institute, Wayne State University, Detroit, MI 48201, USA.

Amy Powers
Cancer Immunology Program, Cardinal Bernardin Cancer Center, Department of Pathology, Loyola Medical School, Maywood, IL 60153, USA.

Jack G. Rabinowitz, MD
Professor of Radiology (Chair Emeritus), Department of Radiology, Mount Sinai School of Medicine, New York, NY 10029, USA.

Paola Rizzo
Cancer Immunology Program, Cardinal Bernardin Cancer Center, Department of Pathology, Loyola Medical School, Maywood IL 60153, USA

Bruce W. S. Robinson, MD
Professor of Medicine, University Department of Medicine, Sir Charles Gairdner Hospital, Monash Avenue, Nedlands, WA 6009, Australia.

William N. Rom, MD
Division of Pulmonary & Critical Care Medicine and Bellevue Chest Service
New York University School of Medicine, New York, NY 10016, USA.

Amanda Segal, MBBS, FRCPA
Consultant Pathologist, Department of Anatomical Pathology, Western Australian
Centre for Pathology and Medical Research, Perth, WA 6009, Australia.

Keith Shilkin, MBBS, FRCPA, FRCPath, FHKCPath
Consultant Pathologist, Western Australian Centre for Pathology and Medical
Research, and Clinical Professor of Pathology, University of Western Australia,
Perth, WA 6009, Australia.

Joseph B. Shrager, MD
Assistant Professor Of Surgery, Section of General Thoracic Surgery, University of
Pennsylvania School of Medicine, Philadelphia, PA, USA.

Daniel Sterman, MD
Assistant Professor of Medicine, Pulmonary and Critical Care Division, Department
of Medicine; and Thoracic Oncology Research Laboratories, University of
Pennsylvania Health System, Philadelphia, PA, USA.

Richard I. Thompson, MD
Director and Consultant Radiologist, Department of Radiology, Sir Charles
Gairdner Hospital, Monash Avenue, Nedlands, WA 6009, Australia.

Alain J. Valleron
Unite de Recheiches Biomathematiques et Biostatistiques. (INSERM) Faculte de
Medicine.Saint Antoine, 27 Rue Chaligny 75571, Paris Cedex 12, France.

† J. Chris Wagner, MD

Darrel Whitaker, PhD, CFIAC, MAIMS, MRCPath
Consultant Cytologist, Western Australian Centre for Pathology and Medical
Research, Perth, WA 6009, Australia.

Neil White, MD
Associate Professor and Senior Specialist, Respiratory Clinic, University of Cape
Town /Groote Schuur Hospital, and Director, Occupational Medicine Clinical
Research Unit, UCT Lung Institute, PO Box 34560, Groote Schuur, South Africa.

Introduction

Malignant mesothelioma is a 20th century phenomenon and as we begin a new century it is timely to review the clinical, research, epidemiological and legal aspects of this disease.

As a medical student studying pathology around 1970 I can recall only minimal attention being given to mesothelioma. In fact I once reviewed my medical student lecture notes and there were only about three lines of notes on mesothelioma This was the case despite the fact that we were already beginning to see mesothelioma cases in Western Australian following widespread exposure to blue asbestos from the Wittenoom Mine. The situation has changed dramatically since then. Now, all our medical students are aware of the disease mesothelioma – the high frequency of the disease in our clinical departments means that students are exposed to many patients suffering from mesothelioma. Indeed when a patient presents with a pleural effusion and chest wall pain, mesothelioma is often assumed to be the diagnosis until proven otherwise. In addition, the community are well aware of the risks of asbestos exposure following many news reports describing the extent of the industrial tragedy of asbestos. This is particularly the case in Western Australia where the widespread exposure to blue asbestos (crocidolite) from the Wittenoom mine, which operated between 1948 and 1966, has been described as an industrial tragedy of the scale of Bhopal in India. It differs from Bhopal, however, in that the duration of morbidity and mortality is spread over many decades.

The epidemic of mesothelioma has been seen throughout the world, not just in Australia. In Europe mesothelioma has risen up the 'league ladder' of cancers, such that it is no longer considered a rare tumour. In some heavily industrialised parts of the world it is likely that mesothelioma occurs frequently but, in the absence of careful record taking, it is difficult to know for certain what is happening to the incidence of the disease, e.g., in some former Soviet bloc countries. The peak incidence of this disease is not expected to be reached until the next decade or so and, even after the peak is reached, thousands of cases will occur in the following decades because of the widespread exposure of individuals in cities to asbestos in various forms. In addition, it is clear that the pleura is somewhat vulnerable to the development of malignancy and it is possible that agents other than asbestos may cause mesothelioma. For example, the incidence of mesothelioma in farmers has always been assumed to be probably due to their incidental exposure to asbestos on the farm but may in fact be related to their use of potentially carcinogenic chemicals which could be absorbed into the pleural cavity. This is yet to be confirmed but when the main asbestos exposure cases have been clarified, other causes may become obvious.

Detailed study of mesothelioma is important not only in its own right but for a number of other reasons. Firstly, it is an example of an occupational lung disease which has frightening rather than nuisance consequences. In that regard the social and medico-legal aspects of the disease are important to discuss. For every patient who develops mesothelioma, thousands of patients live in fear that the 'sword of Damocles' will fall upon them; i.e. the morbidity extends beyond those individuals who get the disease. In fact some patients suffer profound anxiety and depression knowing that they have been exposed to asbestos and may develop malignancy at some time in the future. In Australia we have been fortunate to have a dedicated group of individuals who have formed a society which not only supports the individuals who are at risk of the disease or who have developed the disease but also act as advocates for these individuals medically and legally. Secondly, malignant mesothelioma has a number of features which make it an ideal 'model' for learning about cancer in general. Because most at-risk individuals can be clearly identified, preventative studies, e.g. using vitamin A, can be undertaken. Also, it is possible to study these individuals to determine if there are any early markers of disease, e.g. serological markers. The fact that mesothelioma is largely untreatable by any of the standard therapeutic modalities (surgery, radiotherapy and chemotherapy) means that a number of centres have been compelled to try novel experimental treatments. In this regard mesothelioma has been an excellent target for immunotherapy protocols, with some success, and has been one of the first tumours treated by gene therapy, either suicide gene therapy or immunological gene therapy.

When we began our research into mesothelioma in the mid-1980s there were very few laboratories studying this disease, few cell lines available, few animal models available and little was known about the basic cell biology underlying the disease. The situation has changed dramatically and there are currently a number of groups studying mesothelioma. An impressive degree of international co-operation exists between these scientists who have met together as the International Mesothelioma Interest Group every two years for the past decade to share scientific and clinical information. This degree of co-operation means that it is much more likely that advances in mesothelioma research will be rapidly disseminated to the medical and scientific community and, most importantly, makes it more likely that cross-fertilisation of ideas will occur which will lead to improvements in the diagnosis, therapy and prevention of this disease.

When I think of mesothelioma research into the 21st century what do I predict? Firstly, I have no doubt that we will, within another decade, have unravelled a lot of the underlying questions relating to mesothelioma pathogenesis. This is a tumour in which fresh tumour cells can be accessed (e.g. via pleural fluid) without a major requirement for manipulation and digestion and this, combined with modern technology such as DNA array procedures, should elucidate the basic mechanisms of carcinogenesis and tumour growth and lead to the identification of crucial molecular targets for clinical studies. In terms of treatment, all of the laboratory and clinical studies so far suggest two things. Firstly, that only a multi-modality approach will be effective, i.e. some combination of surgery, chemotherapy, etc. Secondly, that novel approaches will be required – it is unlikely that the enormous resistance of this disease to standard therapies will change. Even when we understand why mesothelioma is resistant to chemotherapy, it is unlikely that we will be able to develop curative chemotherapy regimes. Therefore the use of immunotherapy, suicide gene therapy, etc., need to be further developed and integrated with these existing therapies in the hope that, within 5 years or so, a multi-modality approach can be developed which is effective for a large proportion of patients in terms of disease-free survival and quality of life.

This book summarises the state of the art of mesothelioma. All the authors are experts in their field and have leadership roles within the international mesothelioma community. We hope that the contents of this book will provide the readers with an up-to-date view of mesothelioma and a platform for understanding future laboratory and clinical studies of this unfortunate disease.

Bruce W. S. Robinson

=1=

The North American Experience with Malignant Mesothelioma

Alissa K. Greenberg, Theodore C. Lee and William N. Rom

Incidence

In the United States

In 1890 Biggs[1] reported a case of 'endothelioma' of the pleura. This report may have been the first recognised case of malignant mesothelioma in North America. Since then the incidence of mesothelioma in North America and the world has steadily climbed.

Studies of the incidence of mesothelioma in North America have been hampered by a paucity of data. Before 1988, the United States did not even have a specific code for mesothelioma, so many cases were misclassified on death certificates as lung cancers or abdominal cancers. In the United States, the best estimates of mesothelioma incidence are derived from the Surveillance, Epidemiology and End Results (SEER) Program of the National Cancer Institute. The SEER database[2] includes about 9.5 per cent of the United States population. It covers 10 regional areas, in five states (Connecticut, Iowa, New Mexico, Utah and Hawaii), and five major urban areas – San Francisco–Oakland, New Orleans, Seattle, Atlanta, and Detroit. Although the SEER regions are reasonably representative of the United States population in terms of demographic and epidemiological factors, the programme may not accurately reflect the country as a whole. It includes some shipbuilding areas, but large urban areas where asbestos was used in manufacturing and construction are underrepresented. The database is organised by case; each case is identified by age, sex, race, date of diagnosis and cancer type. The data for mesothelioma are published only intermittently. However, this database provides the most comprehensive national incidence data available for this disease.

In 1997 Price[3] analysed the SEER data for mesothelioma. He divided the data into five-year age groups in each diagnosis year. He found a consistently higher rate of mesothelioma in men than in women. The rate for women remained relatively constant over the years. On the other hand, the rate for men increased until 1992, when it peaked at 1.9

Supported by grant: M01 RR00096.

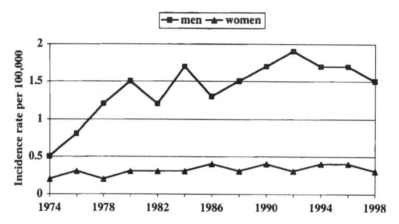

Figure 1.1. *Age-adjusted mesothelioma incidence in the United States. Source: SEER data. Values for 1998 estimated.*

per 100 000 people. Since then the incidence rate in men has been slowly decreasing (Fig. 1.1).[2] This trend is presumably due to occupational asbestos exposure, which was highest during the years 1930–60. The highest lifetime risk was for the 1925–30 birth cohort – a group that would have been at work in shipyards, manufacturing and construction during the years 1930–60. In recent years in the United States, the incidence has been approximately 2000–3000 cases per year, or 11.4 cases per million men and 2.8 cases per million women.[4] The mortality rate in people with prolonged heavy exposure to asbestos varies from 2 to 10 per cent in different studies, and the latency period between initial exposure and manifestation of disease is usually 20–50 years. From 1987 to 1996 an average of 520 people died per year in the United States of malignant mesothelioma.

Data from the United States Department of Health and Human Services[5] show that states with the highest incidence of mesothelioma are all coastal or Great Lakes States. Florida has displaced New York as the State with the highest number of deaths per year from mesothelioma. In 1996, 78 people died of mesothelioma in Florida. The states with the highest age-adjusted mortality rates were Washington and Oregon, probably due to the presence of shipyards. The most frequently recorded occupation on death certificates of people with mesothelioma in the United States was homemaker (10.6 per cent of all deaths), followed by managers and administrators, plumbers, pipefitters and steamfitters, production supervisors, labourers, electricians, farmers, carpenters and machinists. The most common industry was construction, followed by ship building and railroads. Other areas with significant mesothelioma incidence were schools and government.

In Canada

In Canada several large epidemiological studies have provided data for estimates of the incidence of mesothelioma. Morrison and colleagues in 1984[6] looked at all cases of pleural mesothelioma diagnosed in British Columbia from 1973 through 1980 and reported to the National Cancer Incidence Reporting System (NCIRS) of Statistics Canada. They identified 64 cases (54 men and 10 women). Almost all cases were clustered in Cowichan Valley, Capital and Greater Vancouver counties. They noted an overall increasing incidence with age. Among men, but not women, they found an increasing incidence over time, and correlated this with a relatively high level of ship-building and ship repair activity in Vancouver and Victoria thirty to forty years before the study. Similar increased rates of mesothelioma have been observed in shipbuilding centers in the United States and Great Britain. The authors also compared the incidence of mesothelioma obtained from NCIRS data to that obtained by looking at death records. They found that only 60 percent of the cases were identified by looking at mortality data – so death records are therefore a poor substitute for incidence records, since mesothelioma is often not recorded as the cause of death.

In 1985 Churg and colleagues[7] surveyed all pathologists in British Columbia, in an attempt to identify all cases of mesothelioma diagnosed in 1982. Occupational histories were obtained when possible, the pathology slides were reviewed, and when tissue was available the lung was analysed for asbestos content. They identified 19 cases (17 men and 2 women) of confirmed mesothelioma; obtained occupational histories for 16, and analysed lung tissue fibre content in 7. The calculated incidence per year based on their data was 17 cases per million men and 1.9 cases per million women over age 15. Compared with data from 1966–1975, this was a marked increase in the incidence rate for men, but no obvious increase for women – similar to the observations by Price in the United States. Fourteen of fifteen men had a history of occupational asbestos exposure, mostly in shipyards, or in construction or insulation work. In the six men whose lung tissue was analysed, the pulmonary content of chrysotile asbestos was within the range of the general population, but the values for amosite and crocidolite were elevated on average 300-fold compared to a reference population. No commercial amphibole was found in the lungs of the one woman analysed. They concluded that the cases in women may not have been associated with asbestos, and may represent the background non-asbestos associated mesothelioma rate in the general population.

Since the end of 1967, all pathologists in Canada (over 400) have been surveyed periodically to identify all cases of fatal mesothelioma diagnosed at autopsy or biopsy. In 1972 the survey was extended for one year to all pathologists (almost 7000) throughout the United States.[8] On each occasion, nearly all responded. The investigators visited the pathologists and collected material for panel review. They selected a control from the same pathology file with metastatic lung disease from a primary tumor outside the chest, matched for date, sex and age. They also interviewed relatives to obtain detailed residential and occupation histories. As of 1972, there were 344 male cases of mesothelioma; 188 cases compared with 78 controls fell into one of five defined exposure groups. Insulation work showed the highest relative risk at 46.1. Asbestos production and manufacture was next at 6.1. Occupational exposure to asbestos was recorded in only two of 162 female cases, and in no controls. In eight cases and two controls, exposure had been in the home, likely from the clothing of an asbestos worker.

Based on this study, the annual incidence in Canada for 1960 to 1966 was one case per million persons – 1.5 in men and 0.8 in women. For the period 1966–1972 the incidence in Canada was 2.9 per million men and 1.4 per million women; in the United States in 1972 the rates were 2.7 and 0.8 per million. The authors also investigated the effect of neighbourhood exposure. They compared the number of cases and controls who had lived within 20 miles of asbestos mines in Canada and California. They found no increased risk associated with living near chrysotile mines. They also looked at neighbourhoods with asbestos factories. By applying age and sex specific rates found in Canada, the number of mesotheliomas expected was compared with the number observed in various areas. The highest ratio of expected to observed cases was found in the Manville–Somerville area of New Jersey (to be discussed below) where the ratio of observed to expected was 26.5.[9]

Causes of malignant mesothelioma

Asbestos

The adverse effects of asbestos were first observed in the early 1900s and the relationship to mesothelioma was suggested in the 1940s. One of the earliest reports linking mesothelioma to occupational asbestos exposure came out of the medical clinic at an asbestos mine in Canada. At a scientific meeting in 1952 Cartier,[10] then in charge of the industrial medical clinic at Thetford Mines, Quebec, reported eight cases of respiratory cancer, two of which he described as pleural tumors. He declared that two such rare cancers in a small series of only eight cases suggested an occupational origin. By 1960 the scientific community generally recognised asbestos as a cause of mesothelioma.

However, the issue was far from settled. In a national survey of mesothelioma in Canada from 1960 to 1968, McDonald and colleagues[11] found a history of asbestos contact in a relatively small proportion of cases – mostly in insulation and allied trades rather than in the asbestos-producing industry. They surveyed pathologists across the country to find all cases of mesothelioma after 1959. They found 165 cases (111 pleural, 47 peritoneal, 3 both and 4 pericardial). Updates in subsequent years showed a slightly increased association with asbestos exposure, but still lower than expected. When pathologists reviewed the cases[12] the diagnosis was confirmed in only about 50 per cent of the cases, among whom the incidence of asbestos exposure was also higher. A follow-up analysis added a chrysotile mining industry cohort and two small groups of employees in gas mask factories to the survey data. They found 254 fatal cases of mesothelioma (181 men, 73 women) in Quebec from 1960 to 1978. They were able to obtain occupational and residential histories for the majority, and found that only about 40 per cent of the male cases and 5.4 per cent of the female cases were attributable to occupational asbestos exposure (asbestos manufacture, production, insulation, heating trades, shipyards, and construction). Six people probably had household exposure. The intervals between first employment and death from mesothelioma were longer for miners and millers than for manufacturing workers. All the miners and millers had pleural mesothelioma, while the factory workers included 8 with peritoneal mesothelioma. The incidence did not clearly increase over this time period.

Subsequent studies showed an increased percentage of cases attributable to asbestos exposure. Ruffie and colleagues conducted a retrospective study of 332 patients diagnosed with pleural mesothelioma at several teaching hospitals in Ontario and Quebec between 1965 and 1984.[13] They found 396 patients with mesothelioma, including 332 of the pleura. Of the patients with pleural mesothelioma, 262 were men and 70 were women. Ages ranged from 22 to 85 years. About 60 per cent of those with history available had identifiable asbestos exposure. Only 3 were known to have had household exposure and 68 per cent of men and 17 per cent of women had identifiable occupational exposure. With more detailed occupational histories, more exposures may have been found. In Sherbrooke and Quebec City, almost all of the exposed patients came from the asbestos mining areas of Asbestos and Thetford Mines – most working in asbestos processing, as opposed to mining. In Ontario, an important source of exposure was from asbestos-cement factories, where 21 cases were observed in a cohort of 535.[14] Twenty-five per cent of patients with mesothelioma in Ontario were immigrants who had asbestos exposure in their country of origin.

In 1994 Spirtas and colleagues[15] published a study aimed at defining the attributable risk of asbestos exposure in the United States. They used the Los Angeles County Cancer Surveillance Program, the New York State Cancer Registry (excluding New York City), and 39 large Veterans Administration hospitals to identify people diagnosed with mesothelioma from 1975 to 1980. They identified 208 cases of pathologically confirmed mesothelioma. Controls were 533 people who had died of other causes. They interviewed immediate family members to obtain asbestos exposure history. Among men the attributable risk for asbestos exposure was 88 per cent, among women it was 23 per cent (although the confidence interval was very wide at 3–72%). The increasing incidence of mesothelioma in the United States is primarily due to the increased incidence among men, thus probably reflecting more occupational exposure.

Most patients with mesothelioma do have a history of exposure to asbestos, although it may have been brief and remote in time. The variability in percentages of cases with identifiable asbestos exposure may be related to several factors: incomplete history taking, unknown or hidden occupational exposures, or environmental exposure.

Other possible causes

Although it is clear that asbestos causes mesothelioma, other factors also play a role. It is not clear why only a relatively small proportion of people exposed to asbestos develop mesothelioma, or why anywhere from 20 to 60 per cent of people with mesothelioma in different studies lack a known history of asbestos exposure.[16,17] There may be as-yet unidentified cofactors that act as co-carcinogens with asbestos in the induction of mesothelioma.

Evidence that not all cases of mesothelioma are caused by asbestos is threefold. First, we have evidence that a background rate of mesothelioma does exist.[18] Historically, primary malignant tumours of the pleura were recognised by pathologists at autopsy in the late nineteenth century, before the industrial use of asbestos could have been responsible, and without any link to occupation. Epidemiological evidence from mortality statistics for mesothelioma over the past 50 years in the United States and Canada also support a background rate of mesothelioma. Many studies have shown that disease incidence has increased much more rapidly in men than in women, reflecting occupational asbestos exposure among the men. The rate among women has remained relatively stable, indicating that it may be the background rate of mesothelioma. Backward extrapolation suggests that before the diverging pattern began, mortality was about 1–2 per million population in both sexes. This possibility is supported by data from regions with low mesothelioma mortality where both male and female rates are at about this level, and by data for California,[19] after exclusion of occupationally related cases. However, it is also possible that waterborne or airborne fibres originating from naturally occurring asbestos deposits are the cause of this background rate of mesothelioma.

Second, since the latency period after asbestos exposure is normally at least 14 years, the occurrence of malignant mesothelioma in childhood may be evidence of a genetic predisposition, or an environmental exposure which may cause mesothelioma in some cases. In a Canadian survey,[11] from 1960 to 1980, four fatal cases in children were found through systematic inquiry of all pathologists – a rate of about 0.7 per 10 million per annum. A similar figure can be derived from the 13 cases identified by Grundy and Miller[20] from death certificates in the United States from 1965 to 1968. And data from the SEER programme[21] in the United States (1973–84) reveal an incidence among children of about 0.5 per 10 million per year.

Third, lung burden analyses provide some evidence that not all cases are caused by asbestos. In several studies in both the United States and Canada, a certain number of cases could not be attributed to either amphibole or chrysotile fibres. Various other agents have been suggested as additional causes of mesothelioma. A report from India suggested that organic fibres may cause mesothelioma in sugar cane workers. Reports of cases of mesothelioma in sugar cane workers in southern Louisiana[22] provided some support for this hypothesis. After the harvest, the cane is burned off and long, thin, respirable silica fibres form, a process that might also occur after forest fires and other circumstances. Theoretically, these fibres could cause mesothelioma in much the same way that asbestos fibres do.

Reports from Turkey implicate the mineral zeolite, and some suggest there may have been related cases in the region of zeolite deposits in the Rocky Mountain States of North America. The possibility that artificial mineral fibres may play a role in mesothelioma pathogenesis has also been investigated. Three large cohort studies investigated this possibility. They showed no relationship, but exposure levels were very low.

Recently, there has been interest in the possibility that a virus may contribute to the pathogenesis of mesothelioma. Simian virus 40 (SV-40) is a DNA tumour virus that induces tumours identical to mesotheliomas in rodents, and immortalises human mesothelial cells *in vitro*.[23] SV-40-like sequences have been reported in metastatic melanoma, human ependymomas and choroid plexus tumors. In 1994, Carbone and colleagues looked at human mesothelioma, and found SV-40-like DNA sequences in 29 of 48 mesotheliomas studied, and demonstrated simian virus large-T antigen expression in 13 of 16 specimens. Evidence of asbestos exposure was found in 36 of 48 cases. The researchers postulated that an SV-40-like virus might act independently or as a cocarcinogen with asbestos.[24] Several other groups have had similar findings.

This possibility has some significant ramifications for people. SV-40 may have been given to tens of millions of children who received polio vaccines in the 1950s and 1960s. These early polio vaccines, which were produced in Asian macaque kidney cell cultures and were inactivated by formalin, contained variable amounts, usually low titers, of live SV-40 – which is relatively resistant to formalin killing. The oral polio vaccine, mass distributed in the United States in 1963, was SV-40 negative. In addition, recent studies indicate that SV-40 infection may be widespread in the United States population, even among those not exposed to the early polio vaccine.[25] Two recent studies, though not conclusive, suggest that there may be an increased risk of mesothelioma development in the birth cohorts who could have been exposed to the vaccine contaminated with SV-40.[25a] The role of SV-40 in the pathogenesis of malignant mesothelioma is an active area of research, covered elsewhere in this book.

United States and Canadian asbestos use and production

Historically, Canada has been one of the largest asbestos miners, and the United States has been one of the largest asbestos consumers. In 1877 extensive chrysotile asbestos deposits were discovered in eastern Quebec. These areas were developed in the 1880s, and soon half of all the world's asbestos was mined in Canada. A small amount was also mined in the United States. The asbestos industry grew rapidly in the 1930s and 1940s and the use of asbestos in North America was at its peak from the 1950s through 1970. In 1970 the United States used almost a quarter of the asbestos produced throughout the world (Fig. 1.2).

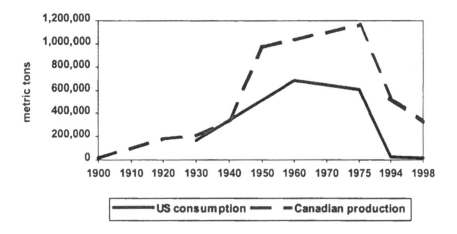

Figure 1.2. *United States consumption and Canadian production of asbestos, 1900–98. Sources: US Bureau of the Census, Natural Resources Canada, Statistics Canada, Quebec Bureau of Mines.*

In contrast to other areas of the world, the United States used predominantly the serpentine chrysotile type asbestos. Approximately 95 per cent of United States consumption has been chrysotile.[26] Currently it accounts for more than 99 per cent of United States asbestos consumption.[27] The United States imported 165 000 tons of chrysotile in 1935 and 650 000 tons in 1962. Crocidolite was used much less, and much later. Less than 500 tons of crocidolite were imported in 1935, and only 20 000 tons by 1962. In 1997, it was reported that 238 tons were imported, but it has been estimated that only 5 tons were used.[27] Small amounts of amosite have also been used in the United States, averaging about 16 000 tons per year in the 1960s.

Starting in 1970, United States consumption of asbestos declined precipitously, largely as a result of mounting evidence of its toxicity. During the early 1970s the number of asbestos lawsuits increased dramatically. World production of asbestos has declined in the 1990s to approximately 2.7 million tons per year – about 50 per cent of the peak production in 1973. Canada is now the second largest miner of asbestos, after Russia. In the United States, consumption of asbestos in 1997 was only 21 000 metric tons.[27]

Workers in various industries in North America were exposed to significant amounts of asbestos. Primary exposure occurred in the mines and mills of Canada, and a few smaller mines in the United States. Secondary exposure occurred for workers involved in the manufacture of asbestos products, including textiles, friction materials, tiles and insulation materials. By far the most significant exposures were in those who then used the asbestos products in construction, insulation work and other capacities. Bystander exposure occurred in those who did not directly work with asbestos but who were present at sites where it was used, as on construction sites. Finally, indirect exposure or household exposure occurred when the asbestos workers wore their dust-covered clothes home and exposed their spouses and children. Particularly significant exposure occurred in the shipbuilding industry during World War II.

Workers born after 1929 may have somewhat lower exposure levels since they have experienced fewer years of exposure at peak asbestos consumption levels, and have benefited from tighter controls on occupational asbestos exposures. Currently the most common uses of asbestos in the United States are in friction products, gaskets and roofing products. The workers most at risk for asbestos exposure now include asbestos removal workers, workers conducting renovations in buildings with asbestos-containing material, and maintenance or custodial workers in buildings with asbestos-containing materials. These exposures, however, are much lower than were the historical occupational exposures.

Occupational exposures and the fibre-type debate

Over the years investigators have looked at the incidence of mesothelioma in different cohorts of workers in North America, attempting to answer several questions about asbestos and mesothelioma. Initially studies were aimed merely at documenting the relationship between asbestos and mesothelioma. Subsequently, debate became heated over whether different types of asbestos fibres were more or less carcinogenic than others – particularly whether the serpentine type (chrysotile) was as carcinogenic as the amphiboles (crocidolite, amosite and tremolite). North America was the perfect forum for this debate, since the mines and mills in Canada seemed to provide a means to study workers exposed only to chrysotile, and in the United States chrysotile has been the predominant exposure. Mossman, Gee, McDonald and Wagner, who favored crocidolite as the sole cause of mesothelioma, squared off against Selikoff, Smith, Cullen and others, who believed that all forms of asbestos were a threat.

Insulators

Asbestos has been used as an insulation material since 1866. In the United States and Canada, until the early 1940s, the only asbestos used was chrysotile, almost exclusively from the Canadian mines. During the 1930s the United States began to use small quantities of amosite asbestos imported from South Africa. Amosite was mixed with chrysotile in making insulation blocks. The insulators likely had heavy though intermittent exposure. Exposures were especially high in shipyards where they ripped out and replaced old asbestos insulation in the confines of boiler rooms and submarine hulls.

The insulators have been a well-organised group. The first insulation workers' union was formed in New York City in 1883 – the "Salamander Association of Boiler and Pipe Felters" (the name came from a story about Marco Polo, who was shown some inflammable cloth while traveling through Siberia, and was told that it was made from salamander's wool). In 1910 the Salamander Association merged with other independent locals in the United States and Canada and became the International Association of Heat and Frost Insulators and Asbestos Workers. The union rolls thus provided the ideal cohort to study the relationship between asbestos and mesothelioma.

In 1962 Selikoff and Hammond conducted a study of a group of 632 asbestos insulation workers in the New York–New Jersey area. These men had been on the union rolls in 1943, and had been exposed to chrysotile asbestos for 20 years or more. They found excess deaths in this group – 253 compared to 195 expected. Mesothelioma had caused 7 deaths. By 1976, 8 per cent had died of mesothelioma. This was one of the first studies providing proof that industrial exposure to asbestos was extremely hazardous.

In 1965 Selikoff and colleagues[28] reviewed the relation between exposure to asbestos and mesothelioma in a study of 307 consecutive deaths among asbestos insulation workers in New York and New Jersey from 1943 to 1964. They surveyed 1522 union members, including every person who had been a member of the local union at any time from 1942 to 1962, and found 10 cases of mesothelioma (4 of the pleura and 6 of the peritoneum) which could be verified by pathological review. The mortality rate was more than 3 per cent. The rate among the general United States population at that time was 3 per million, as determined by a prospective study by the American Cancer Society. They also attempted to calculate the onset and duration of exposure through occupational histories, review of trade practices and union records.

Selikoff and his colleagues then began a prospective study beginning in 1967 of the 17 800 insulators in the United States and Canada who were members of the international union on 1 January 1967. When a member died the investigators were notified and they examined the death certificate and all available clinical data. From 1967 to 1987,[29] of 4951 deaths (3454 expected), they found 458 cases of mesothelioma. The major increase in incidence of mesothelioma occurred more than 20 years after the initial exposure. Almost 10 per cent of deaths were due to mesothelioma, with a particularly high rate of peritoneal disease (173 pleural, 285 peritoneal).

These were landmark studies in occupational medicine, and also lent fuel to the debate over the carcinogenicity of different fibre types. Insulation material initially contained almost exclusively chrysotile from Canada; subsequently amosite was used as well. Crocidolite was not used in insulation materials, although small amounts were used in cement pipes, gaskets and filters. Examination of lung tissue and BAL cells[30] from this group confirmed the absence of crocidolite fibres. Instead, there was a preponderance of chrysotile fibres in mesothelioma tissue, as well as varying amounts of amosite in the rest of the lungs. Therefore the studies in insulators seemed to confirm that fibre types other than crocidolite could cause mesothelioma, and suggested that chrysotile was a potent carcinogen since the rate of malignancy, particularly mesothelioma, among this cohort was so high. However, several questions remained open – the amount of exposure the insulators received was not certain, and whether chrysotile alone could be the culprit in mesothelioma pathogenesis was still unclear.

Miners and millers

The miners and millers of chrysotile asbestos in Canada seemed to be the perfect group in which to pursue these questions, as they were thought to represent a group exposed to only one type of fibre. However, the situation was not so simple. Canada and Russia have produced most of the world's asbestos. Chrysotile asbestos was first mined in 1878 in the Eastern Townships region of Quebec, and is now the overwhelming type mined in Canada. The two main mining areas are now the towns of Asbestos and Thetford. Most of the mines were open pit mines, where 13-metre (40-foot) holes were drilled in asbestos-containing ore deposits, and were then blasted with explosives. Workers loaded the loose ore onto trucks and then transported it to a crushing machine. Moisture was removed by heating the crushed ore in huge dryers. During milling the ore went through stages of screening and vacuum separation in which loose asbestos fibre was lifted from the rock. Conveyor belts, chutes, and vacuum-exhaust pipes transported the ore and fibre through the mills. Most employees worked in the mills, cleaning up spilled asbestos fibre, feeding asbestos into storage bins, and maintaining equipment. Before 1970, only total dust counts were made – asbestos fibre concentrations were not measured separately. Virtually all jobs in this industry were very dusty. In the 1970s asbestos fibre concentrations were measured, and it was found that average asbestos-fibre concentrations were significant, especially in the drying and crushing operation, and greatly exceeded the asbestos standard of 5 fibres per cubic centimetre (5 f/cm^3) of air then in effect in the United States.

Several groups have studied the miners and millers in the Thetford and Asbestos mines over the years. Initially it was thought that this group might reflect exposure only to chrysotile asbestos, and therefore could answer the question of whether chrysotile was carcinogenic by itself. McDonald and colleagues began a comprehensive study of respiratory morbidity and mortality in a cohort of almost 12 000 workers, born between 1891 and 1920, who had worked in the Quebec asbestos industry, including the mines and mills near Asbestos and Thetford. After exclusion of men lost to follow-up, the cohort consisted of 9780 men: 4175 from the main complex of mines and mills of Thetford mines, 4031 in the mine and mill of Asbestos, 708 in the asbestos products factory of Asbestos, and the others from smaller mines in the Thetford region. Initially they found very few deaths due to mesothelioma. Among 2413 male deaths in the cohort as of the end of 1966, there were only three deaths due to mesothelioma.[31] The overall death rate was much lower than that found in other groups.[32,33]

This large cohort of chrysotile miners and millers in Quebec has been followed ever since, with updated results published periodically,[31,34-36] and a review of the data relating to mesothelioma published in 1997.[37] By 1993,[38] almost 80 per cent of the cohort had died, and the youngest survivors were in their mid-70s. From the total of more than 8000 deaths, 38 were probably due to mesothelioma – all except one probably pleural mesothelioma. Thirty-three were miners and millers, and 5 were factory workers. Eight had a history of only minimal known exposure to the asbestos industry, although on further analysis 2 of these were employed in gas mask manufacture, which involved exposure to crocidolite. When the results were analysed further, the investigators found 25 mesotheliomas in Thetford Mines and only 8 in Asbestos. This corresponded to a rate 33.7 versus 13.2 per 100 000 subject years. At the factory in Asbestos where the 708 employees were potentially exposed to crocidolite and/or amosite, there were 5 deaths due to mesothelioma out of a total of 553 deaths – a rate of 46.2 per 100 000 subject years. The cases at Thetford were more common in miners than millers, whereas those at Asbestos were all in millers. Within the Thetford Mines there were geographical differences in the rates of mesothelioma, with a substantially increased risk associated with years of employment in a localised group of 5 mines. The authors felt that this indicated that the explanation might be mineralogical.

Multiple lung tissue analyses were done in some of the cases,[39-42] and revealed that even though these men were exposed overwhelmingly to chrysotile, tremolite fibres predominated in the lungs of the miners and millers, especially those from the region of Thetford mines with the highest incidence of mesothelioma. In the two factory workers and three of the five miners and millers from Asbestos, there were substantial concentrations of crocidolite. The authors concluded that perhaps the chrysotile was not carcinogenic at all, and the cases of mesothelioma were entirely due to the presence of amphiboles – tremolite in the mines and crocidolite in the factory. Churg and colleagues[39] also found high concentrations of chrysotile fibres in the lungs of people with mesothelioma.

However, other studies contradicted the findings of McDonald and colleagues. Begin[43] and colleagues reviewed the 120 cases of mesothelioma that came before the Worker's Compensation Board of Quebec from 1967 to 1990. This was a different database than that used by McDonald and colleagues. The 49 cases from the chrysotile mining and milling area were compared with 50 cases in manufacturing and construction, and

21 cases from industries where asbestos was not a major work material – often an 'incidental' material. The first group had a significantly older mean age with longer exposure time. In the mining towns of Thetford and Asbestos, the incidence of mesothelioma was proportional to the workforce (20 in Asbestos and 29 in Thetford), suggesting that the greater tremolite contamination in Thetford was not a significant factor in causing mesothelioma. Begin reported an incidence of 2.5 cases per year from 1980 to 1990 or 62.5 cases per million per year, and 150–250 cases per million per year among the miners and millers. These numbers were significantly more than those reported by McDonald in his earlier cohort. The number of cases overall increased significantly in the 1960s to 1990s, a time during which most of the McDonald cohort was deceased, suggesting that McDonald's cohort definition may have missed the peak incidence of mesothelioma in Quebec. The longer exposure duration in the cases with mesothelioma is consistent with Churg's finding of increased chrysotile fibres in the lungs of mesothelioma cases.

Nicholson, Selikoff and others[32] also undertook a study of mortality in Canadian miners and millers, in an attempt to determine the carcinogenicity of chrysotile. They tried to define a cohort that would be comparable to previously published cohorts of factory workers and insulation workers. They identified 544 employees who had spent as least 20 years working in the mines and mills in the Thetford area, and found only one case of mesothelioma. The lower rate of mesothelioma found in this study could be due to a variety of factors. Fibre type may play a role, with amphiboles likely somewhat more carcinogenic. However, the difference may also be due to the size or concentration of the fibres inhaled, or it might have just been too early to see the cases of mesothelioma.

Two small cohorts of vermiculite miners in the United States have also been studied,[44] one of which had also experienced substantial exposure to fibrous tremolite. These studies revealed 4 cases among 165 deaths (406 subjects). Notably, these studies were earlier – only 12–21 per cent of the subjects had died.

The shipyards

Currently the highest age adjusted incidence of mesothelioma in the United States is in Washington and Oregon, probably due to the shipbuilding industry. Asbestos exposure in shipyards frequently involves massive exposures of short duration in enclosed spaces, as opposed to the chronic exposure in mining and manufacturing processes. Thus, shipyard workers represent a group where the effects of short-term intense exposure might be seen. Asbestos has been used to insulate the steam pipes and boilers of ships since the turn of the century. The asbestos may be woven in a mattress of cloth and wrapped around piping, applied as a cement-like material, or sprayed as fireproofing. Not only the insulators were exposed – bystander exposure in this situation was probably significant, since the work was done in the enclosed spaces of ship boiler rooms.

Shipyard worker populations fluctuate greatly. In 1918 there were 318 500 shipyard workers in the United States, compared to 75 000 during the 1920s and 1930s. With the approach of World War II, the shipyards underwent a tremendous expansion and shipbuilding became the largest manufacturing industry in the United States for a time. By the end of 1943, 1 722 500 people were employed in shipyards.[45] In some yards between

10 and 20 per cent of these workers were women. Turnover was very high, so it has been estimated that about 4.5 million people were employed in shipyards during World War II. After the war the number of shipyard workers rapidly decreased.

Since no dust counts were taken, no one really knows what levels of asbestos fibre existed. They were likely very high at times. In 1975 the use of asbestos in ship-building and ship repair was largely abandoned. However, ship repair remained a problem because asbestos previously used as insulation on steam pipes and boilers had to be ripped out and replaced during renovation and repair work.

A health survey of 1074 insulation workers in United States shipyards was conducted at the end of World War II. No significant evidence of disease was found. However, this was a little early to come to any conclusion. The risk of asbestos-related disease among shipyard workers was first recognised in England when five cases of mesothelioma were identified among employees of the Royal Navy Dockyard in Devonport. Evidence of asbestos-associated disease has also been reported among workers employed in United States shipyards during and after World War II.

Several studies since have shown high rates of asbestos-associated disease among shipyard workers in Connecticut, San Francisco and Georgia. In the Pacific Northwest, Hinds[46] looked at all death certificates with mesothelioma listed as the cause of death for the years 1968 through 1976 for the Puget Sound region of Washington State. He found 40 cases of mesothelioma, and compared them to matched controls identified from the death files. He found a clear association between mesothelioma and employment in the Puget Sound Naval Shipyard.

Lung burden studies in the Pacific Coast shipyard workers[47] revealed amosite fibres in all cases of mesothelioma. The cases of mesothelioma also seemed to be associated with the presence of low aspect ratio amosite fibres, indicating a possible role for fibre size.

Factory workers

Authors on both sides of the fibre-type debate have investigated factory workers in various industries. In some workplaces, measurements of dust exposure were made, and both the exact fibre type and degree of exposure could be evaluated. Thus these factories proved to be optimal forums to continue the debates over fibre type versus fibre size versus amount of exposure.

In 1967, Enterline and Kendrik[48] conducted a study of the effect of asbestos exposure on factory workers. They recorded the causes of deaths among 21 755 white men aged 15 to 65 who worked in several different asbestos-products plants in the United States at some time during the period 1948 to 1951, identified from social security tax returns filed with the United States Bureau of Internal Revenue for the first quarters of 1948, 1949, 1950 and 1951. Deaths were identified from death claims filed with the social security administration through 1963, and death certificates were reviewed. A cohort of 6281 cotton textile workers was used as a control group for the asbestos textile workers. Among 1853 death certificates examined, only one listed mesothelioma. Although respiratory cancer rates were increased overall, mortality was actually lower than for the general population. At most the follow-up was only 17 years, so the full effect of asbestos exposure had probably not yet been seen.

The amosite factories – Paterson, New Jersey, and Tyler, Texas

Just before the United States entered World War II, an amosite asbestos factory was established in Paterson, New Jersey, to supply the Navy with asbestos insulation for the pipes, boilers and turbines of its ships. Amosite asbestos was used almost exclusively, with very small amounts of chrysotile. Amosite asbestos is mined only in the Transvaal in South Africa, and it had not been studied as much as other fibre types. Thus data concerning its carcinogenic potential were unclear. Since there was no evidence that amosite was carcinogenic, increasing amounts were used to substitute for crocidolite. Before 1930, no amosite was imported into the United States. From 1935 to 1965 imports rose from less than 500 tons to 21 400 tons. Therefore the full effects of exposure to amosite may only be apparent now.

From 1941 through 1945, 933 men worked in the Paterson plant, which continued to operate until 1954. The employees tended to be older, and most worked for only a short time. No dust counts were taken at the factory, but the ventilation system was extremely poor and asbestos fibre concentrations were probably very high. Many of the workers therefore were likely to have had short, intense exposure. These workers were investigated by Selikoff and colleagues beginning in 1972.[49-51] By 1977 they found significantly more deaths than expected, and 14 cases of mesothelioma – 7 pleural and 7 peritoneal. Even those who were employed for short periods were at increased risk of asbestos-related disease.

Longer term follow-up studies for the same factory were published in 1986 and 1988.[52,53] By 1988, of 820 men employed at the Paterson plant for some period between 1941 and 1945, 740 were known to be dead. Mesothelioma was identified in 17 cases (8 pleural, 9 peritoneal), or 2.2 per cent of deaths. The latency period was 20–41 years. The authors noted a rise in incidence until 35 years after exposure, and then a decrease. Those with peritoneal disease tended to have worked longer in the factory. Mortality rate correlated with degree of exposure – both length and intensity.

When the Paterson plant was closed in 1954, the company opened its successor in Tyler, Texas, which remained in operation until 1971. Like the Paterson plant, this factory was one of the few that used only amosite. In this plant, industrial hygiene data are available. Average fibre concentrations ranged from 15.9 to 19.4 f/mL, well above the standard of 5 f/cm^3 then in effect. However, even these levels may not reflect the high levels of dust that existed intermittently. This plant was reported to be one of the dirtiest. In 1971, the National Institute of Occupational Safety and Health inspected the plant and found that thick layers of asbestos dust coated the floors and the ventilation was poor. The dust collection system consisted of canvas bags beneath the roof, which were periodically emptied by shaking, raining huge amounts of asbestos dust inside the plant. Some areas were too dusty to allow accurate fibre counts. The factory was shut down. Employees were followed prospectively to determine adverse effects.

Levin and colleagues[54] found that as of 1993 there were 315 deaths among 1130 former worker from this plant. Six were due to mesothelioma, a rate of 3 per cent, significantly more than in the general population, but less than the rate found in some groups, like Selikoff's insulators.

The experiences at these factories lend support to the concept that the amphiboles have greater ability than chrysotile to cause mesothelioma. But they also indicate that the intensity of exposure is important. Fibre burden analyses have also confirmed the strong association between amosite exposure and mesothelioma. Roggli and colleagues[55] identified amosite asbestos in 81 per cent of 90 cases of mesothelioma. The amosite fibres accounted for 58 per cent of all fibres 5 mm or greater in length.

The chrysotile factories—Manville and Connecticut

One of the largest asbestos plants in the world between 1912 and 1980 was located in Manville, in Somerset County, New Jersey. The plant employed up to 3500 people at one time, and manufactured asbestos products for more than 70 years. The plant primarily used chrysotile asbestos to produce multiple products. Beginning in the 1970s, the factory moved away from using asbestos products. Enterline and Henderson in 1972[56,57] studied a cohort of 1348 men who retired from this company between 1941 and 1967. In the whole group they found only one case of mesothelioma. They published a follow-up report in 1979,[58] which included all deaths up to 1973. For the entire period the cohort had an overall mortality rate 20.4 per cent higher than that of all United States white males. The excess was due almost entirely to cancer and diseases of the respiratory system. They found 5 cases of mesothelioma in the cohort, including one that had been missed previously.

In contrast to Enterline's finding of only a mildly increased incidence of mesothelioma, two reports indicating a marked increase in cases of mesothelioma surfaced from a hospital in the vicinity of the Manville plant. In 1967 a surgeon in Somerset hospital reported 17 cases of mesothelioma (9 pleural and 8 peritoneal) over a three-year period.[59] He explained the high concentration by the close proximity of the asbestos mill, 3 km from the hospital. There was also a large asbestos dump adjacent to a residential area. Radiologists from the same hospital[60] also reported 10 cases, all with some occupational asbestos exposure. Several years later,[61] the surgeons had treated another 36 cases, and searching through the medical records of neighbouring hospitals they found an additional 19 cases, making the total 72. All of the cases where a history was available had an identifiable asbestos exposure in the nearby asbestos mill, except for 2 women who had environmental exposure. Over the years from 1951 to 1972 the incidence increased yearly from 1 per year to 8–9 per year.

The discrepancy between these two studies is easy to explain, and highlights one of the difficulties with epidemiological studies of rare diseases with long latency periods. Enterline's inclusion criteria required that members of the cohort had retired at a certain time, and had lived at least until age 65. They missed all the cases of mesothelioma in people who had already died, or who had not retired.

This plant was also known to be extremely dusty, supporting the theory that the degree of exposure is a determining factor in the incidence of mesothelioma. Employees were quoted in the hospital charts as complaining 'It was like working in a snowstorm', and 'I worked in an asbestos fog 20 minutes daily for 22 years'.[60]

In 1984 McDonald and colleagues[62] conducted a study of 3641 workers employed for one month or more in a friction products plant in Connecticut from 1938 to 1958.

Like the Manville plant, this factory also used almost exclusively chrysotile asbestos. By 1983, of 3513 employees traced, 1267 had died; death certificates were obtained for 1228. No cases of mesothelioma were identified. The authors suggest that these results support the amphibole hypothesis. However, exposures to asbestos in this plant were probably very low since there were no deaths attributed to asbestosis, which is a disease marker for high exposures.

Textile factories

The textile factories present another interesting situation. These factories mostly used chrysotile from Canada, and yet in several studies the workers in these factories had a much higher incidence of lung cancer than the miners and millers in Quebec. The rates of mesothelioma seemed more comparable. Three possible explanations for the discrepancy in cancer rates have been given. First, perhaps the factory workers were also exposed to significant amounts of amphiboles. Second, the chrysotile bundles may be broken up and in a more respirable form by the time they reach the factories. Third, the textile factories may be significantly dustier than the mines and mills of Quebec.

An asbestos textile plant in Charleston, South Carolina, began production of asbestos products in 1896, and of asbestos textiles in 1909. Chrysotile was the only type of asbestos used. In this plant, major engineering controls to reduce asbestos exposures were in place by 1940. Production of asbestos textiles ceased in the late 1970s. Dement and colleagues[63] studied a cohort of 1261 white men employed for one month or more between 1940 and 1965. They followed them until 1991. By that time half the cohort had died, and there were 74 lung cancers, and 3 cases of mesothelioma.[64] This corresponded to a rate of about 3 in 1000 deaths compared with 5 in 1000 in the Quebec miners and millers cohort.[37] On the basis of historical air-sampling data, the investigators found a steep lung cancer exposure–response relationship, and noted that textile fibres appear to be considerably longer than airborne fibres measured in mining and milling.

A similar study was performed at a textile plant in Manheim, Pennsylvania,[65] with the same owners as the Charleston plant. The plant used mainly chrysotile, but also small quantities of amosite and crocidolite. The exposure–response relationship for lung cancer mortality was virtually identical to that in Charleston, but there were at least 14 cases of mesothelioma, as opposed to only one during the same time period in Charleston. This increased incidence of mesothelioma may have been due to the presence of amphiboles in this plant; however, it may also have been related to the significantly dustier conditions in Manheim. It was reported to be very dusty until the 1930s, when wetting, improved handling methods and ventilation hoods were added. Mesothelioma incidences were shown to be higher in the dustier plants and in those with increased levels of amphiboles. So the fibre-type question continued as a point of debate.

Crocidolite factories – cement, gas masks and cigarette filters

Crocidolite asbestos was used sparingly in North America. Three industries, however, were known to use significant amounts of crocidolite, and have been studied to determine the effects of amphibole exposure.

A substantial portion of the asbestos produced worldwide has been used in the asbestos cement industry to make construction products. Exposures in this field have most often been to mixed fibre types – chrysotile, crocidolite and amosite. Hughes and Weill in 1986[66,67] conducted a prospective mortality study on 6931 employees of two asbestos cement plants in New Orleans, Louisiana. In plant 1 there was minimal amphibole exposure; in plant 2 crocidolite was used regularly. Up to 1984, 10 mesotheliomas had occurred, 2 from plant 1, and 8 from plant 2. In plant 2 a case-control analysis found a relation between risk of mesothelioma and duration of employment and proportion of time spent in the pipe areas, thus adding to the evidence of a greater risk of mesothelioma from crocidolite than from chrysotile.

Finkelstein described similar findings in an asbestos cement factory in Ontario.[68,69] In a cohort of 535 workers hired before 1960, employed for at least one year, and followed until 1990, he found 19 pathologically verifiable cases of mesothelioma. This factory began production in 1948, manufacturing asbestos-cement pipe in one shed and rock-wool or fibreglass insulation in another; asbestos cement board was produced in a third building. Both chrysotile and crocidolite asbestos were used, except in the board operation where only chrysotile was used. Incidence of mesothelioma seemed to increase with increasing cumulative exposure in areas of the plant where crocidolite was used.

During World War II a gas mask assembly plant opened in Ottawa, Canada. The masks used crocidolite filter pads. These pads were delivered to the assembly plant in Ottawa, unpacked in a large room, reduced to the correct weight by removing some of the surface layer, put into canisters and tested. There was no special exhaust ventilation. The plant was in operation from 1939 to 1945, but asbestos was used only until 1942. By 1975,[70] of 199 people who worked in this factory during the relevant time periods, there were 56 deaths, 11 from mesothelioma. These results were compared with the cohort of Quebec miners and millers and the rate of malignancy was much higher in the gas mask workers exposed to crocidolite.

In the United States from 1951 to 1957 a company near Boston manufactured cigarette filters using crocidolite asbestos. Using a dry process, the fibres were mechanically mixed with cotton and acetate fibres and then deposited on crêpe paper. This was an extremely dusty process in contrast to the conventional wet process in which asbestos was added to a pulp. This was also a particularly dirty factory with crocidolite asbestos on window sills and in the corners, and 16 years after the plant closed Rom[26] found an open burlap bag half full of crocidolite asbestos in the middle of the plant floor.

Measurements at six production locations in 1952 showed an average of 80 particles of asbestos dust per millilitre of air, which was below the then-current Massachusetts standard but well above current standards. In 1989 Talcott and colleagues published a report detailing the marked excess in mortality and morbidity from asbestos-related diseases in a cohort of 33 workers who made these filters.[71] By the end of the study period in 1988, 28 had died, 5 were diagnosed with malignant mesothelioma, 11 had lung cancer and 19 had asbestosis. Mesothelioma accounted for 18 per cent of the observed deaths. Several factors were probably involved in the high rate of mesothelioma. The predominant exposure to crocidolite, as well as the extremely dusty nature of the industrial process, may have both played roles.

In these two crocidolite factories, the rates of mesothelioma were very high. However, once again, the plants were both extremely dusty with poor ventilation. Again it was difficult to prove whether it was the fibre type or the degree of exposure which produced the markedly increased incidence of mesothelioma.

Construction industry

In the past, the construction industry accounted for an estimated 70–80 per cent of total United States consumption of asbestos fibre, and an enormous number of workers in various construction trades have been exposed to varying amounts of asbestos. From 1958 to 1973, until the Environmental Protection Agency abolished the practice, asbestos fireproofing material was sprayed in more than half the multistoried buildings constructed in the United States. About 25 per cent of the sprayed material would fail to adhere, and was released into the air. All workers on the site during and after the spraying were exposed. Thirty per cent of the water distribution pipe sold in the United States in 1974 was asbestos cement.

A mortality study of the members of the union of plumbers and pipefitters in the United States found significant excesses in proportional mortality ratios for malignancies, including 7 deaths due to mesothelioma.[72] Two studies of sheet-metal workers in New York City found significantly increased mortality, and mesothelioma was recorded on death certificates in 9 out of 716 total deaths (1.3 per cent).[73,74] Studies in construction workers are difficult since specific exposures often are not known, and workers change jobs frequently. Epidemiological studies, however, consistently show that construction workers are one of the groups most at risk for asbestos-related disease and mesothelioma.

Miscellaneous exposed groups

Several other groups in North America have been studied to determine the effects of asbestos exposure. Railroad machinists were exposed to significant amounts of mostly chrysotile asbestos, especially during the application and removal of asbestos insulation on the boilers of steam locomotives. The last steam engine repairs took place in the late 1950s. In 1988 Mancuso[75] published a study investigating the risk of mesothelioma among railroad machinists. His cohort was railroad machinists employed by a company before 1935, and still alive in 1945. He analysed the data for 181 people hired from 1920 to 1929. By 1986, 156 were identified as dead. There were 41 cancer deaths, 14 with mesothelioma. The relative risk was 1 mesothelioma in every 13 machinists hired. Similarly, in 1986 Schenker et al.[76] completed a case-control analysis of mesothelioma among United States railroad employees. The United States Railroad Retirement Board notified investigators of all deaths among male railroad workers occurring in 1981–82. They reported 15 059 deaths during the study year. Twenty cases of mesothelioma were identified. More cases occurred among the workers in asbestos-exposed job categories. The latency period was 30 years or more.

In the jewellery industry, asbestos has been used to make soldering forms. There have been case reports of mesothelioma among jewellery workers.[77] However, Dubrow and Gute[78] reported no cases of mesothelioma among 3141 Rhode Island jewellery workers who died during the decade 1968–78. This may have been a premature conclusion, since asbestos was not used in this industry in any significant amount until the 1940s. A cluster of 5 silversmiths with mesothelioma has also been observed in a Native American pueblo of 2000, where asbestos had been routinely used in the production of silver jewellery.[79]

After years of dispute, many of the investigators have come to some agreement: that amphiboles and particularly crocidolite are probably more carcinogenic than serpentines, but at high enough exposure levels, all the fibre types can cause mesothelioma.

Non-occupational exposure

Several studies have documented that non-occupational exposure to asbestos is also associated with mesothelioma. Given that chrysotile is thought to be less carcinogenic than the amphiboles, the question was then raised as to whether the low levels of exposure seen with non-occupational situations can cause mesothelioma or other asbestos-related diseases.

Researchers at Mt Sinai Hospital in New York City studied the health experience of 679 household contacts of the 1664 workers employed at the Paterson, New Jersey, factory between 1941 and 1954. They discovered 5 cases of mesothelioma in family members of factory workers. Asbestos dust was also found in the homes of former Paterson factory workers 20 years after the factory was shut down. There was some indication that both the occurrence of mesothelioma and the length of the latent period were dose related.

The impact of neighbourhood asbestos exposure has also been investigated in relation to the Paterson factory. In 1979, Hammond and Selikoff[80] traced 2447 men who were living within 800 metres of the factory in 1942, and compared them to residents of a neighbourhood a few kilometres away. They found that dust samples collected from houses located near the asbestos factory contained appreciable amounts of asbestos fibre even many years after the factory closed. So far, however, they have not reported any increased mortality.

In 1996, Berry[81] published a study of the incidence of mesothelioma in Somerville County, New Jersey, the location of the Manville asbestos plant. This plant produced multiple asbestos products, primarily (95 per cent) using chrysotile asbestos. A previous study in 1987 indicated that the rate of mesothelioma was significantly higher in Somerset County than in the rest of New Jersey. Berry expanded on this study. He used the New Jersey State Cancer Registry to identify cases of mesothelioma from 1979 through 1990, and compared the incidence rates in Manville, Somerset County excluding Manville, and the rest of New Jersey. He then excluded all who worked at the Manville plant.

He found that there were 1358 newly diagnosed mesotheliomas reported to the New Jersey State Cancer Registry during this period; 143 were identified as residents of Somerset County, and 55 of those were Manville residents. The total New Jersey rate of mesothelioma was slightly higher than SEER estimates for the nation as a whole, and the rate in Somerset County was four times higher, and the Manville rate about 25 times higher than the state as a whole. Of the 143 cases in Somerset County, 61 were identified as having worked in the Manville plant. This left 82 with no evidence of employment in the plant. Twenty-four of these were residents of Manville. Mesothelioma incidence in Manville residents who did not work at the plant was significantly elevated for both men and women relative to average state rates. Manville women had the highest standardised incidence rate for mesothelioma at 22.4 (95 per cent CI: 9.7–44.2); the rate for men was 10.1 (95 per cent CI: 5.8–16.4).

Presumably these increased incidence rates were due to household exposure as well as ambient air exposure. The study design did not allow for differentiation between the two. Anecdotal information from residents and plant employees indicated that the asbestos-manufacturing operation in Manville produced large quantities of particles that were released daily into the air, regularly coating houses, trees and yards in the surrounding area, like a fresh snowfall.[82] This study clearly showed that relatively high ambient levels of asbestos could also cause mesothelioma.

The mining region of Quebec is an area with high ambient levels of asbestos, and several studies have investigated whether residents of this area who do not work in the mines and mills, or live with someone who does, have an increased risk of asbestos-related disease. Between 1891 and 1980, asbestos dust emissions and fallout were usually visible. Asbestos aerosols were similar in make-up to those found in North American cities today – more than 98 per cent were chrysotile. Measurements of ambient chrysotile asbestos concentrations in these areas[83] have shown them to be approximately 250 to 500 times that of most North American cities.

Fibre-burden studies[84] have shown that long-term (more than 25-year) residents of the Thetford mines area had increased concentrations of chrysotile and tremolite in their lungs, compared with residents of Vancouver who served as controls. Churg compared 7 autopsy lung specimens of long-term residents of Thetford Mines with 20 long-term chrysotile industry workers and 20 male residents of Vancouver older than 50 years autopsied during the same period. He found that the Thetford residents had median concentrations of chrysotile and tremolite of about one-fiftieth of the chrysotile workers, but about 10 times that of the population of Vancouver.

However, in the past, several epidemiological studies of people living in the mining towns of eastern Quebec have not demonstrated an excess of respiratory diseases.[8,83,85,86] Most recently, a study by Camus and colleagues[87] looked at the mortality rates of women in this area in order to evaluate the risk of environmental asbestos exposure. They determined the number of deaths among women older than 30 between 1970 and 1989 in this area, compared with other areas of Quebec, excluding shipbuilding areas and a large city. They estimated asbestos exposure for the study population, looking at neighbourhood exposure resulting from emissions from asbestos mining or milling, household exposure resulting from dust brought home by asbestos workers, and occupational exposure. Their estimates of asbestos exposure were based on multiple sources of information: historical ambient dust measurements, annual mine production information, emission controls and locations of exhaust pipes, topographical maps, directional distribution of winds, a survey of 817 elderly residents, and autopsy studies of asbestos lung burdens. Then an international panel of five experts analysed the data to estimate average neighbourhood exposure levels in the three main mining towns.

They estimated that average annual ambient levels peaked at 1 fibre per millilitre or more (fibres longer than 5 micrometres) between 1940 and 1954. They also estimated that the 3 main towns were 7 to 20 times more polluted than other towns in the mining areas. Cumulative exposure for these women was estimated by multiplying years of exposure by the estimated asbestos levels for the year and town in which each woman had lived. Household and occupational exposures were also calculated. These data were extrapolated to the population as a whole. They estimated that neighbourhood exposure represented about 65 per cent of the population's average cumulative exposure, household exposure about 30 per cent and occupational exposure about 5 per cent. The average cumulative level of exposure was 25 fibre years per millilitre. They found no significant increased risk of lung cancer among the exposed population. However, they did find an increased risk of mesothelioma and asbestosis. There were 7 deaths due to mesothelioma. The authors plan to investigate this more fully. The numbers may be even higher, since historical death certificates reflect the incidence of mesothelioma poorly.

This study still does not settle the question of whether ambient chrysotile was to blame for the cases of mesothelioma. Churg et al.[84] had earlier observed elevated levels of amosite and crocidolite asbestos in three women who died of mesothelioma and who had not worked in the mines or mills. However, 2 had worked in asbestos bag repair. The third had an unknown source of exposure. Other women who did not work in the mills and mines may have worked in gas mask manufacture. So these three actually were likely occupational. And some have argued that this may also be the case for the 7 women in the Camus study.

In the 1980s, after labour union campaigns and government regulations had greatly reduced occupational exposure to asbestos in North America, attention turned to environmental exposure. Concentrations of asbestos in the air of United States cities range from 1 to 100 nanograms per cubic metre (ng/m^3); the average is 3.62 ng/m^3. The highest concentrations have been found in New York City. The fibre type is mostly very short chrysotile fibres. There is no convincing data that this amount of asbestos in general urban air pollution poses any risk. Mortality among women in North America and Western Europe has shown little or no increase during the last 20–30 years, despite the contribution of occupational and household exposure, and the greater awareness by physicians and pathologists of mesothelioma in the same period.

However, some authors and public health authorities have postulated that this degree of environmental exposure is significant. They point to the significant percentages of people in epidemiological studies who have no identifiable occupational exposure. They also base their concerns on extrapolations of dose–response relationships seen in occupational studies. In 1983, Enterline[88] published an estimate, based on these premises, that one-third of all cases of mesothelioma that occur yearly in the United States are related to environmental asbestos exposure, giving a lifetime risk of 100 per million population. The validity of using occupational data to estimate the risk of asbestos-related diseases in the general population is debatable.

Fibre-burden studies have also fueled the concern that ambient levels of asbestos fibres pose a risk, since they have been able to document some cases of mesothelioma with only scant asbestos fibres in the lungs, indicating minimal exposure. Chen and Mottet reported a case of a patient with no known exposure but with a few asbestos fibres identified in the lung at autopsy, indicating that in some people minimal environmental exposure may be sufficient to cause mesothelioma.[89]

Several other issues related to asbestos have created concerns in North America. In 1972 it was discovered that mineral fibres similar to amosite asbestos were contaminating drinking water supplies drawn from Lake Superior. The source was traced to Silver Bay, a town on Lake Superior where taconite ore mined in the Mesabi Range is processed and iron is extracted. The leftover tailings were then dumped as slurry into an artificial delta in the lake. Fibres occur in many other bodies of waters, particularly in mining regions, and have not yet been shown to pose a health risk.[90]

Around the same time warnings surfaced that asbestos might pose a hazard in schools. Asbestos pollution was found in a grade school in Wyoming, a university dormitory in California, and a library at Yale University. As many as 10 000 United States schools may have asbestos products. Again, the degree of threat is not known. However, cases of mesothelioma in young people may reflect exposure in school or at home. In 1972 the National Cancer Institute reported 12 cases of mesothelioma in people under the age of 20 in the United States between 1960 and 1968.

The future

After Selikoff's 1962 study little was done to try to limit workers' asbestos exposure. Asbestos fireproofing material was still sprayed on the steel girders of high-rise buildings, asbestos was still used in ceilings and walls in school buildings, shipyards were still filled with asbestos dust, and the industry made few attempts to control dust in plants and factories. Workers could sometimes be found working in asbestos dust clouds. It was not until the 1970s that asbestos-dust control measures were enforced in the United States and Canada, and around the same time most industries began to switch to alternative materials whenever possible.

Given the latency period of 20–30 years for the development of mesothelioma after asbestos exposure, we should now be passing the peak of mesothelioma incidence in North America. The latest SEER data confirm that mesothelioma incidence is likely decreasing. Based on SEER data, Price[3] estimates that we should now have reached the peak incidence of about 2300 cases per year. He projects that the number of female cases will remain constant at approximately 500 per year in the United States, and that the male cases will begin to decline and reach 500 cases per year by 2055.

Estimating the population at risk for asbestos-related disease is difficult – the precise number of people occupationally exposed at any given time is not known, nor is the level of exposure necessary to increase the risk of mesothelioma. Estimates in the past of what the rate would be in the year 2000 have ranged widely from 900 a year to 3000 per year. The consensus is that the peak incidence of mesothelioma in Canada and the United States is likely past.

However, there is still active debate over whether the buildings constructed with asbestos in the past now pose a significant risk. As these buildings begin to age and crumble, will there be a 'third wave' of asbestos disease among maintenance workers, demolition and construction crews, and the general populace who use these buildings? [91] In addition, although Canada and the United States have markedly reduced their use of asbestos, and instituted tight controls on exposure levels when it is used, this is not the case in the rest of the Americas. Mexico has been using increasing amounts of asbestos in construction products. Their imports of asbestos from Canada have risen markedly over the last few years.[92] Given the limited regulation of the construction industry in Mexico and other Central and South American countries, workers are likely being exposed to significant amounts of asbestos fibres, the results of which will not become apparent for another 2 or 3 decades.

References

1. Biggs, H. *Proc N Y Pathol Soc* 1890; p.119.
2. National Cancer Institute. Surveillance, epidemiology, and end results cases diagnosed 1977–1998. Submission cancer public use database. Bethesda, MD: United States Department of Health and Human Services, 1999.
3. Price, B. Analysis of current trends in United States mesothelioma incidence. *Am J Epidemiol* 1997; **145**: 211–218.
4. Antman, Pass, Delaney, Rect. *Cancer: Principles and Practice of Oncology, 4ᵗʰ ed.* De Vita, V.T., Hellman, S., Rosenberg, S (ed,). Lippincott Press: Philadelphia, 1498–1508.
5. United States Department of Health and Human Services, Public Health Service, Centers for Disease Control and Prevention, Work-Related Lung Disease Surveillance Report 1999.
6. Morrison, H.I., Band P.R., Gallagher, R., *et al.* Recent trends in incidence rates of pleural mesothelioma in British Columbia. *Can Med Assoc J* 1984; **131**: 1069–1071.
7. Churg, A. Malignant mesothelioma in British Columbia in 1982. *Cancer* 1985; **55**: 672–674.
8. McDonald, A.D., McDonald, J.C. Malignant mesothelioma in North America. *Cancer* 1980; **46**: 1650–1656.
9. McDonald, J.C., McDonald, A.D. Epidemiology of mesothelioma from estimated incidence. *Prev Med* 1977; **6**: 426–446.
10. Cartier, P. Abstract of discussion. *Arch Ind Hyg Med* 1952; **5**: 262.
11. McDonald, A.D., Harper, A., El Attar, O.A., McDonald, J.C. Epidemiology of primary malignant mesothelial tumours in Canada. *Cancer* 1970; **26**: 109–112.
12. McDonald, A.D., Magner, D., Eyssen, G. Primary malignant mesothelial tumors in Canada, 1960–1968. A pathological review by the mesothelioma panel of the Canadian tumor reference centre. *Cancer* 1973; **31**: 869–876.
13. Ruffie, P., Feld, R., Minkin, S., *et al.* Diffuse malignant mesothelioma of the pleura in Ontario and Quebec: a retrospective study of 332 patients. *J Clin Oncol* 1989; **7**: 1157–1168.
14. Finkelstein, M.M. Mortality among employees of an Ontario asbestos-cement factory. *Am Rev Respir Dis* 1984; **129**: 754–761.
15. Spirtas, R., Heineman, E.F., Bernstein, L., *et al.* Malignant mesothelioma: attributable risk of asbestos exposure. *Occup Environ Med* 1994; **51**: 804–811.

16. Roggli, V.L. *Malignant Mesothelioma*. Henderson, Shilkin, LeLanglois, Whitaker (eds), The Cancer Series, Hemisphere Press, New York, 1982, pp. 201–250.
17. Shepherd, K.E., Oliver, L.C., Kazemi, H. Diffuse malignant pleural mesothelioma in an urban hospital: clinical spectrum and trend in incidence over time. *Am J Ind Med* 1989; **16**: 373–383.
18. McDonald, J.C., McDonald, A.D. Mesothelioma: Is there a background? *Eur Respir Rev* 1993; **3**: 71–73.
19. Peto, J., Henderson, B.E., Pike, M.C. Trends in mesothelioma incidence and the forecast epidemic due to asbestos exposure during World War II. In: Peto, R., Schneiderman, M., (eds). *Quantification of Occupational Cancer. Banbury Report 9*. Cold Spring Harbor, NY, 1981; pp. 51–72.
20. Grundy, G.W., Miller, R.W. Malignant mesothelioma in childhood. Report of 13 cases. *Cancer* 1972; **30**: 1216–8.
21. Cooper, S.P., Fraire, A.E., Buffler, P.A., *et al*. Epidemiologic aspects of childhood mesothelioma. *Pathol Immunopathol Res* 1989; **8**: 276–86.
22. Rothschild, H., Mulvey, J.J. An increased risk for lung cancer mortality associated with sugar cane farming. *J Natl Cancer Inst* 1982; **68**: 755–760.
23. Ke, Y., Reddel, R.R., Gerwin, B.I., *et al*. Establishment of a human in vitro mesothelial cell model system for investigating mechanisms of asbestos-induced mesothelioma. *Am J Pathol* 1989; **134**: 979–91.
24. Carbone, M., Pass, H.I., Rizzo, P., *et al*. Simian virus 40-like DNA sequences in human pleural mesothelioma. *Oncogene* 1994; **9**: 1781–1790.
25. Rizzo, P., Bochetta, M., Powers, A., *et al*. SV40 and the pathogenesis of mesothelioma. *Semin Cancer Biol* 2001; **11**: 63–71.
25a. Fischer, S.G., Weber, L., Carbone, M. Cancer risk associated with simian virus 40 contaminated polio vaccine. *Anticancer Res* 1999; **19**: 2173–2180.
26. Rom, W.N. Asbestos related diseases. *Environmental and Occupational Medicine*. In: Third Edition. Ed W.N. Rom. Lippincott-Raven Publishers, Philadelphia, 1998.
27. Virta, R.L. Asbestos, US Geological Survey – Minerals Information – 1997.
28. Selikoff, I.J., Churg, J., Hammond, E.C. Relation between exposure to asbestos and mesothelioma. *N Engl J Med* 1965; **272**: 560–565.
29. Selikoff, I.J., Seidman, H. Asbestos associated deaths among insulation workers in the United States and Canada, 1967 to 1987. *Ann N Y Acad Sci*, **643**: 1–14.
30. Kohyama, N., Suzuki, Y. Analysis of asbestos fibers in lung parenchyma, pleural plaques and mesothelioma tissues of North American insulation workers. *Ann N Y Acad Sci* 1991; **643**: 27–52.
31. McDonald, J.C., McDonald, A.D, Gibbs, G.W., *et al*. Mortality in the chrysotile asbestos mines and mills of Quebec. *Arch Environ Health* 1974; **28**: 61–68.
32. Nicholson, W.J., Selikoff, I.J., Seidman, H., *et al*. Long term mortality experience of chrysotile miners and millers in Thetford Mines, Quebec. *Ann N Y Acad Sci* 1979: **330**: 11–21.
33. McDonald, J.C., McDonald, A.D. The epidemiology of mesothelioma in historical context. *Eur Respir J* 1996; **9**: 1932–1942.
34. McDonald, J.C., Liddell, F.D. Mortality in Canadian miners and millers exposed to chrysotile. *Ann N Y Acad Sci* 1979; **330**: 1–9.
35. Liddell, D. Cancer mortality in chrysotile mining and milling: exposure–response. *Br Occup Hyg* 1994; **38**: 519–523.
36. Liddel, F.D.K., McDonald, A.D., McDonald, J.C. The 1891–1920 birth cohort of Quebec chrysotile miners and millers: developments from 1904 and mortality to 1992. *Ann Occup Hyg* 1997; **41**: 13–36.

37. McDonald, A.D., Case, B.W, Churg, A., *et al*. Mesothelioma in Quebec chrysotile miners and millers: epidemiology and aetiology. *Ann Occup Hyg* 1997; **41**: 701–719.
38. McDonald, J.C, Liddell, F.DK., Dufresne, A., McDonald, A.D. The 1891–1920 birth cohort of Quebec chrysotile miners and millers: mortality 1976–1988. *Br J Ind Med* 1993; **50**: 1073–1081.
39. Churg, A., Wright, J.L., Vedal, S. Fiber burden and patterns of asbestos related disease in chrysotile miners and millers. *Am Rev Respir Dis* 1993; **143**: 25–31.
40. Case, B., Churg, A., Dufresne A, *et al*. Lung fibre content for mesothelioma in the 1891–1920 birth cohort of Quebec chrysotile workers: a descriptive study. *Ann Occup Hyg* 1997; **41**: 231–236.
41. Pooley, F.D. An examination of the fibrous mineral content of asbestos lung tissue from the Canadian chrysotile mining industry. *Environ Res* 1976; **12**: 281–298.
42. Churg, A., DiPaoli, L., Kempe, B., Stevens, B. Lung asbestos content in chrysotile workers with mesothelioma. *Am Rev Respir Dis* 1984; **130**: 1042–1045.
43. Begin, R., Guntier, J.J., Desmeules, M., Ostguy, G. Work-related mesothelioma in Quebec, 1967–1990. *Am J Ind Med* 1992; **222**: 531–542.
44. McDonald, J.C., McDonald, A.D., Armstrong, B., Sebastien, P. Cohort study of mortality in vermiculite miners exposed to tremolite. *Br J Ind Med* 1986; **43**: 436–444.
45. Bureau of Labor Statistics, 1945; United States Department of Commerce, 1952.
46. Hinds, M.W. Mesothelioma in shipyard workers. *West J Med* 1978; **128**: 169–170.
47. Churg, A., Vedal, S. Fiber burden and patterns of asbestos-related disease in workers with heavy mixed amosite and chrysotile exposure. *Am J Respir Crit Care Med* 1994; **150**: 663–669.
48. Enterline, P.E, Kendrick, M.A. Asbestos-dust exposures at various levels and mortality. *Arch Environ Health* 1967; **15**: 181–186.
49. Selikoff, I.J, Hammond, E.C., Churg, J. Carcinogenicity of amosite asbestos. *Arch Environ Health* 1972; **25**: 183–186.
50. Selikoff, I.J, Hammond, E.C, Churg, J. Mortality effects of cigarette smoking among amosite asbestos factory workers. *J Natl Can Inst* 1980; **65**: 507–513.
51. Seidman, H., Selikoff, I.J., Hammond, E.C. Short-term asbestos work exposure and long-term observation. *Ann N Y Acad Sci* 1979; **330**: 61–89.
52. Ribak, J., Seidman, H., Selikoff, I.J. Amosite mesothelioma in a cohort of asbestos workers. *Scand J Work Environ Health* 1989; **15**: 106–110.
53. Seidman, H., Selikoff, I.J., Gelb, S.K. Mortality experience of amosite asbestos factory workers: dose–response relationships 5–40 years after onset of short-term work exposure. *Am J Ind Med* 1986; **10**: 479–514.
54. Levin, J.L., McLarty, J.W., Hurst, G.A., *et al*. Tyler asbestos workers: mortality experience in a cohort exposed to amosite. *Occup Environ Med* 1998; **55**: 155–160.
55. Roggli, V.L, Pratt, P.C., Body, A.R. Asbestos fiber type in malignant mesothelioma: an analytical scanning electron microscopic study of 94 cases. *Am J Ind Med* 1993; **23**: 605–614.
56. Enterline, P, DeCoufle, P., Henderson, V. Mortality in relation to occupational exposure in the asbestos industry. *J Occup Med* 1972; **14**: 897–903.
57. Enterline, P.E., Henderson, V. Type of asbestos and respiratory cancer in the asbestos industry. *Arch Environ Health* 1973; **27**: 312–317.
58. Henderson, V.L, Enterline, P.E. Asbestos exposure: factors associated with excess cancer and respiratory disease mortality. *Ann N Y Acad Sci* 1979; **330**: 117–126.
59. Borow, M., Conston, A., Livornese, L.L., Schalet, N. Mesothelioma and its association with asbestosis. *JAMA* 1967; **201**: 93–97.
60. Demy, N.G., Adler, H. Asbestosis and malignancy. *Am J Roentgenol* 1967; **C**: 597–602.

61. Borow, M., Conston, A., Livornese, L., Schalet, N. Mesothelioma following exposure to asbestos: a review of 72 cases. *Chest* 1973; **64**: 641–646.
62. McDonald, A.D., Fry, J.S, Woolley, A.J., McDonald, J.C. Dust exposure and mortality in an American chrysotile asbestos friction products plant. *Br J Ind Med* 1984; **41**: 151–157.
63. Dement, J.M., Harris, R.L. Jr, Symons M.J., Shy C.M. Exposures and mortality among chrysotile asbestos workers. Part I: exposure estimates and Part II: mortality. *Am J Ind Med* 1983; **4**: 399–419 and 421–433.
64. Dement, J.M., Brown, D.P. Lung cancer mortality among asbestos textile workers: a review and update. *Ann Occup Hyg* 1994; **38**: 525–532.
65. McDonald, A.D., Fry, J.S., Woolley, A.J., McDonald, J.C. Dust exposure and mortality in an American factory using chrysotile, amosite and crocidolite in textile manufacture. *Br J Ind Med* 1982; **40**: 368–374.
66. Hughes, J.M., Weill, H., Hammand, Y.Y. Mortality of workers employed in two asbestos cement manufacturing plants. *Br J Ind Med* 1987; **44**: 161–174.
67. Hughes, J.M., Weill, H. Asbestos exposure – quantitative assessment of risk. *Am Rev Respir Dis* 1986; **133**: 5–13.
68. Finkelstein, M.M. Analysis of the exposure –response relationship for mesothelioma among asbestos-cement factory workers. *Ann N Y Acad Sci* 1991; **643**: 85–89.
69. Finkelstein, M.M. Mortality among employees of an Ontario asbestos-cement factory. *Am Rev Respir Dis* 1984; **129**: 754–761.
70. McDonald, A.D., McDonald, J.C. Mesothelioma after crocidolite exposure during gas mask exposure. *Environ Res* 1978; **17**: 340–346.
71. Talcott, J.A., Thurber, W.A., Kantor, A.F. *et al.* Asbestos-associated diseases in a cohort of cigarette-filter workers. *N Engl J Med* 1989; **321**: 1220–1223.
72. Sprince, N.L., Oliver, L.C., McCloud, T.C. Asbestos related disease in plumbers and pipefitters employed in building construction. *J Occup Med* 1985; **27**: 771–775.
73. Michaels, D., Zoloth, S.D. Asbestos disease in sheet-metal workers: proportional mortality update. *Am J Ind Med* 1988; **13**: 731–734.
74. Zoloth, S.D., Michaels, D. Asbestos disease in sheet-metal workers: the results of a proportionate mortality analysis. *Am J Ind Med* 1983; **7**: 315–321.
75. Mancuso, T.F. Relative risk of mesothelioma among railroad machinists exposed to chrysotile. *Am J Ind Med* 1988; **13**: 639–657.
76. Schenker, M.B., Garshick, E., Munoz, A., *et al.* A population-based case control study of mesothelioma deaths among US railroad workers. *Am Rev Respir Dis* 1986; **134**: 461–465.
77. Kern, D.G., Hanley, K.T., Roggli, V.L. Malignant mesothelioma in the jewelry industry. *Am J Ind Med* 1992; **21**: 409–416.
78. Dubrow, R. Gute, D.M. Cause-specific mortality among Rhode Island jewelry workers. *Am J Ind Med* 1987; **12**: 579–593.
79. Driscoll, R.J., Mulligan, W.J., Schultz, D., Candelaria, A. Malignant mesothelioma: a cluster in a Native American pueblo. *N Engl J Med* 1988; **318**: 1437–1438.
80. Hammond, E.C., Garfinkle, L., Selikoff, I.J., *et al.* Mortality experience of residents in the neighborhood of an asbestos factory. *Ann N Y Acad Sci* 1979; **330**: 417–422.
81. Berry, M. Mesothelioma incidence and community asbestos exposure. *Environ Res* 1997; **75**: 34–40.
82. Borow, M., Livornese, L.L. Mesothelioma following exposure to asbestos: a review of 72 cases. *Chest* 1973; **201**: 587–591.

83. Siematycki, J. Health effects on the general population: mortality in the general population in asbestos mining areas. In: *Proceedings of the World Symposium on Asbestos*, Montreal, Asbestos Information Center, 1983: 337–48.

84. Churg, A. Lung asbestos content in long-term residents of a chrysotile mining town. *Am Rev Respir Dis* 1986; **134**: 125–127.

85. Theriault, G., Grand-Bois, L. Mesothelioma and asbestos in the Province of Quebec 1969–1972. *Arch Environ Health* 1978; **34**: 15–18.

86. McDonald, J.C. Health implications of environmental exposure to asbestos. *Environ Health Perspect* 1985; **62**: 319–328.

87. Camus, M., Siemiatycki, J., Meek, B. Nonoccupational exposure to chrysotile asbestos and the risk of lung cancer. *N Engl J Med* 1998; **338**: 1565–1571.

88. Enterline, P.E. Cancer produced by nonoccupational asbestos exposure in the United States. *J Air Pollut Control Assoc* 1983; **33**: 318–322.

89. Chen, W., Mottet, N.K. Malignant mesothelioma with minimal asbestos exposure. *Human Pathol* 1978; **9**: 253–257.

90. Becklake, M.R. Asbestos-related diseases of the lung and other organs: their epidemiology and implications for clinical practice. *Am Rev Respir Dis* 1976; **114**: 187–227.

91. Landrigan, P.J., Kazemi, H. (eds) The Third Wave of Asbestos Disease: Exposure to Asbestos in Place – Public Health Control. Proceedings of the Public Health Control Conference, June 1990; New York: New York Academy of Sciences, 1992.

92. Data from Natural Resources Canada, Stage I to Stage IV, Value of Domestic Exports of Minerals and Mineral Products by Commodity by Destination, 1997.

= 2 =

History and Experience of Mesothelioma in Europe

Jean Bignon, Yunico Iwatsubo, Francoise Galateau-Salle
and Alain J. Valleron

Historical overview of malignant mesothelioma (MM) in Europe

In 1991, Wagner introduced the Mesothelioma Conference in Paris with an historical review, from the 1870s to the 1930s, when European and American pathologists were discussing the exact origin and nature of the so-called primary neoplasms of the pleura.[1]

Mesothelioma as a real pathologic entity

Klemperer and Rabin used the word 'mesothelioma' for the first time in 1931.[2] In this early period, the biphasic pattern of this tumour, epithelial and mesenchymatous, had been demonstrated by different pathologists.[3,4] Thereafter, we have to wait until the 1950s to find case reports of 'primary diffuse pleural mesotheliomas' described by different authors in Europe and in North America.[5-7]

Finally, in the 1960s, the pioneer work of European and North American pathologists reached a consensus for considering that diffuse malignant mesothelioma, located mainly in the pleura and less frequently in the peritoneum, was a primary neoplasm arising from the pluripotential mesothelial cells. The pathological diagnosis of mesothelioma appeared difficult, so that, in most serious epidemiological studies, the diagnosis was ascertained by a panel of national or supranational expert pathologists.[8] At present, most European countries have a mesothelioma panel of trained pathologists.

Discovery of the relationship with asbestos exposure

Another major step in the history of mesothelioma was the studies which demonstrated that asbestos exposure was a strong causal factor for the development of this malignant tumour. In fact, it took about 30 years for this to be demonstrated! While a case of mesothelioma associated with asbestos exposure was published in 1943 by Wedler in Germany,[9] this tumour was very rare in Europe and North America, so its relationship with asbestos exposure was not identified.

After 1950, the frequency of mesothelioma seemed to be increasing in males working in industry, possibly in relation with the growth of asbestos uses. By contrast the tumour was rare in females. Actually, the year 1960 is of historical note as, 5 years after the publication by Richard Doll[10] demonstrating the link between lung cancer and occupational exposure to asbestos, Wagner *et al.* reported 33 cases of MM in Northwest Cape (South Africa) among crocidolite miners and their family contacts.[11] Thus, the causal relationship between mesothelioma and exposure to asbestos was demonstrated. Five years later in France, Turiaf *et al.* reported the first case of pleural mesothelioma in a 54-year-old man with a 30-year history of occupational exposure to asbestos.[12]

Incidence of malignant mesothelioma (MM)

As mesothelioma, whatever its two main locations (pleura and peritoneum), represents a severe disease, highly related to asbestos exposure, all industrialised countries are presently concerned with the evaluation of the true incidence of this cancer and its relationships with the different types of asbestos exposure. This section will cover the incidence of mesothelioma in European countries and the role played by accurate registration of cases for assessing this fundamental parameter.

Incidence in industrialised countries

In industrialised countries, data on mortality from mesothelioma can be obtained from death certificates and incidence rates from cancer registries. Actually, the problem is to know the accuracy of mesothelioma cases registration.

As recently as the 1970s, in order to establish the incidence of this malignancy and its causal relationships, several industrialised countries decided to collect data on pleural and peritoneal cases for the whole country (United Kingdom, Scandinavian countries) or only for some specific areas (USA, Canada). From these studies, the 'background' level of mesothelioma incidence could be estimated at around 1 to 2 per million per year in industrialised countries[13]

Incidence rates vary in different countries, apparently in relation with tonnages and types of asbestos production and/or consumption: 28.3 cases per million among males in Australia[14] and 33 per million in South Africa,[15] both countries being producers of crocidolite and amosite. In European countries, various incidence rates have been observed: for instance, the mortality rate in males was reported to be 17.5 per million in Great Britain[16] and 20.9 per million in the Netherlands.[17]

During the past 30 to 40 years, most industrialised countries (e.g., North America, Europe, Australia) have observed an increase in the annual incidence of MM (at about 7% to 10% per annum), with an obvious predominance among males. Such trends suggested the causal role of specific occupational asbestos exposures (particularly to amphiboles), no other causes having been identified in this early period,[18-22] but possibly also in relation to a real improvement in diagnosis and registration of this rare type of cancer.

In the 1960s, definite mesothelioma cases showed a marked clustering in areas where there was substantial industrial use of asbestos. Thus, in the USA, Connelly *et al.* observed that the highest rate was in shipyard areas (Seattle, San Francisco, Hawaii).[19] However, from the mesothelioma register in Great Britain, Peto *et al.* found that mesothelioma deaths were still increasing and will continue for at least 15 to 25 years.[21] As the deceased's job (probably the last one) was mentioned on United Kingdom death certificates, the authors could calculate the trend of mesothelioma in different jobs; workers in construction and maintenance of buildings containing asbestos accounted for the largest proportion of these deaths. This important finding stresses the usefulness of a nationwide mesothelioma register as the most relevant tool for the surveillance of possible risks of malignancy related to low-dose asbestos exposures, for instance in asbestos-containing buildings.

As a definite diagnosis of MM is difficult to establish with certitude, requiring the opinion of trained clinicians and pathologists, it is probable that estimates from death certificates do not match those obtained from cancer registries. It is probable that presently this tumour is underreported, although the reverse is also possible! Thus, for the period 1967–68, 413 cases from England, Wales and Scotland were notified as mesothelioma to the national register. After revision of the slides by the British panel of pathologists, 246 cases were accepted as definite and 76 cases as definitely not mesothelioma.[23] Such discrepancies have been reported from other industrialised countries where both registry-based incidence data and mortality data were available.[24] In their review, Iwatsubo *et al.* have shown that, for different studies, variations in the percentage of pathologically confirmed diagnosis of mesothelioma ranged from 26% to 96%.[25]

Incidence of mesothelioma in Europe from case registration

The background level of mesothelioma was assumed to be as low as 1 to 2 per million inhabitants,[13] but since the 1950s, this incidence has been increasing in the general population of most industrialised countries.[25,26]

Since mesothelioma is usually a rapidly fatal malignancy, mortality rates based on the underlying cause of death, as recorded on *death certificates*, have often been used as a close approximation of *incidence rates*. But large discrepancies have been observed in some cases,[19] so that we should distinguish the studies according to the origins of the data: either mesothelioma registries, general cancer registries or death certificates.

In non-asbestos-producing European countries, it appears that an accurate evaluation of the true incidence of mesothelioma cases and their causal relationships was the best epidemiological tool for assessing the types (amphiboles versus chrysotile) of imported asbestos and determining the cumulated tonnes of past exposures. Nevertheless, this aim had some limitations, as only a limited number of European countries (Scandinavian countries, United Kingdom) decided early in the 1970s to register all pleural and peritoneal mesotheliomas cases.

In the United Kingdom, a mesothelioma register was set up in 1967.[23] Mesothelioma cases were identified from the death certificates mentioning 'pleural or peritoneal mesothelioma', information provided by registrations from the Cancer Bureaux, the Pneumoconiosis Panel and also from chest physicians, surgeons, pathologists and coroners. A definite diagnosis was made by reviewing histological materials referred to the UICC Panel of Pathologists. For the year 1967–68, 412 cases were notified to the register, of which 245 were considered as definite mesothelioma, leading to a rate of 2.29/million/year for England, Wales and Scotland.

Gardner *et al.* examined the time trend of mortality by pleural cancer, i.e., death coded into the category 163 of the ICD, 9th revision, in England and Wales for the period 1968–78 from the death records (Office of Population Censuses and Surveys).[27] For the entire period, the mortality rate by pleural cancer was 5 per million in men and 2 per million in women.

A later publication of the mesothelioma register concerning the period 1968–83[16] showed an increase of about 10% in men. The mesothelioma mortality in 1983 was 17.5 per million in men and 3.2 per million in women.

In the Netherlands, Meijers *et al.* examined the mortality trend of pleural malignancies between 1970 and 1987.[17] The coded underlying cause of death was provided from the Dutch Central Bureau of Statistics. In men, the average pleural cancer mortality increased from 10.7 per million for the period 1970–78 to 20.9 per million for the period 1979–87. In women, these rates were, respectively, 2.5 per million and 3.6 per million.

In Scandinavian countries (Finland, Sweden, Denmark, Norway), the existence of a national cancer register of all deaths from cancer facilitated the task of examining the time trend of cancer incidence.

In Finland, a nationwide Finnish Cancer Registry was established in the 1950s.[28] This Cancer Registry allowed Karjalainen *et al.* to study the trend of mesothelioma incidence in Finland between 1960 and 1995.[29] In that country, anthophyllite asbestos was produced and widely used from 1918 to 1975. The age-adjusted incidence of mesothelioma was under 1 per million in both sexes around 1960, and then rose steeply in 1975–90. In 1990–94, the age adjusted incidence of mesothelioma was 10 per million in men and 2.9 per million in women. The overall pattern of mesothelioma seems to be stable in the very recent period. This plateauing could be related to a significant decrease in the use of amphiboles. Nevertheless, it seems that the mesothelioma risk related to anthophyllite asbestos is low,[30] but crocidolite was also used from the late 1960s.

In Sweden, Järvholm *et al.* studied the incidence of pleural mesothelioma between 1958 and 1995 with respect to preventive measures taken to reduce occupational exposure to asbestos.[31,32] There were about 10 cases of pleural mesothelioma in men and no case in women in 1958. In 1995, 92 cases in men and 15 in women were observed. An increasing incidence was found in recent birth cohorts in men.

In Denmark, Andersson and Olsen described the time trend and the distribution of MM since 1942.[33] The registration to the National Cancer Registry was based on reports from hospital departments, pathology institutes, notifications from practising physicians and death certificates. For the entire period, the authors observed a regular increase in both sexes. The incidence rates for the latest period, 1978–80, were 14.7 per million in men and 7 per million in women.

In Norway, Mowé *et al.* examined the time trends of mesothelioma incidence between 1960 and 1988.[34] The investigation was based on data from the Cancer Registry of Norway to which all new cases of cancer are reported from hospitals and pathology departments. The age-adjusted incidence of mesothelioma increased during the observed period in men: 4 per million for 1960–69 to 13 per million for 1980–87. In women, mesothelioma incidence remained at the same level, 1 per million, during the whole period.

In several other European countries (France, Germany, Italy), up to now, case registration was limited to some specific areas.

In France, all data obtained from death certificates are collected by the Service Commun N°8 (SC8) of Institut National de la Santé et de la Recherche Médicale (INSERM). Since 1968, information on the underlying medical causes of death mentioned by the practitioners on death certificates has been coded by INSERM SC8 according to the *International Classification of Diseases* (ICD 8 or 9). The numbers of deaths due to pleural malignancies were those classified in category 163 of the ICD 8 (i.e., malignant neoplasm of pleura, stated or presumed to be primary) and category 158 of the ICD 9 (i.e., malignant neoplasm of peritoneum, stated or presumed to be primary).

A 'registration' of mesothelioma cases was set up in 1975.[35] Actually, as death certificates were totally confidential, MM cases could only be collected through pathologists and clinicians. Thus, this 'register' was mainly made up of a panel of French pathologists (still working) trained to confirm the diagnosis of mesothelioma, eventually with the contribution of the EEC mesothelioma panel. From the death certificates, for the period 1968–92, the mortality with mention of pleural malignancies increased from 8.2 per million to 22.5 per million in men and 4.7 per million to 9.2 per million in women. The average increase during this period was 4.3% in men and 2.8% in women.[36]

In such conditions, the French 'register' was not able to provide valid information on the true incidence of MM. In January 1987, the mesothelioma panel interrupted its random case collection on a national basis, to conduct a case-control study in 5 regions of France, with a double objective: evaluation of the dose–response for different occupational exposures and, eventually, identification of other asbestos-related jobs (cf. below).

Recently, Ménegoz *et al.* (Réseau France CIM) examined the trend of mesothelioma incidence from data obtained by 7 departmental registries for the period 1979–93.[37] These registries cover about 9.5% of the French population. For the entire period, the increase was 25% over 3 years. In men, the incidence increased from 7 per million/year for the period 1979–81 to 16 per million/year for 1991–93.

The progression of MM in France was estimated at around 7 to 8% per year.[36] It is worth comparing these data to the trend observed in the UK, the national register of this country indicating a mesothelioma rate about three times higher than F rance. This difference correlates with a much lower consumption of amphiboles in France than in the UK.[21,22]

General trend in Europe

In the countries where registration of mesothelioma was accurate, between the 1950s and now, a linear progression of mesothelioma incidence (about 5–10% per year) was observed (apart from Finland). This increase was parallel to the progression of asbestos imports, but with a delay of 30 to 40 years, due to the long latency period of asbestos-related mesothelioma. Elsewhere, the curve of this progression showed different slopes, in relation to the tonnages of crocidolite and amosite imports.

The incidence of mesothelioma in France seems to be lower than that observed in the other European countries. This could be due to a later widespread use of asbestos in France compared to other European countries.

Two classical sources of bias should be discussed in the estimation of the disease rate: false-positive diagnosis leading to an overestimation of disease rates and incomplete registration leading to an underestimation.

Since mesothelioma is usually a rapidly fatal malignancy, mortality rates based on the underlying cause of death, as recorded on *death certificates*, have often been used as a close approximation of *incidence rates*. But large discrepancies have been observed in some cases in the USA (Connelly *et al.*, 1987), so that we should distinguish the studies according to the origins of the data: either mesothelioma registries, general cancer registries or death certificates.

In non-asbestos-producing European countries, it appears that an accurate evaluation of the true incidence of mesothelioma cases and their causal relationships was the best epidemiological tool for assessing the role played by types (amphiboles versus chrysotile) of imported asbestos and for determining the cumulated tonnes of past exposures.[21,22] Nevertheless, at present such a tool has serious limitations in Europe, since a limited number of European countries (Scandinavian countries, United Kingdom) had decided early in the 1970s to register all pleural and peritoneal mesothelioma cases.

Mesothelioma being defined on specific pathological criteria, the certainty of diagnosis requires pathological proof, eventually confirmed by a panel of experienced pathologists.[8] The confirmation rate shows a large variation according to studies.[18,23,38-41] Thus, according to the Cancer Surveillance Program in the USA, in Los Angeles County, the lowest rate was 26% between 1972 and 1979,[38] while in Australia the highest rate was 96%.[40] A confirmation rate as low as 26% emphasises that it may be extensively underestimated. Indeed, it has been suggested that some cases diagnosed as lung cancer might actually correspond to mesothelioma.[41,42]

The validity of the method using mortality from pleural malignancies as an approximation of mesothelioma incidence has been examined in several studies. In the United Kingdom, Newhouse and Wagner published a study carried out with the aim to validate the diagnosis mentioned on the death certificates of more than 400 past workers of an asbestos factory.[43] After revision of the pathological slides by the UICC Panel of Pathologists, by reviewing histological material they demonstrated that the incidence of mesothelial tumours was underestimated; thus, for the years 1967–68, 19 further mesothelioma cases were identified as the cause of death. Another study has shown that 90% of the death certificates in males and 70% in females coded for pleural malignancy (ICD 163) mentioned mesothelioma as the cause of death.[27]

In the Netherlands, Meijers *et al.* found that the number of deaths from pleural malignancies, as recorded on death certificates (193 deaths) in 1986, was relatively close to the number of cases either notified to the mesothelioma panel or reported by surveying all Dutch pathologists (171 cases).[17]

A recent study conducted in France suggested that only 45.5% of death certificates classified into category 163 of the ICD WHO, 9th revision, during the period 1992–93 were confirmed as definite or probable mesothelioma. On the contrary, in 75% of males and 70% of females, the histologically confirmed pleural mesotheliomas were correctly coded into the category 163 of the ICD WHO, 9th revision (Iwatsubo et al., 1995, personal communication).

These validation studies have shown that there may be a large discordance between pleural mesothelioma incidence and recorded mortality rates by pleural cancer, the extent and the direction of which vary largely according to the studies.

After the 1950s, in industrialised countries where registration of mesothelioma cases was accurate, a linear progression of incidence was observed (about 5–10% per year). This increase was parallel to the progression of asbestos imports, but with a delay of 30 to 40 years, due to the long latency period of this cancer. Elsewhere, the curve of this progression shows different slopes, apparently in relation with tonnages of crocidolite and amosite imports.

Relationship of mesothelioma to asbestos exposure

As underlined by Howell et al., there are several routes of exposure to asbestos fibres: occupational, paraoccupational (domestic contamination from asbestos workers), residential contamination near dusty industrial sources, incidental, related contact with asbestos products for domestic uses or hobbies, and general environmental exposure from asbestos sediments at the surface of soil.[44,45]

Occupational exposures

In Europe, most mesothelioma cases are related to asbestos exposures in occupational activities in various industries, some of them not apparent. However, staff in two industries were particularly exposed to asbestos dusts: shipyard workers and construction workers.

The excess number of mesothelioma cases in coastal areas of European countries is consistent with shipyard-related exposures (workers involved in shipbuilding and repair). The situation applied in the Scandinavian countries (Sweden, Norway, Finland, Denmark), The Netherlands,[46] the United Kingdom, [1] the Loire–Atlantique and Normandy areas of France,[47-49] and the Province of Trieste in Italy.[50]

On the other hand, recently, Peto et al.[21] identified from the UK mesothelioma register an excess of mesothelioma in workers involved in construction and building maintenance, particularly plumbers, gas fitters, carpenters and electricians, who appeared as the largest high-risk group.

Dose–response relationships

Several authors, when evaluating cohort studies[20,51-54] and case-control studies[42,55,56] focusing on mesothelioma, have reported a dose–response relationship.

Jones *et al.* examined the occurrence of respiratory malignancies among workers in a gas-mask factory in the UK.[51] The production of gas masks lasted 4.5 years from September 1940. Crocidolite as well as chrysotile was used in production. A total of 951 women were known to have worked in this job. Up to the end of 1978, 17 cases of mesothelioma were observed, 16 in those exposed to crocidolite only and one in those exposed to both crocidolite and chrysotile. Among the 16 cases exposed to crocidolite only, a dose–response relationship was observed with duration of exposure.

Raffn *et al.* studied the incidence of cancer and the mortality among employees in the asbestos cement industry in Denmark for the period 1943–84.[53] Subjects included were those exposed between 1928 and 1984. The estimated exposure levels varied greatly during the study period: in 1948, between 50 and 800 fibres per millilitre (f/mL); in 1957, between 10 and 100 f/mL; in 1973, 41% of the measurements were above 2 f/mL. Among the 7996 men and 517 women studied, 10 pleural mesotheliomas were observed. The incidence of pleural mesothelioma increased with the duration of exposure among subjects with 15 years or more of latency (SIR=3.77 for less than 5 years of exposure versus 13.56 for more than 5 years of exposure).

Peto *et al.* observed that the risk of mesothelioma in an occupationally exposed cohort (north American insulators) was best described by a mathematical model in which the risk increases with the third or fourth power of time since first exposure;[20] their data were compatible with a linear dose–response relationship. Peto *et al.* found also this type of relationship when considering the mortality of subjects (men and women) employed at the Rochdale asbestos textile factory.[21] A total of 18 mesothelioma cases in men (7 in the first group and 11 in the third group) were observed during the study period. Despite the small number of deaths observed (10 occurred in the main cohort), the observed and predicted numbers were in reasonable agreement for different times since first exposure.

Newhouse *et al.* studied the mortality of asbestos factory workers (asbestos textiles and others asbestos products such as asbestos cement) in east London.[52] The population concerned 3000 male factory workers, 1400 laggers and 700 women factory workers. The men were first exposed between 1933 and 1964 and the women between 1936 and 1942. Crocidolite asbestos as well as amosite and chrysotile was used in the factory. Exposure to asbestos was classified into 4 categories according to degree (light or moderate versus severe) and duration (<2 years versus ≈ 2 years). During the study period, 38 pleural and 35 peritoneal mesotheliomas were observed in men and 14 pleural and 11 peritoneal mesotheliomas in women. Among factory workers, the mesothelioma death rates increased according to both duration and severity of asbestos exposure.

Albin *et al.* studied the mortality and cancer morbidity in cohorts of asbestos cement workers (predominantly chrysotile) and referents in Sweden.[54] All male employees registered in the asbestos company between 1907 and 1977 were included. Status was determined until 31 December 1986. The estimated median cumulative exposure was 2.3 f/mL-years. A significant dose–response relationship with asbestos exposure was found for cumulative exposure: RR=1.9 for each f/mL-year among employees with 40 years or more of exposure.

Tuomi *et al.* studied the relative risk of mesothelioma associated with different levels of exposure to asbestos in a case-control study.[56] Cases were hospital patients from departments of pulmonary medicine at the university central hospitals of Finland in 3 cities (Helsinki, Tampere and Turku), observed between 1985 and 1988. Asbestos exposure was evaluated from occupational history and the lung asbestos fibre burden. The comparison of 31 male mesothelioma and 43 lung cancer patients showed a dose–response relationship with the level of retention of asbestos fibres (OR=3.1 95%, confidence interval [CI] 1.3–7.5 for $\approx$ one million fibres/g dry tissue; OR=7.2 95%, CI 2.5–23.4 for more than 10 million fibres/g of dry tissue).

In a large case-control study conducted in France since 1987, three of us examined the dose–response relationship using several types of exposure parameters and studied the role of time-related exposure patterns (intermittent compared to continuous exposure). Between 1987 and 1993, 405 cases and 387 controls were interviewed. The job histories of these subjects were evaluated by a group of 5 experts for exposure to asbestos fibres according to probability, intensity and frequency. A cumulative exposure index was calculated, as the product of these three parameters and the duration of the exposed job, summed over the entire working life. Among men, the odds-ratio (OR) increased with the probability of exposure and was 1.2 [95% CI 0.8–1.9] for possible exposure and 3.6 (95% CI 2.4–5.3) for definite exposure. A dose–response relationship was observed with the cumulative exposure index (CEI): the OR increased from 1.2 (95% CI 0.8–1.8) for the lowest exposure category to 8.7 (95% CI 4.1–18.5) for the highest.

In this study, we used several surrogate parameters for dose to examine dose–response relationship. We considered separately the intensity, frequency and duration of exposure, and each parameter was significantly related to mesothelioma. The relative risk increased together with each parameter. In addition, when each of these parameters was adjusted for the others, the relative risk of each, although lower, remained significant. These results suggest that each exposure parameter contributed to some extent to the mesothelioma, although the dose–response relationship seemed to be described best by the CEI.

Very few studies have focused on the time-related pattern of occupational exposure as a significant factor in the occurrence of mesothelioma. Our study examined the temporal exposure pattern according to the frequency of exposure and the CEI. We observed a dose–response relationship with cumulative exposure for both intermittent and continuous patterns of exposure. Much more attention to the role of these temporal patterns is needed, adjusting for cumulative exposure. Our results suggested that intermittent exposure does not entail as high a risk of mesothelioma as continuous exposure

Other routes of asbestos exposure

A major concern is the significance of mesothelioma cases without any definite occupational asbestos exposure, which represent around 25–30% of the total.[13,57] Are these cases due to hidden or environmental exposures to asbestos or are they related to other causes?

Environmental and neighbourhood exposure to asbestos

It seems likely that mesothelioma may arise from domestic and environmental exposures, either natural or para-occupational. This is of concern particularly among family members of asbestos workers but also in the general population who inhale fibres in the vicinity of asbestos plants.

In the mesothelioma series of the London area published by Newhouse and Thompson, there were 25 cases without evidence of any exposure to asbestos.[58] Among them, 11 cases used to live within 800 metres of an asbestos factory, a number significantly greater than among a control group of patients without mesothelioma. However, at that early time, the authors seemed to be reluctant to accept this relationship, waiting for more evidence in the future.

Subsequently, the same kinds of observation have been made in other European countries: in Finland, in relation with dwelling in the vicinity of an anthophyllite mine;[59] and in north-western Italy, where an increased incidence of histologically confirmed mesothelioma was reported in the vicinity of a large asbestos cement factory at Casale Monferrato, in operation from 1907 to 1985.[60]

Endemic cases of mesothelioma have been also observed in rural areas in several European countries, Metsovo in Greece[61] and Corsica in France,[62] and also, far from Europe, New Caledonia, with a high incidence of mesothelioma, particularly in rural areas.[63] The asbestos fibres concerned are mainly of the tremolite type, except in Finland, where anthophyllite was invoved. Those cases are related to outdoor and indoor contamination from environmental geologic sources of asbestos dusts.

Mesothelioma cases related to indoor exposures are well known, particularly among family members of asbestos workers coming home with contaminated clothes. This issue might also be relevant to indoor contamination by fibres in buildings with asbestos containing materials, fibres being eventually released at very low concentrations (0.001–0.0001 f/mL of air). Presently, there is no sufficiently large epidemiological survey to confirm such a relationship.[64] We must refer with caution to the mathematical projections published in the two documents: HEI-AR, 1991 and INSERM, 1997.[26,36]

Role of fibre types

Numerous epidemiological studies, discussed at length in HEI-AR, have compared the incidence of lung cancer and mesothelioma in various situations. Moreover, the ratio of mesothelioma/lung cancer numbers has been compared according to fibre types. However, the observed discrepancies between cohorts may be due to the fact that it was retrospectively difficult to know exactly what types of asbestos have been used in these plants.

McDonald et al. (Table 2.1) had the opportunity to evaluate the incidence of mesothelioma deaths in different contrasted cohorts:[24]

i) workers exposed only to crocidolite during gas mask manufacture;
ii) miners exposed to pure chrysotile;

Table 2.1. Summary of incidence and mortality studies on mesothelioma (meso) in Europe.

Type of Study	Country/ reference	Study period	Diseases included	Annual rate/10⁶ in men	in women
Population-based cancer registries	Denmark Anderson[33]	1978–80	pleural meso	14.7	7
	Norway Mowé[34]	1960–69	pleural meso	4	1
		1970–79		8	1
				13	1
	Finland Karjalainen[28]	1980–87	pleural and peritoneal meso	10	2.9
		1990–94			
Population-based meso registries	United Kingdom Greenberg[23]	1967–68	pleural or peritoneal meso	2.3 for both sexes	
	France Bignon[35]	1982	pleural meso	1.8	0.25
		1983		1.8	0.28
		1984		2.5	0.36
		1985		2.5	0.54
National rates of meso (mortality data)	United Kingdom Gardner[27]	1968–78	pleural malignancies	5	2
	Jones[16]	1968–71	pleural of peritoneal meso	4.9	1.5
				7.1	1.7
		1972–75		11.4	2.4
				15.3	3.2
	Netherlands Meijers[17]	1976–79	pleural malignancies	10.7	2.5
		1980–83	20.9	3.6	
		1970–78			
		1979–87			

iii) workers in a textile manufacture exposed to a mixture of chrysotile, amosite and crocidolite.

The proportional mortality due to mesothelioma (per 1000) increased from pure chrysotile to pure crocidolite, being intermediate for the mixed fibres. We can deduce from Table 2.1 comparing different cohorts that those where workers had been exposed to commercial amphiboles (crocidolite, amosite, anthophyllite), or to a mixture of amphiboles with chrysotile, were associated with a high mortality rate from mesothelioma (20 to 86 per thousand), compared with the much lower proportional mortality ratios for workers exposed to pure chrysotile.

However, at present there is no consensus on that point, as reported in the HEI-AR document: 'The evidence that chrysotile rarely causes pleural mesothelioma is not conclusive'.[26] There are only two cohorts of heavily exposed workers, but only to chrysotile fibres (in the Quebec mines and in the South Carolina plant), where mesothelioma was absent or, if observed, was considered as related to tremolite, as a geological contaminant of chrysotile. Such an explanation might be supported by the results of the electron microscopic study carried out by Sebastien *et al.*, which showed that the lung of Quebec chrysotile miners and millers contained a significant proportion of long (greater than 5 microns) tremolite fibres,[65] although this fibre type represents only a 1% contaminant of the Quebec chrysotile mines.

The presence of fibres in the parietal pleural tissue, where mesothelioma usually starts, has rarely been studied. Recently, Boutin *et al.* have demonstrated the presence of a significant amount of fibres in biopsies of parietal pleura.[66] The electron microscopic analysis of tissue samples obtained through thoracoscopy has shown high focal concentrations of asbestos, mainly long crocidolite fibres and also, in one case, tremolite fibres in a man possibly environmentally exposed in Corsica. The hypothesis of a focal accumulation of long durable fibres in close contact with the target mesothelial cells is worthy of serious examination.

Although a majority of studies considered that mesothelioma was more related to significant exposure to amphibole fibres (+ +) than to chrysotile (+ ou -), we must mention that there are some exceptions or some disagreement:

i) Woitowitz and Rôdelsperger published a different opinion when reporting a study of 615 samples of respirable air collected by the German Institute of Occupational Safety.[67] In the friction lining industry, only chrysotile was present in 611 samples; by contrast, crocidolite was discovered only four times in a single plant between 1981 and 1982. Thus, the authors reported to have observed an increased incidence of mesothelioma cases among car mechanics who have been exposed only to chrysotile, with a mean dose of less than 1 f/mL-years.

ii) Smith and Wright published a paper entitled 'Chrysotile asbestos is the main cause of pleural mesothelioma', which is not convincing.[68]

iii) The mathematical model used recently by Nicholson and Raffn on cancer due to asbestos in the USA and Denmark reached the conclusion that the 'data speak strongly that much of the mesothelioma risk is predominantly from exposure to chrysotile'.[69]

However, in the context of mesothelioma, in France, an electron microscopic analysis of lung tissue samples[70] showed that crocidolite fibres were found at higher concentrations than chrysotile in mesothelioma cases compared with lung cancer patients or control cases (cardiac surgery). Edward *et al.* made the same observation.[71]

Low-dose exposure to asbestos fibres

The significant relationship observed between likely low-dose asbestos exposure (0.5 to 1 f/mL-years) and pleural mesothelioma[72] raises the following question: are the cases where we failed to identify any significant occupational asbestos exposure related to other situations?

i) *Occult para-occupational or domestic exposures* to asbestos at significant concentrations? Such situations were illustrated by the publication of conjugal or familial cases.[73,74]

ii) *Environmental outdoor exposures.* Since the historical publication of Kiviluoto describing pleural calcifications in an area of Finland related to non-occupational endemic exposure to anthophyllite asbestos,[75] numerous similar observations, including cases of mesothelioma, have been made in rural areas where superficial

Table 2.2. *Odds ratios for relations between pleural mesothelioma and asbestos exposure parameters among men: French mesothelioma case-control study, 1987–93, with a latency period of 20 years (table from Iwatsubo et al.[75])*

Asbestos exposure parameters	Cases	Controls	OR*	95%CI
Highest probability of exposure				
Not exposed	95	154	1.0	
Possible	51	71	1.2	0.8–1.9
Definite	184	87	3.6	2.4–5.3
Highest intensity of exposure				
Low	55	74	1.2	0.8–1.8
Medium	106	66	2.8	1.8–4.3
High	74	18	7.1	3.9–12.9
Highest frequency of exposure				
Sporadic	56	86	1.0	0.7–1.6
Irregular	94	46	3.3	2.1–5.1
Continuous	85	26	5.5	3.4–9.7
Duration of exposure (years)				
1–7	63	64	1.7	1.1–2.6
8–19	74	60	2.0	1.3–3.1
>20	98	34	5.4	3.2–8.9
Time since exposure (years)				
20–37	77	53	2.3	1.4–3.6
38–48	83	47	2.8	1.8–4.5
49 or more	75	58	2.2	1.4–3.6
Age at first exposure (years)				
<16	66	55	1.9	1.2–3.1
16–22	96	52	3.0	1.9–4.6
23 or older	73	51	2.3	1.5–3.7
Cumulative exposure ('f/mL-year')†				
0.001–0.49	77	109	1.2	0.8–1.8
0.5–0.99	29	12	4.2	2.0–8.8
1–9.9	80	27	5.2	3.1–8.8
10+	49	10	8.7	4.1–18.5

*OR adjusted for age and socioeconomic category.
† Cumulative exposure index was based on subjective assessment, that is, semiquantification of exposure by the experts and selected weighting factors assigned to each category of exposure, with no objective measurement of airborne asbestos levels. Thus, the exposure unit, f/mL-years is expressed in quotation marks.

rocks are more or less fibrous. In Europe, mesothelioma related to such exposures has been observed in Bulgaria, Cyprus,[76] Greece,[61] and Corsica in France,[62] and in New Caledonia.[63] Usually in such environmental exposures, the dwellers of both sexes have been exposed since childhood to airborne dusts derived from the soil contaminated with fibres, mostly of the tremolite type. There is one exception in two villages of Cappadocia (Turkey) where the highest incidence of MM observed was caused by a volcanic fibrous dust, zeolite-erionite, which is the most potent carcinogenic fibrous mineral.[77]

These findings have been an important step in the natural history of mesothelioma.[35,78] More recently, cases of mesothelioma have been related to *environmental industrial exposures*, for instance in Italy in the neighbourhood of an asbestos plant.[60]

iii) Mesothelioma related to *passive indoor exposure at very low concentrations in asbestos-containing buildings*. Such contaminations have been held by some authors[79] to be responsible for asbestos-related diseases, mainly pleural plaques. In such buildings, concentrations of fibres in air samples rarely exceed 0.001 f/mL, but fibre counts in different countries suggest that substantially higher levels may sometimes occur. In order to investigate a possible health hazard for building occupants in relation with airborne mineral fibre exposure, in the 1980s, we started an epidemiological follow-up of volunteers among the permanent staff of the huge University of Paris Jussieu.[80] So far, only pleural plaques have been observed, but mainly in a few maintenance workers or laboratory technicians. For such exposures at very low doses, theoretically, it is barely impossible to demonstrate the reality of such a dose–response relationship.[64] However, evidence of damage in many buildings suggests possible peaks at high concentrations of fibres, that may have exceeded 1 f/mL for short periods of time. If we integrate such concentrations in our dose–response relationship,[72] we can deduce the possibility that such exposure may generate mesothelioma, particularly if an hypothetical cofactor exists.

What about the future?

Prediction of mortality from mesothelioma

A major concern in public health is to know the trend of the incidence rate of mesothelioma: is it decreasing, stable or increasing? What about the evolution in the next 20 years?

Recently, three publications have provided estimates of the mortality from mesothelioma in both sexes which can be predicted in the next few years.

In 1995, Peto *et al.*, analysing the data from the British Mesothelioma Register, forecast a peak of deaths in 2020.[21] They estimated the total size of the 1996–2020 epidemic of deaths due to mesothelioma in males as 62 000 (which extrapolates to 166 males per million male inhabitants of Britain).

In 1997 Price, analysing current trends of mesothelioma incidence in the USA,[81] concluded that the peak of mesothelioma was just going to appear (1997) and that the projected number of future mesothelioma cases suggests a peak in the annual number of cases at 2300 for males, before the year 2000. Then, the number of male cases will drop during the next 50–60 years toward 500.

In 1998, from the available data in France, Gilg Soit Ilg *et al.* predicted that the nationwide peak will occur between 2020 and 2060, and, for men, the total size of the epidemic will be 20 000 over the period 1998–2020, which extrapolates to 43 per million.[22]

Such studies are important, because it is the death toll which predominantly builds the perception of the risk in the general population. They are necessarily based on the past and present mortality data. They face three difficulties: i) the low quality of death certificates, especially for the oldest subjects, for whom it is difficult to code principal, underlying and associate causes of deaths; ii) the lack of mortality codes in ICD 9 related to pleural and peritoneal mesothelioma; iii) the fact that mortality from mesothelioma is just a component, but the most specific, of cancer mortality associated with asbestos exposure.

The published methods of forecasting share the same methodological approach: essentially, they assume that the mortality at age 'a' for persons of the cohort born in year 'c' can be expressed as a simple product of two factors: the first one is the factor age A (a), the second one is the factor cohort C (c). In all the three aforementioned studies, it has been shown that this very simple assumption provided an excellent fit to the observed data. Therefore, the principle of the method is to estimate the unknown factors A(a) and C(c) on the past data and then to use these estimates to forecast the future: for example, the mortality of men 85 years old in 2020 can be predicted by multiplying the factor A (85) and the cohort factor C (2020–85 = 1935) which were both evaluated on the past data when possible. As recent cohort factors cannot be estimated from data of the past [e.g. C (2000)], assumptions are necessary. These assumptions are highly questionable. For instance, Peto *et al.* assumed that all the cohort factors after 1953 will be half of those of the 1944–48 birth cohort.[20,21] In France, we choose four hypotheses, which, unfortunately, cannot be tested at present. The statistical methods of estimation provide confidence intervals of the different predictors.

The most available results concern the predictions of the number of mesothelioma deaths in men, extrapolated from data of the past. As previously seen, they depend strongly on hypotheses that are impossible to test.

Two series of results, which are less discussed in public, are certainly more important.

The first concerns the estimated lifetime probabilities of dying from mesothelioma in recent generations, compared with the older ones. For instance, we found that, in France, these lifetime probabilities were increasing in the new generations (we estimated a lifetime risk of 0.8% for men born in 1965–68), while these lifetime probabilities were found to be decreasing in UK and US studies. This might be explained by the different patterns of asbestos consumption in these three countries;

The second concerns the analysis of mortality in women. We did not find any trend in the mortality in females, which is in line with the results of Price in USA[81] (Peto did not study women's mortality). This is certainly reassuring, as the opposite would be expected if environmental exposures to asbestos played a significant part in the mortality from mesothelioma.

Significance of mesothelioma without asbestos exposure?

Although familial cases of MM have been reported, there is no valid proof allowing us to demonstrate that genetic factors might predispose to the development of this type of malignancy. In most familial cases, it was found that one family member was occupationally exposed to asbestos, and may have contaminated the whole family. Nevertheless, a genetic factor remains possible.[57]

Two years after the review by Peterson *et al.* on 'Non-asbestos-related malignant mesothelioma',[82] McDonald and McDonald[18] stated that aetiological studies carried out in most series of registered mesothelioma cases usually failed to find a well defined past asbestos exposure in about 20–30% of the cases. In 1982, we tried to compare a series of exposed and unexposed mesothelioma cases, but the differences were small and not significant.[83] Others have published cases where the search for other aetiological factors was not contributive. Those cases seem to correspond to the background of this malignancy, estimated in our countries at around 2 per million per year, with a sex ratio around one. In the absence of unequivocal data, the question of the possible impact of environmental or indoor exposure remains, as demonstrated in specific areas, for instance in the vicinity of asbestos plants, as previously mentioned.

Detection of other causal factors or cofactors

Apart from the endemic production of mesotheliomas related to erionite fibres[77] and cases related to exposure to radiation or associated with the SV-40 virus (which will be discussed later), failure to identify asbestos exposure in about 20–30% of cases of ascertained mesothelioma, with a low pulmonary asbestos fibre burden, led to a search for other possible factors in humans (see the review by Peterson *et al.*,[82]).

The only causes identified have been the few cases as follows:

Radiation: thoracic irradiation, for the treatment of mediastinal malignancies and use of thorium dioxide as a radiographic contrast medium, have been implicated in the pathogenesis of mesothelioma in several patients.[84-87]

Many *chemicals*, given by different routes of administration and at different doses, have been shown to induce mesothelial tumours in rodents.[88] Among those chemicals, 3-methyl cholantrene appeared particularly potent. Moreover, in our laboratory, it has been shown that benzo-a-pyrene was able to transform rat pleural mesothelial cells *in vitro*, but without any synergy with asbestos.[89] It is noticeable that rat pleural mesothelial cells exhibit cytochrome P-450 activity. Despite these positive results in rodents, no chemical has been clearly identified as a possible causal factor in man, except for two cases probably related to common ingestion of paraffin oil.[82]

It remains to say that we had the opportunity to observe *non-asbestos-related mesothelioma cases*,[83] a situation extensively reviewed by Peterson *et al.*[82] The conclusion of these authors was 'that sufficient evidence exists to suggest that non-asbestos-related agents can induce malignant mesothelioma in man and additional epidemiological studies in this area are needed'.

At present, for European industries producing man-made fibres as substitutes for asbestos, the main concern is to develop and commercialize safe products. Among the man-made vitreous fibres, ceramic fibres might be dangerous in humans, since they have produced mesothelioma by inhalation in rodents and were responsible of pleural plaques in workers involved in their production.[16]

The role of the SV-40 virus?

The discoveries by Carbone *et al.*[90] i) that SV-40 virus gave 100% mesothelioma after direct injection into hamsters; and ii) the presence of SV-40-like virus sequences in the DNA extracted from tumour cells found in 28 cases from a series of 48 human pleural mesothelioma, raised several questions.

From whence came the virus? Is it a simian virus? Carbone has suggested that the contamination might have been possible through the Salk vaccine. In France, this seems questionable, because the Salk vaccine was not used extensively.

Are we dealing with a cofactor for mesothelial cell transformation? The contamination of mesenchymatous cells by an oncogenic virus (the origin of which has to be elucidated) might suggest a more logical mechanism for mesothelial carcinogenesis; indeed, in the absence of identified cofactor(s), so far asbestos was considered as a complete carcinogen at the level of the pleura (Peto, Barrett, Jaurand, others), as opposed to the model for asbestos-related lung carcinogenesis, where fibres work in synergy with chemical carcinogens, particularly those in tobacco smoke.

However, recently, SV-40 associated with malignant mesothelioma in humans has not been confirmed in all laboratories. Indeed, Strickler *et al.* did not confirm the significant association of SV-40 with mesothelioma or with osteosarcoma:[91] antibodies to SV-40 were detected in only 3 of 50 mesotheliomas, in one of 33 osteosarcomas tested and in one of 35 controls. These scientists concluded: 'These findings call into question the association of SV-40 with mesothelioma.'

In Europe, research is in progress in that field.

In the UK, Gibbs *et al.* have demonstrated the presence of SV-40 DNA sequences in 44% of British mesothelioma cases, but in none of the adenocarcinomas or reactive pleura.[92]

At the University of Caen (France), the group of Françoise Galateau-Salle has carried out a study to determine whether SV-40-like DNA sequences were also present in bronchopulmonary carcinoma and in non-malignant lung samples and to compare these results with those obtained in mesothelioma cases.[93] Thus, 157 frozen pleural and pulmonary samples (including 15 mesotheliomas, 63 bronchopulmonary carcinomas, 8 other tumours, 71 non-malignant samples) and 6 mesothelioma cell lines were studied for the occurrence of SV-40-like DNA sequences by PCR amplification followed by hybridation with specific probes. This study has shown that sequences related to SV-40 large T antigen (Tag) were present in 28.6% of bronchopulmonary carcinomas, 47.6% of mesotheliomas and 16% of cases with non-tumour pleural and pulmonary diseases. No statistically significant difference in the occurrence of these DNA sequences was found between malignant mesothelioma and bronchopulmonary carcinoma. However, a significantly higher number of mesothelioma cases exhibited SV-40-like DNA sequences in comparison with cases having non-malignant pleural or pulmonary diseases ($p < 0.04$). Eight of ten mesothelioma cases positive for SV-40 had a history of asbestos exposure. Of the bronchopulmonary carcinomas that were positive for SV-40, 3 of 12 had a history of asbestos exposure. Immunohistochemistry using monoclonal antibodies directed against Tag did not demonstrate nuclear staining. The DNA sequences were not related to BK virus sequences, but three samples were positive with probes hybridizing with JC virus DNA sequences. Thus, these French data demonstrating that the presence of SV-40-like DNA is not unique to cancer need further studies in order to determine the exact nature and origin of those SV-40-like DNA sequences and their eventual oncogenic potential in human pleural and pulmonary malignancies.

Attitude of European nations toward the use of asbestos – opposing the European Economic Commission (EEC) directives?

Countries that produce and use asbestos, such as Canada, Australia, South Africa and the USA, aware of the dangers of asbestos (particularly asbestosis, lung carcinoma and mesothelioma), decided early in the 1980s to enact strict controls.

Meanwhile, in Europe, the EEC Commission of Brussels adopted the political decision of a 'controlled uses of asbestos'. However, it seems important to show the contrasts in attitude between the different European nations toward the three successive EEC regulations concerning the use of asbestos (83/478, 85/610 and 91/659), aimed at protecting workers and the general population against the risk of asbestos-related diseases, particularly malignancies. Thus, only the use of chrysotile was allowed (except for 14 categories of products), with the reservation of the appropriate labelling.

This attitude was different between nations, particularly between North and South, probably mainly for economic reasons (see Table 2.3).

Scandinavian nations and the UK

As early as the 1960s, the Scandinavian nations, not satisfied with the 'controlled use of asbestos' recommendations of the EEC directives, published more strict regulations, with transitory exemptions for a limited number of industrial products as a step toward a complete ban on all kinds of asbestos. However, the successive steps were a little different in these countries.

• *Sweden*. In 1964, Sweden published the first regulation concerning the use of asbestos, mainly aimed at reducing the risk of lung fibrosis, and recommending that asbestos be replaced wherever possible. There was not yet a limit set for occupational exposure. The first permissible exposure level (PEL), at 2 f/mL, was introduced in 1975, then reduced successively to 1 f/mL in 1976, 0.5 f/mL in 1985, and 0.2 f/mL in 1988. The use of crocidolite was prohibited in 1975, followed in 1976 by the prohibition of asbestos cement products. In 1978, import of raw asbestos had decreased dramatically. In 1982, there was a general prohibition of the use of other types of asbestos. On 1 October 1992, it was forbidden to use, transform and treat chrysotile, with only a few exceptions (friction materials) when substitutes were not available.[31]

• *Denmark*. On 1 January 1986, production, importation and use of raw asbestos or all types of asbestos-containing products were forbidden, but with some delay (up to 31

Table 2.3. General attitude of European Community Nations toward asbestos regulations. Present threshold limit values (TLV) for chrysotile (8 hours work time) and for crocidolite (4 hours or 1 hour work time).*

European country	General attitude in asbestos regulation	Chrysotile (f/mL)	Crocidolite (f/mL)
Austria	All uses forbidden 31.12.90	0.15	0.15
Denmark	All uses forbidden since 1980	0.30	0.30
Finland	All uses forbidden 1.1.94	0.30	0.30
France	Total interdition 24.12.96	0.10	0.10
Germany	All uses forbidden 31.12.94	0.15	0.15
Italy	Total interdiction 13.4.93	0.60	0.20
Luxembourg	No interdiction, only regulation	0.60	0.30
Netherlands	Total interdiction 1.7.93 (crocidolite forbidden in 1978)	0.30	0.10
Portugal	No interdiction	0.60	0.30
Spain	No total interdiction (chrysotile allowed)	0.60	0.25
Sweden	Total interdiction 1.7.92	0.20	No TLV
United Kingdom	No total interdiction 8.12.92	0.50 for 4h	0.20 for 4h

No data for Belgium, Greece or Ireland.
* From the report of Le Deaut and Revol[90] and AFNOR document, 1998.

December 1989) according to types of asbestos and products. Crocidolite and amosite were forbidden.

•*Finland.* On 1 January 1993, importation of raw asbestos as well as asbestos-containing products was prohibited; on 1 January 1994, it was forbidden to sell and use raw asbestos and asbestos-containing products, with few exceptions (friction products and gaskets).

• *Norway.* The use of asbestos peaked around 1970 and import of asbestos has been banned since 1982.[34]

•*United Kingdom.* The first regulation on asbestos in the workplace was published in 1969, specifying a fibre limit in the workplace: the control limit for crocidolite was lowered to 0.2 f/mL. The limit for both chrysotile and amosite was set at 2 f/mL. In 1977, in order to improve further regulations, an Advisory Committee on Asbestos was set up, with J. Peto and M. Turner-Warwick as experts.

In October 1979, new control limits for asbestos were recommended.

• Crocidolite: ban on new applications; publication of new exposure limits – 0.2 f/mL for dust sampling of 4 hours.

• Chrysotile and amosite: exposure limits reduced to 1 f/mL for chrysotile and 0.5 f/mL for amosite (4 hours sampling).

In 1988, HSE published guidelines for the use of asbestos – exposure to all forms of asbestos should be reduced to the minimum practicable. The following limits in the workplace were effected:

1. From August 1984: for a 4-hour period, 2 f/mL for crocidolite and amosite and 0.5 f/mL for other types of asbestos.

2. From March 1988, new regulations on dust control at work were published (10 minute periods): amosite and crocidolite: 0.6 f/mL; other types of asbestos: 1.5 f/mL.

In central Europe

• *West Germany*. In 1979, the German authorities agreed to a compromise with the local asbestos industries as a step to a total ban on asbestos in the forthcoming 10 years. In 1990, all types of asbestos fibres were classified in the group of carcinogenic substances. Industrial production and use of asbestos-containing commercial products were forbidden, with only short-term exemptions for a few industrial articles, such as large asbestos cement boards and canalisation.

• *Austria*. In 1988, the use of asbestos in brake linings was forbidden, with some exceptions. In June 1990, all products containing amphiboles were banned. In January 1994, asbestos-cement products were banned.

• *Switzerland*. The use of asbestos was prohibited on 1 September 1986, but with many exceptions up to 1995.

• *France*. The first permissible exposure level (PEL) to asbestos at 2 f/mL was published in 1977 (décret n° 77-949 of August 17). This decree has been abrogated in order to introduce more severe regulations in 1983 and in 1987, reducing the PEL to 1 f/mL for all types of asbestos. But the PEL was different according to fibre types: 0.5 f/mL for crocidolite and 0.8 f/mL for mixtures of asbestos-containing crocidolite. In 1992, according to the 25/6/1991 EEC directive, PEL was reduced to 0.6 f/mL for chrysotile and 0.3 f/mL for all other varieties of asbestos. Although these limits (PEL) are still recommended by the European Union, numerous European countries had already lowered their own limits for asbestos fibres in the workplace. Thus in France, the décret n° 96-1132 (24 December 1996) lowered the limit for chrysotile, to 0.1 f/mL for 8 hours at work; for other fibre types, to 0.1 f/mL for 1 h at work.

Immediately after the publication of the Expertise Collective INSERM,[36] the Ministery of Social Affairs published décret n° 96-1133 (24-12-1996) prohibiting the use of all types of asbestos fibres, with few exceptions.

• *Italy*. This country has been a producer of asbestos. The Balangero mine (presently closed) produced only pure chrysotile. Among the workers, mesothelioma has been shown to be rare or absent,[94] but lung cancer was the same as for those exposed either to amphiboles or to chrysotile contaminated with amphibole fibres.[35]

On 27 March 1992, a law was passed which prohibited the importation and use of all kinds of asbestos.

Thus, in 1996, in most European countries, the limit values for asbestos fibres were lower than those recommended by the last European Directive, but in general higher than the 0.10 recommended by the French legislation (Table 2.3). However, it seems that seven European countries (United Kingdom, Ireland, Belgium, Luxembourg, Greece, Spain and Portugal) have adopted their legislation in conformity with the EEC directives (83/478, 85/610 and 91/659) permitting the 'controlled use' of asbestos.

On 26 July 1999, the European Community Commission published the directive 1999/77/EC forbidding new applications of asbestos in countries that are members of the European Community.

References

1. Wagner, J.C. The discovery of the association of mesothelioma and asbestos exposure. *Eur Respir Rev* 1993; **3, 11**: 9–11.
2. Klemperer, P., Rabin, C.B. Primary neoplasms of the pleura. A report of five cases. *Arch Pathol* 1931; **11**: 385–412.S.
3. Maximov, A. Ueber das Mesothel und die Zellen der serosen exudate. *Arch Exp Zellforschen* 1927; **4**: 1– 42.
4. Stout, A.P., Murray, M.R. Localised pleural mesothelioma. Investigations of its characteristics and histogenesis by the method of tissue culture. *Arch Pathol* 1942; **34**: 951–964.
5. Campbell, W.M. Pleural mesothelioma. *Am J Pathol* 1950; **26**: 473–483.
6. Leibow, A.N. Armed forces of pathology. *Atlas Tumour Pathology*. 1952; **section v, fasc 17**: 176.
7. Tobiassen, G. Pleural mesotheliomas. *Acta Pathol Microbiol Scand* 1955; **Suppl. 105**: 198–218.
8. Craighead, J.F., Abraham, J.L., Churg, A., Green, F., Kleinerman, J., Pratt, P.C., Seemayer, T.A., Vallyathan, V., Weill, H. The pathology of asbestos-associated diseases of the lungs and pleural cavities: diagnostic criteria and proposed grading schema. *Arch Pathol Lab Med* 1982; **106**: 544–596.
9. Wedler, H.W. Asbestos und Lungenkrebs. *Dtsch Med Wochenschr* 1943; **69**: 575.
10. Doll, R. Mortality from lung cancer in asbestos workers. *Br J Ind Med* 1955; **12**: 81–86.
11. Wagner, J.C., Sleggs, C.A., Marchand, P. Diffuse pleural malignant mesothelioma and asbestos exposure in the North Western Cape Province. *Br J Ind Med* 1960; **17**: 260–271.
12. Turiaf, J., Basset, F., Battesti, J.P., Calvet, J.M. Le role de l'asbestose dans la provocation des tumeurs malignes diffuses de la plèvre «mesotheliome pleural ». *Presse Med* 1965; **73**: 2199–2204.
13. McDonald, A.D., McDonald, J.C. Epidemiology of malignant mesothelioma. In: Antman K, Kaisner, M.J., eds. *Asbestos-Related Malignancy*. New York; Grune and Stratton, 1986; pp 31–55.
14. Leigh, J., Hendrie, L., Berry, D. The incidence of mesothelioma in Australia 1993 to 1995. *Australian Mesothelioma Register, National Occupational Health and Safety Commission* 1998. Sydney, GPO Box 58, Sydney 2001, Australia.
15. Zwi, A.B., Reid, G., Landau, S.P., Kiekowski, D., Sitas, F., Becklake, M.R. Mesothelioma in South Africa, 1976–84: Incidence and case characteristics. *Int J Epidemiol* 1989; **18**: 320–329.
16. Jones, R.D., Smith, D.B., Thomas, P.G. Mesothelioma in Great Britain in 1968–1983. *Scand J Work Environ Health* 1988; **14**:145–152.
17. Meijers, J.M.M., Planteyd, H.T., Slangen, J.J.M., Swaen, G.M.H., Vilet, C.V, Sturmans, F. Trends and geographical patterns of pleural mesothelioma in the Netherlands 1970–1987. *Br J Ind Med* 1990; **47**: 775–781.
18. McDonald, A.D., McDonald, J.C. Malignant mesothelioma in North America. *Cancer* 1980; **46**: 1650–1659.
19. Connelly, R.R., Spirtas, R., Myers, M.H., Percy, C.L., Fraumeni, J.F. Demographic patterns for mesothelioma in the United States. *J Natl Cancer Inst* 1987; **78**:1053–1060.

20. Peto, J., Seidman, H., Selikoff, I.J. Mesothelioma mortality in asbestos workers: implications for models of carcinogenesis and risk assessment. *Br J Cancer* 1982; **45**: 124–135.
21. Peto, J., Hodgson, J.T., Matthews, F.E., Jones, J.R. Continuing increase in mesothelioma mortality in Britain. *Lancet* 1995; **345** (i): 535–539.
22. Gilg Soit Ilg, A., Bignon, J., Valleron, A.J. Estimation of the past and future burden of mortality from mesothelioma in France. *Occup Environ Med* 1998; **55**: 760–765.
23. Greenberg, M., Lloyd-Davies, T.A. Mesothelioma register 1967–68. *Br J Ind Med* 1974; **31**: 91–104.
24. McDonald, J.C., McDonald, A.D. The epidemiology of mesothelioma in historical context. *Eur Respir J* 1996; **9**:1932–1942.
25. Iwatsubo, Y., Pairon, J.C., Archambault de Beaune, C., Chammings, S., Bignon, J., Brochard, P. Pleural mesothelioma: a descriptive analysis based on a case-control study and mortality data in Ile de France, 1987–1990. *Am J Ind Med*. 1994; **26**: 77–88.
26. HEI-AR. Asbestos in public and commercial buildings: a literature review and synthesis of current knowledge. *Health Effects Institute-Asbestos Research*, Cambridge, MA, 1991; 317 pages.
27. Gardner, M.J., Acheson, E.D., Winter, P.D. Mortality from mesothelioma of the pleura during 1968–78 in England and Wales. *Br J Cancer.* 1982; **46**: 81–88.
28. Huuskonen, M.S., Ahlman, K., Mattsson, T., Tossavainen, A. Asbestos disease in Finland. *J Occup Med* 1980; **22**: 751–754.
29. Karjalainen, A., Pukkala, E., Mattson, K., Tammilehto, L., Vainio, H. Trends in mesothelioma incidence and occupational mesotheliomas in Finland in 1960–1995. *Scand J Work Environ Health* 1997; **23**: 266–270.
30. Meurman, L.O., Pukkala, E., Hakama, M. Incidence of cancer among anthophyllite asbestos miners in Finland. *Occup Environ Med* 1994; **51**: 421–425.
31. Järvholm, B., Englund, A., Albin, M. Pleural mesothelioma in Sweden: an analysis of the incidence according to the use of asbestos. *Occup Environ Med* 1999; **56**: 110–113.
32. Järvholm, B., Sandén, A. Lung cancer and mesothelioma in the pleura and peritoneum among Swedish insulation workers. *Occup Environ Med* 1998; **55**: 766–770.
33. Anderson, M., Olsen, J. Trend and distribution of mesothelioma in Denmark. *Br J Cancer* 1985; **51**: 699–705.
34. Mowé, G., Andersen, A., Osvoll, P. Trends in mesothelioma incidence in Norway. *Toxicol Ind Health* 1991; **7**: 47–52.
35. Belloni, G., Boro, G. Il mesothelioma pleurica. *Acta Med Pathol* 1957; **3**: 31–37.
35. Bignon, J., Brochard, P., Pairon, J.C. Mesothelioma: causes and fibre-related mechanisms. *In*: Aisner, J., Arriagada, R., Green, M., Martini, N., Perry, N.C. Comprehensive *Textbook of Thoracic Oncology*. Williams and Wilkins, 1996; pp 735–756.
36. INSERM. Effets sur la santé des principaux types d'exposition à l'amiante. Expertise Collective. 1997. 1 volume Les Editions INSERM. Paris.
37. Ménegoz, F., Grosclaude, P., Arveux, P., Henry-Amar, M., Schaffer, P., Raverdy, N., Daures, J.P. Incidence du mésothéliome dans les registres des cancers français; estimations France entière. *BEH* 1996; **12**: 57–58.
38. Wright, W.E., Sherwin, R.P., Dickson, E.A., Bernstein, L., Fromm, J.B., Henderson, B. Malignant mesothelioma: incidence, asbestos exposure, and reclassification of histopathology. *Br J Ind Med* 1984; **41**: 39–45.
39. Spirtas, R., Beebe, G.W., *et al*. Recent trends in mesothelioma incidence in the United States. *Am J Ind Med* 1986; **9**: 397–407.
40. Ferguson, D.A., Jelihovsky, T., Andreas, S.B., Rogers, A.J., Chung Fung, S., Grimwood, A., Thompson R. The Australian Mesothelioma Surveillance Program 1979–1985. *Med J Aust* 1987; **147**: 166–172.

41. Selikoff, I., Seidman., H. Use of death certificates in epidemiological studies, including occupational hazards: variations in discordance of different asbestos-associated diseases on best evidence ascertainment. *Am J Ind Med* 1992; **22**: 481–492.

42. Teta, M.J., Lewinsohn, H.C., Meigs, J.W. Mesothelioma in Connecticut 1955–1977. Occupational and geographic association. *J Occup Med* 1983; **25**: 749–456.

43. Newhouse, M.L., Wagner, J.C. Validation of death certificates in asbestos workers. *Br J Ind Med* 1969; **26**: 302–307.

44. Howel, D., Arblaster, L., Swinburne, L., Schweiger, M., Renvoize, E., Hatton P. Routes of asbestos exposure and the development of mesothelioma in an English region. *Occup Environ Med* 1997; **54**: 403–409.

45. Howel, D., Gibbs, A., Arblaster, L., Swinburne, L., Schweiger, M., Renvoize, E., Hatton, P., Pooley F. Mineral fibre analysis and routes of exposure to asbestos in the development of mesothelioma in an English region. *Occup Environ Med* 1999; **56**: 51–58.

46. Stumphius, J. Epidemiology of mesothelioma on Walcheren Island. *Br J Ind Med* 1968; **28**: 59–66.

47. De Lajartre, M., De Lajartre, A.Y. Mesothelioma on the coast of Brittany, France. *N Y Acad Sci* 1979; **330**: 323–332.

48. Chailleux, E., Pioche, D., Choppra, S., Dabouis, G., Germaud, P., De Lajartre, A.Y., De Lajartre, M. Epidemiologie du mesotheliome pleural malin dans la region de Nantes-Saint NazaiRe. Evolution entre 1956 et 1992. *Rev Mal Respir* 1995; **12**: 353–357.

49. Letourneux, M., Galateau, F., Legendre, C., Leclerc, A., Beck, A., Launoy, G., Raffaeli, C., Bazin, B. Malignant mesothelioma diagnosed in lower Normandy between 1980 and 1990. *Eur Respir Rev* 1993; **3**: **11**: 87–88.

50. Giarelli, L., Bianchi, C., Grandi, G. Malignant mesothelioma of the pleura in Trieste, Italy. *Am J Ind Med* 1992; **22**: 521–530.

51. Jones, J.S.P., Smith, P.G., Pooley, F.D., *et al.* The consequences of exposure to asbestos dust in a wartime gas-mask factory. In: Wagner JC, ed. *Biological effects of mineral fibers. Lyon France: International Agency for Research on Cancer* 1980; 637–653. IARC Scientific Publication N° 30.

52. Newhouse, M.L., Berry, G., Wagner, J.C. Mortality of factory workers in east London 1933–80. *Br J Ind Med* 1985; **42**: 4–11.

53. Raffn, E., Lynge, E., Juel, K., *et al.* Incidence of cancer and mortality among employees in the asbestos cement industry in Denmark. *Br J Ind Med* 1989; **46**: 90–96.

54. Albin, M., Jakobsson, K., Attewell, R., Johansson, L., Welinder, H. Mortality and cancer morbidity in cohorts of asbestos cement workers and referents. *Br J Ind Med* 1990; **47**: 602–610.

55. Rogers, A.J., Leigh, J., Berry, G., Ferguson, D.A., Mulder, H.B., Ackad, M. Relationship between lung asbestos fiber type and concentration and relative risk of mesothelioma. A case-control study. *Cancer* 1991; **67**: 1912–1920.

56. Tuomi, T., Huuskonen, M.S., Virtamo, M., *et al.* Relative risk of mesothelioma associated with different levels of exposure to asbestos. *Scand J Work Environ Health* 1991; **17**: 404–408.

57. Gardner, M.J., Saracci, R. Effects on health of non occupational exposure to airborne mineral fibres. Bignon, J., Peto J., Saracci R. *Non-occupational exposure to mineral fibres. IARC* 1989; **90**: 375–397.

58. Newhouse, M.L., Thompson, H. Mesothelioma of pleura and peritoneum following exposure to asbestos in the London area. *Br J Ind Med* 1965; **22**: 261–269.

59. Meurman, L.O., Kiviluoto, R., Hakama, M. Mortality and morbidity among the working population of anthophyllite asbestos miners in Finland. *Br J Ind Med* 1974; **31**: 105–112.

60. Magnani, C., Terracini, B., Ivaldi, C., Botta, M., Mancini, A., Andrion, A. Pleural malignant mesothelioma and non-occupational exposure to asbestos in Casale Monferrato, Italy. *Occup Environ Med* 1995; **52**: 362–367.
61. Constantopoulos, S.H., Goudevenos, J.A., Saratzis, N., *et al.* Metsovo lung: pleural calcification and restrictive lung function in northwestern Greece. Environmental exposure to mineral fiber as etiology. *Environ Res* 1985; **38**: 319–331.
62. Rey, F., Viallat, J.R., Boutin, C., *et al.* Les mésothéliomes environmentaux en Corse du Nord-est. *Rev Mal Respir* 1993; **10**: 339–345.
63. Goldberg, P., Goldberg, M., Marne, M.J., Hirsch, A., Tredaniel, J. Incidence of pleural mesothelioma in New Caledonia: a 10-year survey (1978–1987). *Ann Environ Health* 1991; **46**: 306–309.
64. Valleron, A.J., Bignon, J., Hughes, J.M, Hesterberg, T.W., Schneider, T., Burdett, G.J., Brochard, P., Hémon, D. Low dose exposure to natural and man-made fibres and the risk of cancer: towards a collaborative European epidemiology. *Br J Ind Med* 1992; **49**: 606–614.
65. Sebastien, P., McDonald, J.C., McDonald, A.D., Case, B., Harley, R. Respiratory cancer in chrysotile textile and mining industries/exposure inferences from lung analysis. *Br J Ind Med* 1989; **46**: 180–187.
66. Boutin, C., Dumortier, P., Rey, F., Viallat, J.R., De Vuyst, P. Black spots concentrate oncogenic asbestos fibers in the parietal pleura. Thoracoscopic and mineralogical study. *Am J Respir Crit Care Med* 1996; **153**: 444–449.
67. Woitowitz, H.J., Rodelsperger, K. Chrysotile asbestos and mesothelioma. *Am J Ind Med.* 1991; **19**: 551–3.
68. Smith, A.H., Wright, C.C. Chrysotile asbestos is the main cause of pleural mesothelioma. *Am J Ind Med* 1996; **30**: 252–266.
69. Nicholson, W.J., Raffn, E. Recent data on cancer due to asbestos in the USA and Denmark. *Med Lav* 1995; **86**, 5: 393–410.
70. Gaudichet, A., Janson, X., Monchaux, G., Dufour, G., Sebastien, P., De Lajartre, A.Y., Bignon, J. Assessment by analytical microscopy of the total lung fibre burden in mesothelioma patients matched with four other pathological series. *Ann Occup Hyg* 1988; **32**(Suppl 1): 213–223.
71. Edward, A.T., Whitaker, Browne, K., Pooley, F.D., Gibbs, A.R. Mesothelioma in a community in the north of England. *Occup Environ Med* 1996; **53**: 547–552.
72. Iwatsubo, Y., Pairon, J.C., Boutin, C., Ménard, O., Massin, N., Caillaud, D., Orlowski, E., Galateau-Salle, F., Bignon, J., Brochard, P. Pleural mesothelioma: dose-response relation at low levels of asbestos exposure in a French population-based case-control study. *Am J Epidemiology* 1998; **148**: 133–142.
73. Lillington, G.A, Jamplis RW, Differding JR. Conjugal malignant mesothelioma. *N Engl J Med* 1974; **291**: 583–584.
74. Vianna, N.J., Polan, A.K. Non-occupational exposure to asbestos in malignant mesothelioma in females. *Lancet* 1978; **1**: 1061–1063.
75. Kiviluoto, R. Pleural calcifications as roentgenologic sign of non-occupational endemic anthophyllite-asbestosis. Thesis, Stockholm, 1960.
76. McConnochie, K., Simonayo, L., Mavrides, P., Pooley, F.D., Wagner, J.C. Mesothelioma in Cyprus: the role of tremolite. *Thorax* 1987; **42**: 342–347.
77. Baris, Y.I., Saracci, R., Simonato, L., Skidmore, J.W., Artvingli, M. Malignant mesothelioma and radiological chest abnormalities in two villages in central Turkey. *Lancet* 1981; **ii**: 984–987.
78. McDonald, J.C. Health implications of environmental exposure to asbestos. *Environ Health Perspect* 1985; **62**: 319–328.

79. Omenn, G.S., Merchant, J., Boatman, E., *et al.* Contribution of environmental fibers to respiratory cancer. *Environ Health Perspect* 1986; **70**: 51–56.
80. Cordier, S., Lazar, P., Brochard, P., Bignon, J., Ameille, J., Proteau, J. Epidemiologic investigation of a respiratory effects related to environmental exposure to asbestos inside insulted buildings. *Arch. Environ Health* 1987; **42**: 303–309.
81. Price, B. Analysis of current trends in United States mesothelioma incidence. *Am J Epidemiol* 1997; **45**: 211–218.
82. Peterson, J.T., Greenberg, S.D., Bufler, P.A. Non-asbestos-related malignant mesothelioma. *Cancer* 1984; **54**: 951–960.
83. Hirsch, A., Brochard, P., De Cremoux, H., Erkan, L., Sebastien, P., Di Menza, L., Bignon, J. Features of asbestos-exposed and unexposed mesothelioma. *Am J Ind Med* 1982; **2**: 413–422.
84. Maurer, R., Egloff, B. Malignant peritoneal mesothelioma after cholangiography with thorotrast. *Cancer* 1975; **36**: 1381–1385.
85. Stock, R.J., Fu, Y., Carter, J. Malignant peritoneal mesothelioma following radiotherapy for seminoma of the testis. *Cancer* 1979; **44**: 914–919.
86. Babcock, T.L., Powell, D.H., Bothwell, R.S. Radiation-induced peritoneal mesothelioma. *J Surg Oncol* 1976; **8**: 369–372.
87. Hofmann, J., Mintzer, D., Warhol, J. Malignant mesothelioma following radiation therapy. *Am J Med* 1994; **97**: 379–382.
88. Warren, S., Brown, C.E., Chute, R.N., Federman, M. Mesothelioma relative to asbestos, radiation, and methylcholantrene. *Arch Pathol Lab Med* 1981; **105**: 305–312.
89. Paterour, M.J., Bignon, J., Jaurand, M.C. In vitro transformation of rat pleural mesothelial cells by chrysotile fibres and/or benzo(a)pyrene. *Carcinogenesis* 1985; **6**: 523–529.
90. Carbone, M., Pass, H.I., Rizzo, P., Marinetti, M., Di Muzio, M., Mew, D.J.Y., Levine, A.S., Procopio, A. Simian virus 40-like DNA sequences in human pleural mesothelioma. *Oncogene* 1994; **9**: 1781–1790.
90. Rubino, G.F., Scansetti, G., Donna, A. et al. Epidemiology of pleural mesothelioma in northwestern Italy (Piedmont). *Br J Ind Med* 1972; **29**: 436–442.
91. Strickler, H.D., Goedeert, J.J., Fleming, M., Travis, W.D., Williams, A.E., Rabkin, C.S., Daniel, R.W., Shah, K.V. Simian virus 40 and pleural mesothelioma in humans. *Cancer Epidemiol, Biomarkers Prev* 1996; **5**: 473–475.
92. Gibbs, A.R., Jasani, B., Pepper, C., Navabi, H., Wynford-Thomas, D. SV40 DNA sequences in mesotheliomas. In: Simian virus 40 (SV40), a possible human Polyomavirus. Brown F, Lewis AM eds. *Dev Biol Stand* 1998; **94**: 41–45.
93. Galateau-Salle, F., Bidet, P.H., Iwatsubo, Y., Gennetay, E., Renier, A., Letourneux, M., Pairon, J.C., Moritz, S., Brochard, P., Jaurand, M.C., Freymuth, F. SV40-like sequences in pleural mesothelioma, bronchopulmonary carcinoma, and non-malignant pulmonary diseases. *J Pathol* 1998; **84**: 252–257.
94. Le Déaut, J.Y., Revol, H. L'amiante dans l'environnement de l'homme: ses conséquences et son avenir. Rapport N°329 de l'Assemblée Nationale et N° 41 du Sénat. 16 Oct 1997. 172 pages.

= 3 =

The History of Mesothelioma in Australia 1945–2001

James Leigh and Bruce W. S. Robinson

Asbestos was mined in Australia for over one hundred years and Australia was the world's highest user per capita of asbestos in the 1950s. It is thus no surprise that in the 1980s and 1990s Australia has had the world's highest incidence of malignant mesothelioma. While this is not something to be proud of, it has probably led to one of the most complete studies of the disease in the world. It is the purpose of this chapter to describe the history of mesothelioma in Australia as a whole, with special reference to the Wittenoom crocidolite mining operation in Western Australia. Material will be drawn from research studies conducted over the last 20 years by the Australian Mesothelioma Program and Register (National Occupational Health and Safety Commission and University of Sydney) and the University of Western Australia. The chapter updates and enhances previous reviews.[1-3]

History of asbestos production and use in Australia

Between 1880 and 1889 approximately 47 tonnes of amphiboles were mined at Jones' Creek, near Gundagai, New South Wales, and between 1890 and 1899 about 35 tonnes of chrysotile was mined at Anderson's Creek, Tasmania. South Australia was the first State to mine crocidolite, at Robertstown in 1916.

Over the present century there was a gradual increase in asbestos production, with more chrysotile than amphiboles mined until 1939. With the commencement of mining at Wittenoom, Western Australia, in 1937, crocidolite dominated production, until final closure in 1966. New South Wales, the first State to mine asbestos, also produced the largest tonnages of chrysotile (until 1983) as well as smaller quantities of amphiboles (until 1949).

With the closing of the crocidolite mine at Wittenoom in 1966, Australian asbestos production declined to a pre-1952 level. Exports declined from 1967. Imports of chrysotile also started to decline. The earliest records of asbestos imports date from 1929. The main sources of raw asbestos imports were Canada (chrysotile) and South

Africa (crocidolite and amosite). About twice as much chrysotile was imported as was mined and half as much crocidolite was imported as was mined. After Wittenoom was closed, a small amount (122 tonnes) of crocidolite was mined in South Australia.

In New South Wales, the chrysotile mine at Baryulgil continued production. In 1971 the chrysotile deposits at Woodsreef near Barraba, New South Wales, began to be exploited and exports of asbestos fibre expanded as production increased. This operation was open-cast with dry milling.

Australian production of asbestos fibre decreased in 1981 because of the drop in world demand for asbestos and the increased operating costs at the Woodsreef mine. This mine ceased production in 1983 when the dry milling plant could not meet dust control regulations.

Details of Australian asbestos production and imports are shown in Tables 3.1 and 3.2. Australian asbestos (crocidolite and chrysotile) was exported to the USA, Japan, UK and Europe. In particular, Wittenoom crocidolite was exported to the USA and Europe.[3a]

In addition to imports of asbestos fibre, Australia also imported many manufactured asbestos products, including asbestos cement articles, asbestos yarn, cord and fabric, asbestos joint and millboard, asbestos friction materials and gaskets. The main sources of supply were the UK, USA, Federal Republic of Germany and Japan. Apparent consumption of asbestos, the difference between production and imports, and export is shown in Table 3.3 and Figure 3.1. This gives a crude estimate of overall exposure. However, the export process itself, bagging, transport and wharf labour caused much exposure. In Australia over 60% of all production and 90% of all consumption of asbestos fibre was by the asbestos cement manufacturing industry.[4] From about 1940 to the late 1960s all three types of asbestos were used in this industry, crocidolite then being phased out. Amosite use in this industry continued until about 1983. Much of this industry output remains in service today in the form of 'fibro' houses and water

Table 3.1. Asbestos production – Australia.*

Years (10)	Crocidolite tonnes	Chrysotile tonnes	Amosite tonnes	Total tonnes
1880–1889	—	—	26	26
1890–1899	—	20	—	20
1900–1909	—	61	21	80
1910–1919	22	580	23	625
1920–1929	18	3 577	54	3 649
1930–1939	422	1 151	51	1 624
1940–1949	5 619	2 967	750	9 338
1950–1959	63 227	11 511	1	74 739
1960–1969	86 566	8 855	—	95 421
1970–1979	—	394 361	—	394 361
1980–1983	—	160 408	—	160 408
Totals	**155 874**	**583 491**	**927**	**740 293**

*Based on figures supplied by Bureau of Mineral Resources.[4]

Table 3.2. Asbestos imports – Australia (tonnes). *

Year	Chrysotile	Amosite	Crocidolite	Other	Total
19??–1930	—	—	—	—	2 568
1930–1940	—	—	—	—	51 554
1940–1949	—	—	—	—	139 987
1950–1959	186 855	107 509	2 778	16 938	314 080
1960–1969	329 129	81 432	—	24 112	434 674
1970–1979	388 003	87 901	—	79 683	555 587
1980–1983	64 672	8 338	—	4 188	77 198
Total	**968 659**	**285 180**	**2 778**	**124 921**	**1 575 648**

*Based on figures supplied by Bureau of Mineral Resources.[4]

Table 3.3. Apparent consumption of abestos – Australia. *

Year	Production tonnes	Imports tonnes	Exports tonnes	Apparent consumption tonnes
1880–1889	26	—	—	26
1890–1899	20	—	—	20
1900–1909	82	—	—	82
1910–1919	625	—	—	625
1920–1929	3 649	2 568	—	6 217
1930–1939	1 624	51 554	1 196	51 982
1940–1949	9 338	139 987	2 410	146 915
1950–1959	74 739	314 080	51 413	337 406
1960–1969	95 421	434 674	44 703	485 392
1970–1979	394 361	555 587	45 523	704 425
1980–1985	160 408	104 324	9 786	154 946
Totals	**740 293**	**1 602 774**	**455 031**	**1 888 036**

*Based on figures provided by Bureau of Mineral Resources.[4]

and sewerage piping. By 1954 Australia was number four in the world in gross consumption of asbestos cement products, after USA, UK and France, and clearly first on a per capita basis. After World War II to 1954, 70 000 asbestos cement houses were built in the State of New South Wales alone (52% of all houses built). In Australia as a whole, until the 1960s 25% of all new housing was clad in asbestos cement.

Longer chrysotile fibres were used in fireproof textiles, insulation materials, packing and woven brake linings, among other products. Medium length fibres were used mainly as fillers in various linings, facing, floor tiles and asphalts. Crocidolite, because of its high tensile strength, was used in conjunction with chrysotile in the manufacture of asbestos cement pressure pipes. The long fibres were also used for weaving into fabrics for use in boiler laggings and acid-resistant gaskets. It was also used in lining pipes, tanks and other vessels in the chemical industry and as a strengthening agent in epoxy and phenolic resins.

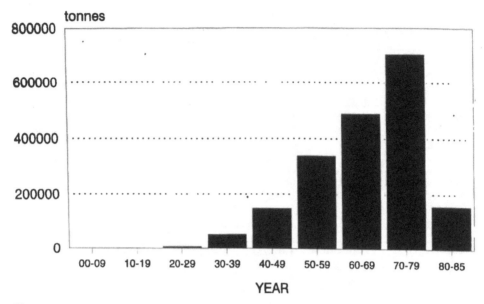

Figure 3.1. *Asbestos consumption in Australia, 1900–85.*

The main attribute of amosite, apart from heat resistance, is its low density. It was therefore used for internal linings in multi-storey buildings, in domestic house ceilings and in ships. It was also used as a support for heavy refractory powders in refractory tiles for the steel industry and in loosely compacted form as a covering for marine engines and aircraft jet engines.

Australia still imports about 1500 tonnes a year of chrysotile fibre, and about $A13.5m worth of asbestos products a year, over half as friction material but also fabricated yarn, fabric, jointing, gaskets, millboard and asbestos cement products.[5,6] However, a planned phase out of new (chrysotile) asbestos use is in place. Handling of asbestos in place and removal operations are subject to a strict National Code of Practice. A series of regulations adopted in the late 1970s and early 1980s by the various States now impose exposure limits of 0.1 fibre/mL for crocidolite, amosite and mixtures and 0.1, 0.5 or 1.0 fibre/mL for chrysotile (TWA 8 hr membrane filter method light microscopy, WHO fibres). The chrysotile limit is currently under review.

Exposures in the past were very high in some industries and jobs – up to 150 fibre/mL (e.g., 25 million particles per cubic foot in asbestos pulverisers and disintegrators in the asbestos cement industry.[7] High concentrations of fibres in mining occupations were also recorded (up to 600 fibre/mL in baggers at Wittenoom).[8]

With this background, it was almost certain that Australia would suffer a mesothelioma epidemic of a severe nature.

The first reported case, from Wittenoom, was in 1962.[9] Three more cases were reported from Victoria in 1966,[10] two from Queensland in 1968[11] and a further nine from Victoria in 1969.[12]

Australian Mesothelioma Surveillance Program

The Australian Mesothelioma Surveillance Program (the program), as it finally became known, endeavoured to correct most of the weaknesses identified in the 1960s and 1970s in other such schemes throughout the world, viz, under-reporting of cases, uncertain diagnosis, poor elucidation of the role of occupational and environmental asbestos exposure and less than comprehensive coverage.[13]

The program began on 1 January 1980 after preliminary work from 1977. Formal voluntary notification of cases was actively sought from a network of respiratory physicians, pathologists, general and thoracic surgeons, medical superintendents, medical records administrators, State and Territory departments of occupational health, cancer registries, compensation authorities or any other source. Notifications from other than the diagnosing physician were confirmed with him or her. After gaining the appropriate consents a full occupational and environmental history was obtained for each case, from either the patient or next-of-kin. The history taking was non-directive but included specific questions on asbestos exposure at the end. These histories were coded by two occupational hygienists, who naturally could not be blinded to case status. They also discussed cases together and were thus not independent. The diagnosing pathologist was requested to provide slides and/or tissue specimens. These were circulated among a pathology panel for confirmation of diagnosis. Post-mortem examination was actively sought for in every case in order to confirm diagnosis and to obtain lung tissue free of tumour for lung fibre content analysis.

Occupational and environmental exposure was classified as definite, probable and possible, based on the subjective opinions of the two hygienists. Occupation and industry classifications were based on the Australian Bureau of Statistics Industry and Occupation Codes. Further grading of intensity of exposure was also very subjective in many cases and duration depended on recollection.

Year of presumptive diagnosis was the year in which mesothelioma was first suspected clinically. Year of definitive diagnosis was the year when pathology panel diagnosis was finalised. The panel of five members of the Royal College of Pathologists of Australasia reported individually on the diagnosis as definite, probable, possible and not mesothelioma. The level of consensus was good, with exact agreement or disagreement of only one category in 94% of cases. A scoring system of 1 (definite), 0.75 (probable), 0.5 (possible) and 0 (not mesothelioma) was used and the definitive score taken as the score nearest the mean of five. Panel members also classified mesothelioma cell type as epithelial, sarcomatous, mixed or not agreed.

Lung fibre content was assessed by a local modification of a sodium hypochlorite digestion and filter method. Both light and electron microscopy (with energy dispersive x-ray analysis) were used. Fibres were counted by asbestos type and length but not diameter. All fibre lengths were recorded but because of uncertainties about filter contaminants by <2 micron fibres, only fibres >2 micron (EM) or >5 micron (LM) were considered in analyses. These methods gave a sensitivity, corresponding to one fibre counted, of 15 000 fibre/g dry lung (LM) and 200 000 fibre/g dry lung (EM). Assuming a Poisson distribution of fibres in the counting units, the upper limit of the 95% confidence interval for the population mean, given a zero count obtained, is 3.69. Thus the EM 'detection limit' is about 740 000 fibre/g.[14] Reports on lung fibre content levels were sometimes used for medico-legal purposes in a fallacious way in that counts were reported as being 'within the normal range' as if this excluded an occupational asbestos exposure and liability. The 'normal' range was in fact taken from urban hospital patients without mesothelioma and, where fibres were counted, exposure obviously had been received (and not always environmental only as judged by fibre length distribution, i.e., it must have sometimes been occupational – no work histories were available). It was not realised until later that these patients should rather be treated as non-cases (referents) in a case-referent study.

Australian Mesothelioma Register

From 1 January 1986, a less detailed notification system has operated, with a short questionnaire history, albeit followed up assiduously; no pathology panel diagnosis and only sporadic lung fibre counts. In the case of Western Australia and New South Wales (60% of all notifications), histories are obtained by direct detailed questioning by compensation authorities or cancer registries. However, only histologically confirmed cases are accepted and full reconciliation with all state cancer registries and compensation authorities is carried out. This is now known as the Australian Mesothelioma Register but is a continuation of the program. A copy of the current register notification form is shown as Figure 3.2.

The incidence of mesothelioma in Australia

Incidence rates are periodically calculated on cases notified to the program. An annual report series is produced (NOHSC, 1989–2000[6]). Cases accepted by the pathology panel in the program as definite, probable or possible are included. Because of delays in definitive diagnosis being received, incidence rates have been calculated up to end 1996 only, because of the up to two year delay in notification experienced while awaiting confirmed diagnosis and reconciliation with the state cancer registries. Figure 3.3 shows age-specific incidence for males and females >20 years of age for the year 1996. Figures 3.4 and 3.5 show age-specific incidence trends over time for males and females. Figures 3.6–3.8 show trends in world population >20 years of age standardised mesothelioma incidence by State, sex and site for recent years. Table 3.4 shows notifications up to December 2000.

From 1 January 1980 to December 2000, a total of 5671 notifications had been received by the program and register. Notifications show a continuing upward trend. The Australian population has increased from 14.5 million in 1980 to 19 million in 2000. Mesothelioma incidence rates, standardised to the world population >20 years have increased from 11.8 per million per year in 1982 to 30 per million per year in 1996 (males and females combined), 51.8 per million per year (male) and 5.9 per million per year (female). The notifications prior to 1982 were probably the result of bedding in of a new program and are artificially low (1980:16; 1981:104), although a smooth curve of increasing notification rate starting from the early 1960s has since been demonstrated by retrospective search (Figure 3.9). Between 1945 and 1979 there were 658 cases (535 male, 123 female) in Australia.[15] Thus the total number of mesotheliomas in Australia from 1945 to 31 De-

NATIONAL OCCUPATIONAL HEALTH AND SAFETY COMMISSION

AUSTRALIAN MESOTHELIOMA REGISTER NOTIFICATION

Please direct all correspondence to:

The Registrar
Australian Mesothelioma Register
National Occupational Health and Safety Commission
GPO Box 58 Sydney NSW 2001
Telephone: (02) 9577 9304

Patient details - please supply <u>ALL</u> available information

SURNAME: .... FIRST NAMES . ...

ADDRESS: ....

STATE: .... POSTCODE: .... GENDER: M / F   DATE OF BIRTH: /   /

IF DECEASED, DATE OF DEATH: /   /   PLACE OF DEATH:
   . . ..

DATE OF INITIAL DIAGNOSIS: Month   Year: HISTOLOGICAL: YES / NO

HOSPITAL DIAGNOSED: .... PRIMARY SITE: ....

CLINICIAN'S NAME: .... NAME OF LOCAL GP: ....

ADDRESS: .... ADDRESS . ...

   ....

Please describe briefly main occupation(s) of patient's worklife.

OCCUPATION   INDUSTRY   YEAR

1 .... 1. .... 19 - 19

2. .... 2. ... ... 19 - 19

3. .... 3. ...   . 19 - 19

KNOWN ASBESTOS EXPOSURE: YES / NO

If "YES" please indicate circumstances and duration: ....

.. ..

. .   .   .

Details of person completing this form.

NAME: .... SIGNATURE: .   .   ..

ADDRESS .. .. DATE   .   . ..

Please circle the appropriate category CLINICIAN PATHOLOGIST CANCER REGISTRY MEDICAL RECORDS ADMIN
                                         DUST DISEASES BOARD OTHER   ..   ..

Office Use Only
Date Received:
                                 REGISTRATION NO:

27

Figure 3.2. *Australian Mesothelioma Register notification form.*

Table 3.4. Mesothelioma notifications in Australia, 1980–99.

Year	NSW	VIC	QLD	WA	SA	TAS	NT	ACT	Total
1980	15	1	0	0	0	0	0	0	16
1981	51	3	18	22	5	5	0	0	104
1982	90	20	9	0	20	2	0	1	142
1983	53	23	26	46	19	6	0	0	173
1984	76	38	20	26	14	1	1	2	178
1985	71	39	27	30	19	1	0	2	189
1986	46	34	38	32	18	2	1	1	172
1987	54	40	26	28	32	0	0	2	182
1988	57	28	45	23	36	1	0	2	192
1989	124	25	35	44	22	3	0	1	254
1990	111	82	43	26	25	1	0	1	289
1991	105	44	46	66	55	10	0	2	328
1992	117	45	40	37	39	3	1	1	283
1993	99	34	42	47	25	5	0	0	252
1994	151	41	74	32	30	8	0	1	337
1995	124	89	49	33	43	11	1	3	353
1996	87	157	53	127	30	4	1	4	463
1997	107	32	64	82	24	5	0	4	318
1998	160	84	65	66	21	8	0	1	405
1999	252	113	73	79	20	7	0	7	551
2000	168	106	99	47	60	7	0	3	490
All	**2118**	**1078**	**892**	**893**	**557**	**90**	**5**	**39**	**5671**
	37.3%	**19.0%**	**15.7%**	**15.7%**	**9.8%**	**1.6%**	**0.1%**	**0.7%**	**100%**

cember 2000 is 6329. Notifications to 31 May 2001 are 6630. If the 1981 figure is accepted it can be claimed that mesothelioma incidence rates have increased fourfold in 18 years in Australia. Both male and female rates have increased but the male rate is over eight times the female rate. These are the highest reported rates in the world and in terms of mortality equal to kidney cancer in males and uterine cancer in females.[16] Western Australia has the highest incidence (total persons, males and females) but contributes only 15% of the

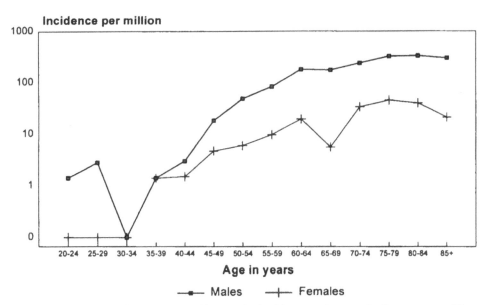

Figure 3.3. Australian age-specific crude incidence of mesothelioma per million persons, by age and sex, 1996.

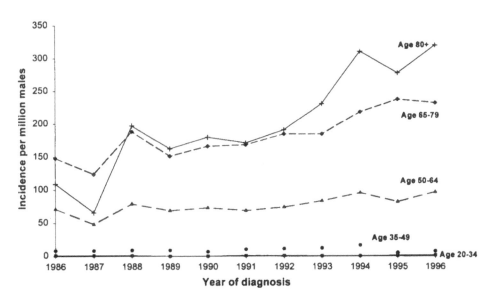

Figure 3.4. Age-specific incidence rates of malignant mesothelioma in Australian men, 1986–96.

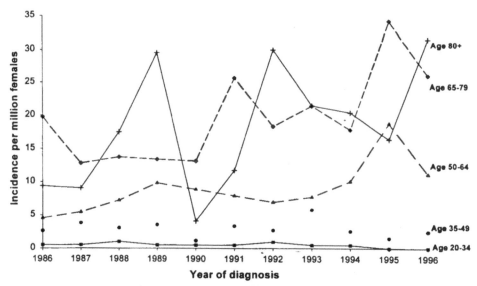

Figure 3.5. *Age specific incidence rates of malignant mesothelioma in Australian women, 1986-1996.*

total cases. Wittenoom contributes about 5% of the Australian cases yet is certainly the most publicised and best known internationally. Most of the cases come from the two most populous and industrialised States, New South Wales and Victoria.[17]

In 93.2% of all program cases the mesothelioma was pleural in site, 6.5% peritoneal and only 0.3% of cases in other sites. Among men 94.3% were pleural, 5.3% peritoneal; among women 86.3% pleural, 13.7% peritoneal. These proportions have been maintained in register cases, with a slightly higher proportion of site not known being reported. The female peritoneal proportion has dropped to 10.4%. Of the cases that underwent pathology panel review, 96% were confirmed as mesothelioma (73% definite, 17% probable and 6% possible). The most common occupational exposures were repair and maintenance of asbestos materials (18%), shipbuilding (11%), asbestos cement production (7%), asbestos cement use (7%), railways (6%), Wittenoom crocidolite mining/milling (6%), insulation manufacture/installation (4%), wharf labouring (3%), power stations (3%), boilermaking (2%), and para-occupational/hobby and environmental (15%). When the earlier cases classed as 'no history of exposure' were reviewed it was found that 57 of the 203 so classified actually had history of some exposure recorded. Thus only around 18% had no known history. Moreover, of this 'no known history' group, 81% had fibre counts detected in the lungs, 30% with more than 10^6 fibre/g >2 micron including 'long' (>10 micron) fibres, suggesting that nearly all cases have been exposed. Indeed, absence of fibres in the lungs does not negate exposure as fibres may have initiated mesothelioma and then been cleared before death. The shortest duration of exposure was 16 hours. Three per cent of cases had exposure less than three months. According to history assessment of the first exposure of 530 cases by the two hygienists, most cases (55%) had mixed amphibole–chrysotile exposure, 13% amphibole only, 7% amphibole, plus pos-

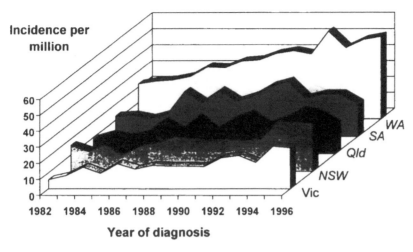

Standardised to World Popn > 20 years

Figure 3.6. *Trends in Australian incidence of mesothelioma per million persons, by State, 1982–96.*

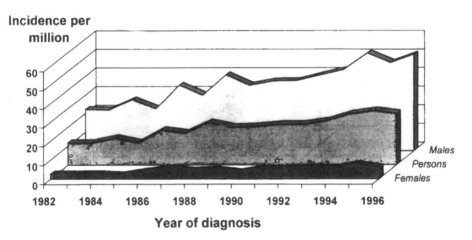

Standardised to World Popn > 20 years

Figure 3.7. *Trends in Australian incidence of mesothelioma per million persons, by sex, 1982–96.*

sible chrysotile, 6% chrysotile, with possible amphibole, and 4% chrysotile only, with 15% unknown fibre type.[18] Mean latency from first exposure to presumptive diagnosis was 37.4 years.[13] The range of latencies was 4–75 years.

In the cases reported since 1 January 1986, when less detail of history of exposure was sought, 89.9% of males responding to questionnaire and 61.2% of females gave a history of asbestos exposure (overall 86.4% – non-response 22% males, 30%

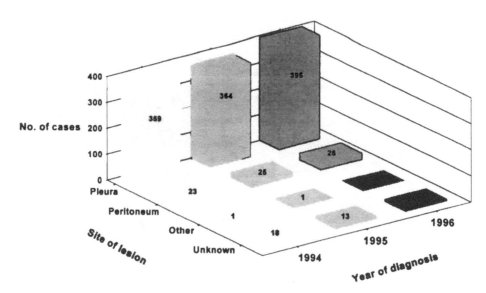

Figure 3.8. Cases of mesothelioma in Australia, 1994–96, by site of primary lesion.

females). The pattern of exposure history is changing, and more product, domestic, environmental and para-occupational exposure is apparent, compared to the older traditional industries. Table 3.5 shows the circumstances of exposure in cases from 1986–2000. This is a combination of occupation and industry or domestic or environmental circumstance. Some common exposure histories were repair and maintenance of asbestos materials (13%), shipbuilding (3%), asbestos cement production (4%), railways (3%), power stations (3%), boilermaking (3%), Wittenoom (5%), wharf labour (2%), para-occupational, hobby, environmental (4%), carpenter (4%), builder (6%), navy (3%), plumber (2%), brake linings (2%) and multiple (12%).

Relationships between mesothelioma site, cell type, lung fibre content and survival

Studies on the relationship of lung fibre concentration and mesothelioma site, cell type and survival were also carried out. Fibre content in the lung depends on the amount of fibre deposited and the amount cleared. The amount deposited depends on the duration and intensity of exposure in the occupational or general environment. The clearance rate is thought to be dependent on the amount deposited at any particular time, i.e., clearance is exponential,[19] although fast and slow clearance compartments have been identified.[20] Thus, the same fibre content in the lung at death or time of resection may be achieved from a high initial deposition, followed by absence of deposition and absence of clearance over a long time, or by a continuous deposition of a lower level, with or without clearance. Because detailed mechanisms of mesothelioma induction are not yet completely understood, dose as estimated by final lung fibre content may not relate to the dose required to

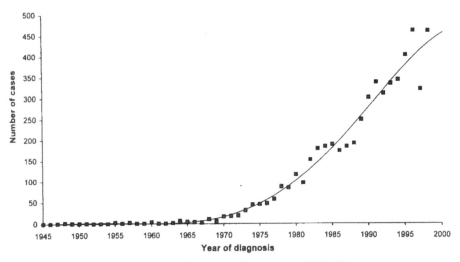

Figure 3.9. Australian mesothelioma incident cases 1945–98.

induce mesothelioma. Thus a high lung fibre content in a mesothelioma case may represent continuing accumulation of fibres after a lower level of fibres has induced malignant change. It is more probable, however, that the malignant change did not occur until the fibre content reached a sufficiently high level. Despite these difficulties in interpretation, lung fibre content is a more certain index of exposure than retrospectively obtained work histories and estimates of occupational and general environmental levels, as shown above.

To examine these questions, an analysis was undertaken of pathology data, lung fibre content data, and survival data obtained from the program to determine: (1) the relationship between lung fibre content and type and cell type of mesothelioma; (2) the relationship between lung fibre content and type and primary site of mesothelioma; (3) the relationship between cell type of mesothelioma and site of tumour; and (4) the relationship between cell type, primary site, and survival.[21]

For each case, the date of provisional diagnosis (PD) was available. For known deceased cases, the date of death was obtained. Tissue for histologic examination was available in 777 cases. Post-mortem examination was done on 226 cases, and formalin-preserved tissue obtained for analysis of lung fibre content.

Histological classification of tumour type and cell type was made in the 777 cases by the pathology panel. The staining techniques used included Haematoxylin and eosin, special stains for reticulin and mucus (such as mucicarmine, periodic acid-Schiff after diastase, and the Alcian blue stain with and without prior digestion with hyaluronidase), and the immunoperoxidase stain for carcinoembryonic antigen (and in selected cases for keratin and epithelial membrane antigen). Both light and electron microscopy were used. A total of 565 cases were definite, 131 probable, 50 possible, and 31 not possible.

The panel corresponded if it appeared that further stains or discussion could help resolve a final diagnosis of probable or possible mesothelioma. Controversial cases were also

Table 3.5. Asbestos exposures as documented in the Australian Mesothelioma Register from 1 January 1986 to 31 October 2000.

	Number exposed		Total
	Single*	Multiple†	exposures
Acoustic engineer	1	–	1
Air-conditioning	12	14	26
Aircraft	11	3	14
Armed forces /wartime	28	16	44
Armed forces /peacetime	6	2	8
Asbestos bagging (not Wittenoom)	8	4	12
Asbestos bags – handled which had contained	8	–	8
Asbestos clothing worn	9	4	13
Asbestos covers for cooking	3	–	3
Asbestos dwelling/fence – built/renovated	70	13	83
Asbestos dwelling – lived in	29	8	37
Asbestos products – lived near	11	2	13
Asbestos products factory – worked near	11	–	11
Asbestos mine – worked/lived near (not Wittenoom)	12	6	18
Asbestos product handled in the workplace	42	8	50
Asbestos product manufacturer – worked	106	36	142
Asbestos product part of workplace or surrounds	26	9	35
Asbestos tailings – played on as a child	8	4	12
Asbestos /or products worker – lived with/washed clothes	42	6	48
Bakery (ovens)	3	–	3
Boilermaker/cleaner/attendant /installer/welder	79	54	133
Brake linings – made/repaired	58	19	77
Brewery	1	–	1
Bricklayer	15	4	19
Brickworks	8	3	11
Builder/ builder's labourer	185	40	225
Carpenter/ joiner	224	42	266
Cement factory worker	20	1	21
Chemical engineer	1	–	1
Civil engineer	7	–	7
Concreting	5	3	8

Table 3.5. continued.

| | Number exposed | | Total |
	Single*	Multiple†	exposures
Construction worker	12	2	14
Demolition	5	2	7
Design engineer	2	1	3
Diesel engineer	–	1	1
Dockyard worker	40	23	63
Electrical engineer	5	7	12
Electrical fitter	15	4	19
Electrical mechanic	3	–	3
Electrician	55	12	67
Electroplater	–	1	1
Engineer	26	1	27
Fireproofing	5	–	5
Firedoors	5	–	5
Firefighter	5	3	8
Fitter/ turner	51	20	71
Foundry	6	2	8
Furnace	6	–	6
Glassworks/ glaziers	6	–	6
Industrial chemist	4	-	4
Industrial engineer	2	-	2
Instrument technician	1	-	1
Insulation	18	4	22
Jeweller	6	2	8
Laboratory technician	6	2	8
Labourer	33	15	48
Lagger	31	16	47
Lagging in workplace	24	4	28
Laundry/ dry-cleaners	14	5	19
Linesman	9	4	13
Locksmith	1	-	1
Machine fitter	3	1	4
Machine inspector	2	-	2
Machine operator	1	3	4
Machinist	3	-	3
Maintenance carpenter	3	1	4
Maintenance electrician	2	1	3
Maintenance engineer	3	1	4
Maintenance fitter	13	4	17
Maintenance mechanic	3	2	5
Maintenance worker	12	3	15
Marine engineer	9	7	16
Mechanical engineer	5	–	5
Mechanical fitter	7	3	10

continued over

Table 3.5. continued.

	Number exposed		Total
	Single*	Multiple†	exposures
Metal fabrication	2	–	2
Metal trades	3	1	4
Metallurgy	1	–	1
Moulder	4	–	4
Navy/ merchant navy	160	64	224
Oil refinery	7	2	9
Painter/ decorator	37	8	45
Panel beater	9	1	10
Papermill	3	2	5
Patternmaker	6	3	9
Pipes – handled/cut/stored/drilled	24	5	29
Plasterer	16	7	23
Plumbing	56	27	83
Power station worker	86	51	137
Pre pak manufacturer	1	–	1
Printing	10	–	10
Radiographer	2	–	2
Railways	101	49	150
Renovations/maintenance/lagging in workplace	21	5	26
Roofing	16	4	20
Sheetmetal	14	11	25
Ships – building/repairing/on	75	57	132
shop fitter	1	–	1
Site visits/inspections	8	7	15
Smelting	1	–	1
Steelworks	13	8	21
Storeman	15	–	15
Stoves	2	–	2
Sugar mill	6	4	10
Tannery	2	–	2
Telephone technician	6	3	9
Tiler	11	1	12
Toolmaker	4	2	6
Trades assistant	17	3	20
Transporting asbestos	14	6	20
Transporting asbestos product	15	2	17
Tyre factory	10	4	14
Waterside worker	94	13	107
Weighing trucks	1	–	1
Welder	22	9	31
Whitewash – Greece/Cyprus	4	1	5
Wine making (filters)	1	–	1
Wittenoom (former mining area in WA)	193	51	244
Wood machinist	3	–	3

Table 3.5 *continued*

Summary of asbestos exposures

Asbestos exposure			
single	2608		
multiple	400		
possible	274		
No apparent asbestos exposure	457		
No response to questionnaire	<u>1099</u>		
Total cases from 1/1/86 – 31/10/2000	4838		
Proportion of respondents with	<u>3282</u>	=	87%
asbestos exposure	3752		

* With no other form of exposure.
† With other forms of exposure.

discussed at periodic meetings of the panel. Cell type was classed as epithelial, sarcomatous, mixed, or not agreed. The primary site of the tumour was classed as pleural (including pericardial) or peritoneal (including tunica vaginalis). This was known in 759 cases of 762.

Site of tumour

There were 685 (91%) pleural cases, and 74 (9%) were peritoneal in origin. There were significant associations between fibre content and tumour site for all fibre contents measured, except chrysotile. High fibre content was associated with peritoneal tumours.

Cell type

Of the 746 cases classed histologically, 331 (44%) were epithelial, 162 (22%) mixed, 63 (9%) sarcomatous, and 190 (25%) not agreed. Epithelial tumours were more likely with lower exposures, sarcomatous with higher exposures, and mixed cell tumours intermediate. This trend was most apparent for total uncoated fibres (light).[21]

Survival

Figure 3.10 shows the distribution of survival time (in known deceased cases) from PD. The distribution is skewed sharply to the left (positive skew). Mean survival time from PD was 11.3 months (standard deviation [SD], 11.3; median, 8 months). Only three cases of the 746 who had histologic examination were known definitely to be alive.

Because mesothelioma is almost always fatal, survival analysis by methods taking account of those still alive was thought to be unnecessary, and direct comparison of survival times according to cell type, site and treatment was regarded as a valid means of assessing the effects of such variables. Treatment does not appear to affect survival significantly and any differences in survival time between cell type and site are thus

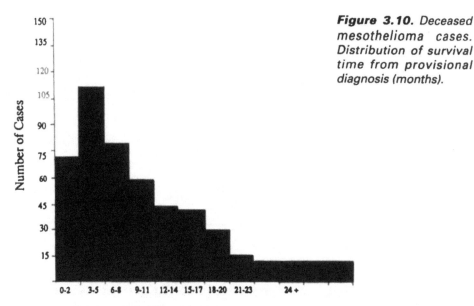

Figure 3.10. *Deceased mesothelioma cases. Distribution of survival time from provisional diagnosis (months).*

Survival from date of provisional diagnosis (months)

not confounded by treatment. Because survival time was approximately log-normally distributed, an analysis of variance was done to compare mean $\log_{10}$ (survival time) (in months) for the three different cell types. The cell type had a significant effect on $\log_{10}$ (survival time) ($F_{2,512} = 16.2$, $P < 0.001$). The arithmetic mean survival times (months) were epithelial, 13.0 (SD, 12.8; median, 9); mixed, 10.2 (SD, 8.7; median, 7); and sarcomatous, 5.8 (SD, 6.5; median, 3.5).

Student's t tests for planned comparison showed that the differences in $\log_{10}$ (survival time) between epithelial and sarcomatous and between mixed and sarcomatous cell types were statistically significant ($P<0.0001$ and $P<0.0001$, respectively). There was no significant difference in survival time between epithelial and mixed cell types. Of the 556 cases with known cell type, 43 had not yet had their date of death confirmed.

Survival time also depended on tumour site. The arithmetic mean survival time for pleural tumours was 11.4 (SD, 13.4) months compared with peritoneal tumours 8.6 (SD, 12.5) months. The difference was highly significant ($P<0.005$, by two-sided unpaired t test on $\log_{10}$ survival time).

Relationship between cell type and site

There was a strong association between cell type and primary tumour site. There were no sarcomatous tumours among the peritoneal mesotheliomas, and only 14% mixed peritoneal mesotheliomas compared with 31% mixed pleural mesotheliomas. An analysis of a series of log-linear models showed that the saturated log-linear model omitting the three-way interaction term (site × dose × cell type) gave the best fit to the data (χ^2=

0.09). This suggested that the site–cell type, dose–cell type, and dose–site relationships are independent of each other and account for the apparently anomalous finding that sarcomatous tumours, although associated with high exposure, were never peritoneal

The results showed that there was an association between lung fibre content and the site of mesothelioma. Higher doses were associated with the peritoneal type of tumour, and this was consistent with previously proposed hypotheses that: (1) heavy accumulation in lung tissue is first required before fibres can penetrate sufficiently to the peritoneal cavity; and (2) malignant change requires physical proximity of the fibre to the cell.[22,23] That the associations are also seen with coated fibres is consistent with these hypotheses, as is the lack of association with chrysotile content, which, because of clearance, is not necessarily as good an index of accumulated dose as is the case for other fibre types.

The association between fibre content and cell type, seen for all fibre content measures except coated fibres, is consistent with the hypothesis that there is a progressive malignant change of mesothelial cells from an epithelial, through mixed, to a sarcomatous neoplasm and that this change is dose dependent. That is, after an initial dose has initiated neoplastic change, continued exposure promotes further dedifferentiation, and coated fibres are not active in this process. This is consistent with the findings of McLemore *et al.*[24] in respect of fibre toxicity to alveolar macrophages, and Vorwald *et al.*[25] in respect of asbestotic fibrogenesis.

The association between dose and cell type appears to be a new finding, but it should be noted that both the site and cell type associations with fibre content are most obvious at levels corresponding to heavy exposure. These associations are not dependent on fibre length.[26]

The association of survival time with site and type of tumour could be explained by later onset of symptoms for peritoneal tumours and by greater invasiveness of sarcomatous tumours.

The findings of others[27] were confirmed in that there was better survival time with the epithelial and mixed types, and shorter survival times with peritoneal tumours.[28,29] Median survival times in this study were comparable to the findings of Adams *et al.*[27] (epithelial, 9 months versus 12 months; mixed, 7 months versus 8 months; sarcomatous, 3.5 months versus 3.6 months). The independent site–cell type association also was consistent with previous reports.[30] These authors also found fewer sarcomatous tumours among peritoneal tumours.

Dose-response relationships between mesothelioma risk and asbestos exposure, by fibre type and length

An outstanding question in human mesothelioma is the dose–response relationship for different fibre types. Using program data, it was possible to approach this by a case-referent study in order to relate relative risks of mesothelioma to dose of fibre as measured both by lung content and estimated airborne exposure. In particular the question of whether chrysotile alone can cause human mesothelioma could be addressed.

Dose–response relationships are best determined by means of a retrospective or prospective cohort study and it is only by this method that absolute risk (cumulative incidence), in relation to estimated exposure can be assessed. However, in diseases of low incidence like mesothelioma, accurate exposure data are not often available for the higher levels of exposure prevailing in the past which have generated most current cases. Also, exposure at current levels is likely to be too low to produce sufficient cases for statistical analysis in a prospective cohort study. Dynamic population studies can directly measure incidence rate ratios, but also depend on quantification of past exposures and sufficient cases.

As an alternative to a cohort study, a case-referent approach can be used, with either history of general environmental or occupational asbestos exposure ('quantified' or categorised) or, better, lung asbestos fibre content in post-mortem or resected lung specimens as the exposure variable. By comparing odds ratios for different exposure levels compared with zero exposure, an estimate of the dose-effect on relative risk of mesothelioma can be obtained, as in cumulative incidence sampling of cases and referents (the program situation). Mesothelioma is a sufficiently rare disease and the sampling fractions of cases and referents are independent of exposure.

Furthermore, the relative effects of different fibre types and sizes on mesothelioma risk can be separately quantified by appropriate statistical modelling, even when, as is usually the case, exposure to multiple fibre types is found.

The Australian study[31] quantified the dose–response relationship between risk of mesothelioma and asbestos exposure by comparing lung fibre content, by type, and by length, in the cases collected in the program, with that in a referent group of lung tissue samples collected over the same period as the cases. The method was similar to that used in other reported studies, e.g., McDonald *et al.*,[32] but a much larger series of cases (221) was analysed and only definite or probable mesothelioma cases were accepted.

The total number of definite or probable mesothelioma cases diagnosed in the period 1 January 1980 to 31 December 1985 was 697. In 221 of these cases (209 definite, 12 probable) formalin-preserved post-mortem lung tissue material was available for fibre analysis. Post-mortem material from five possible cases was also available but was excluded from the current study. Two hundred and seven cases were pleural and 14 were peritoneal. In general, $5 \times 5 \times 5$ cm blocks from the lower lobe of the uninvolved lung were analysed.

Formalin-preserved lung tissue was obtained from 391 consecutive necropsy specimens or lung resection specimens performed at the Royal Prince Alfred Hospital (Sydney, Australia) within the same period. Cases with pneumoconiosis, emphysema, pneumonia, or gastrointestinal cancer were excluded. About half the referents had bronchial cancer. No statistically significant difference in fibre count distributions could be demonstrated between bronchial cancer referents and other referents.

This left 359 referent tissue samples available for study (276 men, 83 women). The design was thus an unmatched case-referent study with reasonable frequency matching for age and sex. The light microscopic referent group included 23% women compared with 9% women among the cases.

Lung fibre content was measured in 0.5 g samples of lung tissue after digestion in sodium hypochlorite. Digests were filtered onto Millipore 0.8 micron (Millipore,

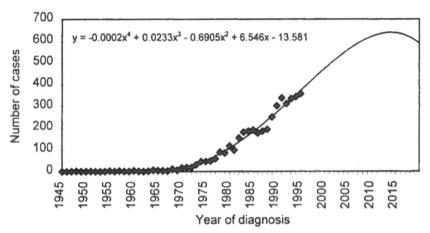

Figure 3.11. *Incident cases of malignant mesothelioma in Australia 1945–96 and extrapolation to 2020 assuming maximum at 2010.*

Bedford, MA) filters for light microscopic study and Nuclepore 0.4 micron filters (Nuclepore, Pleasantown, CA), carbon coated, for transmission electron microscopic (TEM) study using the methods of Rogers.[14]

For light microscopic (LM) analysis, 200 fields of view at LM × 500 were counted using differential interference contrast. Fibre lengths were estimated with a Walton-Beckett graticule. For TEM (JEOL 100CX, JEOL, Tokyo, Japan) and Philips CM12 (Philips, Eindhoven, The Netherlands), 40 grid areas (ten grid areas from four separate grids) were examined at × 8300. Fibre length was estimated from the proportions of the photographic screen or the Nuclepore hole replicas. Fibre type was identified by comparing the energy dispersive x-ray analysis (EDAX) spectrum of the fibre with those of the International Union Against Cancer (UICC) asbestos specimens prepared in the same manner.

Only fibres >2 micron (TEM), >5 micron (LM) in length were counted. As above, analytical sensitivity was 15 000 fibres per gram of dried lung (fibre/g) for light microscopic study and 200 000 fibre/g for TEM (corresponding to one fibre counted).

Light microscopic fibre counts were made on all 221 cases and 359 controls. Electron microscopic fibre counts, EDAX, and fibre length measurements were made on all 221 cases and 103 male controls, drawn randomly from the total group of 276.

Dose–response analysis of relative risk was carried out by grouping fibre content levels into strata and calculating the relative risk (estimated by odds ratio) for each stratum of exposure compared with zero exposure (defined as <15 000 fibre/g by light microscopic study, or <200 000 fibre/g by TEM). Where no referents were exposed, categories were pooled, as otherwise odds ratios are infinite. The Mantel χ^2 test, with one degree of freedom for trend, was used to test the significance of linear trends of relative risk with dose.

A progressive increase in relative risk with increasing fibre content could be seen for all fibre content measures. Tests for trend were are highly significant in all cases.

The increase in relative risk was apparent at the lowest dose levels, suggesting a no threshold effect but relative risk increased more rapidly for dosage greater than 3×10^5 ($10^{5.5}$) fibres/g (light microscopic study) and 10^6 to $10^{6.5}$ fibres/g (TEM). At the higher dose levels, there were often no exposed referents and many exposed cases.

The relative risks for >10 micron chrysotile, crocidolite, and total amphibole fibres were greater than the corresponding risks for fibres <10 micron.

When cases and referents were compared in relation to exposure to single-fibre types only, the numbers of cases and referents for analysis were much lower. However, increased relative risks for lung fibre contents greater than 200 000 fibres/g (all lengths) were still seen for single-fibre type lung contents of chrysotile and crocidolite. Fifteen of 30 cases had >$10^{5.5}$ fibres/g crocidolite only compared with four referents of 39. In cases and referents where amosite only was found in the lungs, six of 20 cases had >$10^{5.5}$ fibres/g in the lung compared with one of 36 referents.

In cases and referents where only chrysotile was found in the lungs (i.e., zero amphibole concentration), seven of 25 cases (two peritoneal) and three of 31 referents had >$10^{5.5}$ fibres/g in the lung). The fact that peritoneal mesotheliomas can occur with chrysotile only exposure appears to be a new finding.

Of the 25 cases with zero concentrations of amphibole found in the lung, 11 had a history of mixed exposure, according to the occupational hygienists, two had a definite history of exposure only to chrysotile, and ten had no ascertainable history of exposure to asbestos. No history was available in two cases. Eleven cases had no fibres (chrysotile or amphibole) detected in the lung. Time from last exposure varied between 7 and 46 years. Occupational histories of the referents were not available.

There was a generally linear relationship between log odds ratio and log fibre content. Accordingly, a series of multiple logistic regression models of the form:

$$\log_e \frac{(P)}{(1-P)} = b_0 + \sum_{i=1}^{n} b_i \log_{10}(\text{fibre content}) + b_{n+1} \text{age}$$

where P = probability of having mesothelioma, and n = number of different fibre types and lengths, were fitted using SAS 6.03 CATMOD (SAS Institute, Cary, NC). Only TEM fibre contents were used in this model. Age was included as a potential confounding variable for which cases and referents were approximately frequency matched. Since a log transformation was used, zero fibre contents were set to 0.2 fibres/μg (200 000 fibre/g, the TEM detection limit). There were some significant correlations between the explanatory variables ($\log_{10}$ fibre contents, age). As would be expected, fibre contents >10 micron were highly correlated for all fibre types. Crocidolite and amosite were correlated and chrysotile <10 micron was correlated with amosite and crocidolite <10 micron. Age was significantly correlated only with chrysotile <10 micron (negative correlation, r = –0.13 P<0.02). Unidentified amphiboles were correlated with all other fibres. Unidentified amphiboles almost universally had a spectrum between amosite and crocidolite. No tremolite was found.

The final model chosen to best represent the data included crocidolite >10 micron, amosite <10 micron, and chrysotile <10 micron. Chrysotile <10 micron was significantly correlated with chrysotile >10 micron but gave a better fit.

Table 3.6. Coefficients in model of form: $R = 1 + \Sigma b_i x_i$.

Predictor variable (all fibre concentrations in fibre/μg)	Model 1 b	Model 1 95% CI	Model 1 P	Model 2 b	Model 2 95% CI	Model 2 P
Crocidolite ≥10 micron	9.1	2.7–23.1	<0.0001	9.4	2.7–24.1	<0.0001
Amosite ≥10 micron	5.2	0.4–21.7	0.004			
≤10 micron				1.9	0.1–6.4	<0.011
Chrysotile <10 micron	7.0	3.5–12.3	<0.0001	7.6	3.9–13.3	<0.0001
–2 log L		305.3			307.1	

The regression coefficients in the final model gave the log (odds ratio) for an increase of one logarithmic unit of fibre dose (i.e., × 10 fibre/μg). The $\log_e$ (odds ratio) ($\log_e$ relative risk) for × 10 fibre/μg crocidolite >10 micron was thus 3.38 + 1.96 × 1.07 (95% confidence interval [CI]). The multiplicative increase in relative risk was thus exp (3.38 + 1.96 × 1.07) = 29.4 (95% CI 3.6 - 241). Corresponding effects of amosite <10 micron and chrysotile <10 micron were as follows: amosite <10 micron 2.3 (1.0–5.3), chrysotile <10 micron 15.7 (6.1–40).

The logistic regression model is inherently a multiplicative risk model. Inspection of the data showed that, although the risk of all fibre type concentrations was more than additive of those of single fibre types, it was not completely multiplicative. Accordingly, a series of additive relative risk models of the form

$$\frac{P}{1-P} = 1 + \sum_{i=1}^{n} b_i x_i$$

were also fitted using GLIM 3.77 (Numerical Algorithms Group, Oxford, UK). This model also has the merit of readily interpretable scale changes in fibre concentration measures (e.g., if clearance effects are to be considered).

Regression coefficients of the two best models are shown in Table 3.6. Ninety-five per cent CI for regression coefficients were obtained by finding values at which –2 log L increased by 3.84 (the likelihood profile method).

It can be seen that the relative importance of the various fibre types and lengths remain similar, with crocidolite >10 micron and chrysotile <10 micron being most important. Amosite >10 micron has a slightly larger relative effect.

The results were thus consistent with the hypotheses that amphiboles are primarily responsible for mesothelioma and that longer fibres have a relatively greater effect. The dose–response relationships suggested that risk was related to dose. However, analysis of a small group of cases and referents with only chrysotile found in the lungs also showed a statistically significant trend (P<0.005) of an increasing relative risk of mesothelioma with increasing fibre content in lungs.

Previous workers have estimated the relative risk (as approximated by odds ratio) for total amphibole lung content. In comparison with their results, the Australian study found an odds ratio of 2.36 (Cornfield 95% CI 1.38 to 4.05) for $>10^6$ fibre/g compared with $<10^6$ fibre/g for fibres <10 micron and 16.63 (3.86 to 100.0) for fibres >10 micron. McDonald et al.[33] compared lung fibre contents in 99 cases of mesothelioma with available tissue, incident in Canada and the USA in 1972, with 100 age and sex matched referents. The numbers of cases and referents at differing lung fibre content levels were tabulated but odds ratios were not reported, nor were tests for trend carried out. Reanalysis of their data[19] in fact shows an odds ratio of 3.8 (95% CI 1.8–8.0) for $>10^6$ fibre/g compared with $<10^6$ fibre/g amosite and crocidolite combined and an increasing gradient of odds ratio with fibre content for amosite, crocidolite, and anthophyllite in men and women. This gradient was apparent for chrysotile only in the high ($>10^6$ fibre/g) amphibole subgroup of those exposed to both chrysotile and amphibole. The dose–response relationship for tremolite was U-shaped. Similarly, reanalysis of the data of Wagner et al.[34] (a study of 86 mesothelioma cases and 56 age-matched referents) gave an odds ratio of 7.4 (95% CI 3.5–16) for $>10^6$ versus $<10^6$ fibre/g combined amosite and crocidolite. A dose–response gradient was not reported or recalculated.

Mowé et al.,[35] in a study of 14 mesothelioma cases and 28 matched referents in Norway, showed an odds ratio of 8.5 (95% CI 2.3–31) for lung content $>10^6$ fibre/g compared with $<10^6$ fibre/g.

Gaudichet et al.,[36] in France, compared fibre content in 20 mesothelioma cases to four different age and sex matched referent sets (squamous cell carcinoma of lung, adenocarcinoma of lung, metastatic carcinoma in lung, cardiovascular disease). Increased amphibole content was found in cases compared with referents for each referent comparison, particularly with crocidolite and amosite and especially crocidolite and amosite >8 micron in length. No difference in chrysotile content between cases and any referent series was found. There were increased numbers of coated fibres in cases compared with referents. Dose–response relationships were not reported.

In a one–one matched case-referent study on 78 cases identified by pathologists in Canada over the period 1979 through 1984, McDonald et al.[32] showed a clear dose–response relationship between mesothelioma risk and lung concentrations of long (>8 micron) and short (<8 micron) crocidolite, amosite and tremolite. However, multiple binary regression analysis showed that the relative risk was related only to fibres >8 micron in length. From their Table 1, it can be computed that the relative risk (odds ratio) for total amphiboles in concentration >1 fibre/µg (10^6 fibre/g) compared with concentration less than 1 fibre/µg is 2.2 (95% CI 1.1–4.4) for fibres <8 µg and 6.6 (3.0–14.6) for fibres >8 micron. Although a detailed matching procedure was used in this study, it is unfortunate that the criterion for inclusion of a case in the analysis on pathologic grounds was not more stringent. Cases classed as definite, probable, possible, doubtful and unclassifiable were all included. Among these only 33 were definite and 25 probable. This wide inclusion criterion may have resulted in tumours which were not mesotheliomas, and with low lung fibre counts, being included, with a resulting bias in the results against any asbestos effects, thus underestimating relative risks.

In making comparisons with the slightly different analysis of McDonald *et al.*,[32] in which linear multivariable risk models for long (>8 micron) and short (<8 micron) fibres were separately fitted, it can be seen that the Australian study found lower coefficients for crocidolite and amosite and a higher coefficient for chrysotile. However, the Australian coefficients were estimated with greatly shortened confidence intervals. The Australian study confirmed that long amphibole fibres were more important than short in the epidemiological relationship, but differed somewhat in the estimates of the relative effects of crocidolite, amosite and chrysotile.

In the study of Tuomi *et al.*[37] from Finland, 51 mesothelioma cases were compared with general autopsy referents and lung cancer referents. Total EM fibre contents at death were compared. All fibre lengths were included and a 3:1 aspect ratio defined fibre. The odds ratio (relative risk) for $>10^6$ fibre/g was 14.4 (90% CI 2.5–178) compared to general autopsy referents and 3.1 (90% CI 1.3–7.5) compared to lung cancer referents. Crocidolite/amosite in combination and anthophyllite/chrysotile in combination were common exposure patterns. Many people in Finland had been exposed to anthophyllite. It was concluded that a no threshold dose–response relationship existed. However, no attempt was made to quantify this or to separate individual fibre type risks.

In the USA, Roggli *et al.*,[38] considering only fibres >5 micron length and >0.2 micron diameter, compared the frequency of occurrence of different fibre types in the lungs of mesothelioma cases. Their analysis could not give a dose–response relationship as no referents were used and no quantitative analyses done. However, based on frequency of occurrence of fibre types at death, they concluded that the 'order of importance' in the USA was amosite>tremolite>chrysotile=crocidolite.

There was a clear dose–response relationship in the Australian study. Although the negative correlation of chrysotile <10 micron with age was consistent with a clearance effect, there was a significant dose–response effect for short chrysotile independently of long amosite and long crocidolite. This was consistent with the analysis of the small group of cases and referents with only chrysotile found in the lungs, which showed a statistically significant trend (P<0.005) of relative risk of mesothelioma with lung fibre content.

In the Australian study, there was also the ability to examine a much larger (light microscope) case-referent analysis of coated fibres (asbestos bodies), and to examine long (>10 micron) coated fibres separately. There was a very clear gradient of relative risk with coated fibre lung content, clearer still with fibres >10 micron. This gradient was of the same order as for amosite and for crocidolite and is consistent with the hypothesis that long amphiboles are preferentially coated.[39] However, it has been suggested by these authors that this epidemiological relationship may also be consistent with the short uncoated fibres being responsible.

There were several possible selection biases operating in the Australian study. First, not all mesothelioma cases came to post-mortem. The distribution by state of post-mortem cases was closely comparable to the distribution by State of notification but there may have been other selection factors giving an increased chance of post-mortem, e.g., likelihood of compensation for relative.

Secondly, the referent group were patients coming to post-mortem in one large referral hospital serving the whole of one State, New South Wales (NSW). New South Wales is the most populated State, with the largest number of mesothelioma notifications (426 in the study period). Whereas all referents would have been included as cases in the study, had they developed mesothelioma, their exposure background is more likely to have been that pertaining to NSW rather than to Australia as a whole. However, since most Australians live and work in cities with a similar mixture of industries and environments where asbestos exposure may occur, any bias due to this effect was likely to be small. Indeed, there would have been more opportunity for industrial and environmental exposure in NSW, so the restriction of referents to NSW would have tended to underestimate relative risks.

This study showed that, for Australia as a whole, the greatest risk of mesothelioma was associated with exposure to crocidolite >10 micron in length. It was difficult to assess the risks associated with chrysotile alone, due to almost universal assessed mixed exposure to amphibole and chrysotile, and the possibility of differential clearance effects. However, in a subset of cases and referents with only chrysotile found in the lungs a significant dose response trend was found.

An attempt was made to estimate relative clearance rates of different asbestos fibre types in man by comparing 'quantified' exposure scores derived from histories with lung fibre contents in order to adjust the above additive relative risk model to express relative carcinogenicities in terms of airborne exposure rather than residual lung burden.[40] This can only be done with the additive relative risk model, not the multiple logistic regression model, because of its multiplicative nature. Unfortunately, estimating relative clearance by this method is very approximate. As noted above, the occupational hygienists' estimates of 'exposure' contain a large subjective element, the weighting system is arbitrary and no statistically significant regression relationship was obtained for estimated mixed exposure and lung chrysotile content. A line fitted by eye is very subjective and open to observer bias. No account was taken of time since last exposure and death in this study. Nor was any account taken of the different clearance of different fibre lengths. In addition, primate and rodent animal studies of relative crocidolite/chrysotile clearance now suggest a ratio of lung/airborne fibre content more like 1:15–20 averaged over all fibre lengths and lifetimes, rather than 1:500–1:1000 as suggested by this study. In rats, Muhle et al.[41] found mean clearance half times of 301 days for crocidolite and 236 days for chrysotile based on fibre number and 827 for crocidolite and 198 for chrysotile based on mass. Oberdörster estimated retention half times in baboons of 90 days for chrysotile and 200–1500 days for amphibole fibre.[42] Wagner et al.[43] found for the same airborne exposure, approximtely 15 times as much amphibole as chrysotile accumulating after 24 months in rats. Finkelstein and Dufresne, in human clearnace studies,[20] concluded that the slow compartment clearance rates for amphiboles and chrysotile >10 micron length were comparable, with half times of about 8 years, similar to the findings in Western Australian crocidolite miners,[44] although according to Churg[45] fast compartment clearance is much greater for chrysotile, being of the order of months. In guinea pigs Churg et al.[46] found clearance of amosite to be only about 40% slower than that of chrysotile. Furthermore, expressing relative risk in terms of lung fibre burden at death begs the question of the relevant carcinogenic dose. One could argue that it is the initial level which may either be reduced by clearance or enhanced by non-significant extra dose. It is fair to state from a regulatory point of view that the risk in terms of airborne levels is relevant but if treatments designed to reduce carcinogenicity in the already exposed are used the lung tissue dose must be considered in more detail.

Assuming a 1:20 relative clearance for amphibole and chrysotile, and rescaling the coefficients in the additive relative risk model (Table 3.6) the estimates of the relative mesothelioma carcinogenicity would become crocidolite:amosite:chrysotile = 9:5:0.35 or 26:14:1. This is generally consistent with longitudinal (cohort) studies of single fibre type exposures which alone can directly assess cumulative incidence and hence absolute risk.[47,48]

The Wittenoom experience

Wittenoom is a town in the beautiful Karijini region of the Pilbara in north-western Australia. The beauty of the mountains and red gorges is blackened by the knowledge that Wittenoom has generated one of the worst industrial disasters in human history.[49]

In the late 1930s prospectors were attracted to the Wittenoom region because of high asbestos prices and they bagged it and carried it out by donkey to the coast. Early industrialised mining under the directorship of Lang Hancock and Peter Wright was replaced by the establishment of Australian Blue Asbestos Limited (ABA), a subsidiary of Colonial Sugar Refining Co (CSR) in the mid-1940s. They managed the Wittenoom mine and mill until it was closed in 1966. The Wittenoom mine and mill attracted many short-term labourers throughout the 1950s and 1960s such that by the early 1950s Wittenoom had become the largest town north of the Tropic of Capricorn in Western Australia. The tremendous value of asbestos in industry, particularly for its insulation and fire-resistant qualities, meant that the Federal and State Governments encouraged, appropriately, the development of this venture. In fact at one stage asbestos was considered by the State Government to have the potential to eclipse the value of gold in the State's economy. 1962 was the peak year of Australian asbestos production, with 18 416 short tons mined, 95% of which was crocidolite from Wittenoom. In context, however, it is important to realise that this represented less than 10% of the crocidolite mined in South Africa in the same year. The Western Australia State Government established the townsite of Wittenoom along with the required infrastructural facilities. The Australian Federal Government also assisted by providing workers' housing, road and shipping subsidies. The majority of the workforce were transient, most working for less than 6 months. The stopes in the mine were only 105 cm and the heat and dust were unattractive for long-term employment. CSR recruited labour from Perth and from Europe, the latter signing two-year contracts and providing most of the underground workforce. Recruitment drives in Italy and Holland were particularly successful. A total of approximately 7000 people worked for ABA although generally there were never more than between 300 and 500 individuals employed at any one time. Most of the workforce was young with 57% less than 30 years of age.

Whilst the underground work in the mine was difficult with the low stope, heat and dirt, clearly the most appalling working conditions were to be found in the mill.

Dust levels were so high that workers would often have difficulty seeing the other side of the mill. More sinister, however, was the fact that whereas the underground dust included a lot of silica and unmilled asbestos, the dust in the mill contained a substantial amount of fine, lethal crocidolite fibres. It is therefore no surprise to note that the mortality amongst mill workers is extremely high.

The level of industrial hygiene at Wittenoom was low. Numerous medico-legal cases have identified the fact that the management at Wittenoom were slow to respond to the published warnings of the dangers of asbestos. Dr Eric Saint, later to become the foundation Professor of Medicine at the University of Western Australia Medical School, visited Wittenoom and prophetically predicted in a letter to the State Government that many of these individuals would suffer from asbestos-related lung disease. Even when the link between crocidolite exposure and mesothelioma was described in the early 1960s, efforts to improve industrial hygiene in the Wittenoom plant were slow and inefficient. The combination of remoteness from the head office, the non-immediacy of asbestos-related pulmonary diseases, the linguistic difficulties and transient nature of the workforce, and the economic pressure under which the always-marginal mine operated combined to ensure that the workers were not given a high standard of occupational hygiene. Indeed, even when the mine was closed in 1966 the decision was made on economic rather than on health grounds.

Equally sadly, the partners and children of workers were exposed to large amounts of crocidolite in what, at the time, seemed like innocuous circumstances. To deal with the problem of the dry red dust at Wittenoom, which was capable of penetrating any door or window, asbestos-containing tailings were transported from the mine site to the township 7 kilometres away and used to cover the school playground, the airport runway, driveways of houses and other areas in which children played. Many of these children have since died of mesothelioma in their 20s, 30s and 40s. Many of their mothers have also died of mesothelioma.

Notwithstanding the above, it would be wrong to give the impression that the town of Wittenoom was some sort of gulag. The Wittenoom residents generated an active social life of picnics, barbecues, dances, games and carnivals. In fact the strong sense of community generated by the longer-term residents has been important in the highly successful Asbestos Diseases Society, a support and lobby/advocacy group formed in Western Australia.

Although the mine was closed in 1966, and the town of Wittenoom removed its essential services in the 1990s, the legacy of Wittenoom lives on. Hundreds of Wittenoom workers and residents have fallen victim to mesothelioma. Many thousands more have suffered the anxiety of knowing that they or their children may die of mesothelioma. One former resident, whose son died of mesothelioma, made the statement 'I went to Wittenoom to earn money to give my family a good start in life and all I've done is kill my son'. Two years later his wife also developed mesothelioma and died.

In the midst of the tragedy of Wittenoom and the inevitable confrontation and anxiety of litigation, a number of positive things need to be highlighted. Firstly, the ex-Wittenoom workers have formed the core of an extremely effective social support and lobby group, the

Asbestos Diseases Society, as a model of organised community care. In a context of anxiety and tragedy in a non-wartime situation, it would be difficult to find a better model. Secondly, the relatively brief periods of exposure to blue asbestos that occurred in this population have provided an excellent basis for studying the epidemiology of asbestos-related cancers, which will hopefully lead to a better understanding, and in the future, prevention of such diseases.[50-52] Thirdly, the large number of cases of asbestos-related diseases that are found in Western Australia have meant that scientists, clinicians, pathologists, epidemiologists, radiologists and others have been able to study this disease in some depth and provide important contributions to the world literature (in other places mesothelioma cases are too infrequent to provide a basis for such studies).[53,54]

Conclusion

The high and increasing incidence of mesothelioma in Australia is due to high asbestos use in the past, combined with poor hygiene practice, relatively high amphibole use in asbestos cement products, slow recognition of chrysotile mesotheliomagenicity and excessive focus on Wittenoom to the exclusion of other more common exposures. The expected total number of cases from 1945 to 2020 is estimated to be about 18 000, based on models by Berry[55] and de Klerk *et al.*[56] for Wittenoom, extrapolated for Australia as whole (assuming Wittenoom contributes 5% of cases), and direct extrapolation from the best fit to the empirical incidence curve, constrained to have a maximum value at 2010, following a 40-year latency from the time of maximum exposure (1970) (Fig. 3.11). This will create a heavy clinical and compensation load. The impact on non-occupationally exposed individuals is another major issue.[57] The various Australia State and Federal government authorities are now developing a national strategy for dealing with this problem.

References

1. Leigh, J. (1994). The Australian Mesothelioma Program 1979–1994. In: Peters GA, Peters BJ (eds). *The Current Status of the Asbestos Public Health Problem* (Vol 9, Sourcebook on Asbestos Diseases) NH, Butterworth, pp 1–74.
2. Leigh, J., Davidson, P., Hull, B. (1997). Malignant mesothelioma in Australia 1945–1995. *Proc Inhaled Particles VIII Ann Occup Hyg* **41** (Supp 1): 161–167.
3. Leigh, J., Davidson, L.P., Hull, B. (1998). Malignant mesothelioma in Australia (1945–1997). Excerpta Medica Supp 53. *Adv Prev Occup Respir Dis*, pp 299–302.
3a. The Colonial Sugar Refining Company Limited. (1956). South Pacific Enterprise. Sydney, Angus and Robertson.
4. Hughes, R.J. (1978). Asbestos. Australian Mineral Industry Annual Review 1976 (including information to June 1977). Bureau of Mineral Resources Geology and Geophysics. Canberra: Australian Government Publishing Service, pp 61–62.
5. Victorian Occup Health and Safety Commission (1990). Asbestos Usage in Victoria, Substitutes and Alternatives.
6. National Occupational Health and Safety Commission (National Institute of Occupational Health and Safety). Australian Mesothelioma Register Report. The Incidence of Mesothelioma in Australia. 1989, 1990, 1991, 1992, 1993, 1994, 1995, 1996, 1997, 1998, 1999 (Annual Report Series).

7. Roberts, C.G., Whaite, H.M. (1952). A survey of dust exposure and lung disease in the asbestos-cement industry in New South Wales. Studies in Industrial Hygiene No 24, NSW Dept of Health.

8. Major, G. (1968). Asbestos dust exposure. In: *Proc 1st Aust Pneumoconiosis Conf* (Sydney), 467–474.

9. McNulty, J.C. (1962). Malignant pleural mesothelioma in an asbestos worker. *Med J Aust* 2: 953–954.

10. Riddell R.J. (1966). Three cases of mesothelioma. *Med J Aust* 2: 554–559.

11. Mortimer, R.H., Campbell, C.B. (1968). Asbestos exposure and pleural mesotheliomas. *Med J Aust* 2: 720–722.

12. Milne, J. (1969). Fifteen cases of pleural mesothelioma associated with occupational exposure to asbestos in Victoria. *Med J Aust* 2: 669–673.

13. Ferguson, D.A., Berry, G., Jelihovsky, T., Andreas, S.B., Rogers, A.J., Fung, S.C., Grimwood, A., Thompson, R. (1987). The Australian Mesothelioma Surveillance Program 1979-1985.

14. Rogers, A.J. (1984). Determination of mineral fibre in human tissue by light microscopy and transmission electron microscopy. *Ann Occup Hyg* 28: 1–12.

15. Musk, A.W., Dolin, P.J., Armstrong, B.K., Ford, J.M., de Klerk, N.H., Hobbs, M.S.T. The incidence of malignant mesothelioma in Australia 1947-1980. *Med J Aust* 1989: 150: 242–3, 246.

16. Hillerdal, G. (1999) Mesothelioma: cases associated with non-occupational and low dose exposures. *Occ Env Med* 56:505–513.

17. Leigh, J., Corvalan, C.F., Grimwood, A., Berry, G., Ferguson, D.A., Thompson, R. (1991). The incidence of malignant mesothelioma in Australia 1982-1988. *Am J Ind Med* 20: 643–655.

18. Grimwood, A. (1988). Mesothelioma and asbestos in Australia. MPH Treatise (University of Sydney).

19. Berry, G., Rogers, A.J., Pooley, F.D. (1989). Mesotheliomas: asbestos exposure and lung burden. In: Bignon J, Peto J, Saracci R (eds). *Non-Occupational Exposure to Mineral Fibres*, IARC Sci Publ 90: 486–496.

20. Finkelstein, M.M., Dufresne, A. (1999). Inferences on the kinetics of asbestos deposition and clearance among chrysotile miners and millers. *Am J Ind Med* 35: 401–412.

21. Leigh, J., Rogers, A.J., Ferguson, D.A., Mulder, H.B., Ackad, M., Thompson, R. (1991b). Lung asbestos fiber content and mesothelioma cell type, site, and survival. *Cancer* 68: 135–141.

22. Browne, K., Smither, W.J. (1983). Asbestos-related mesothelioma: factors discriminating between pleural and peritoneal sites. *Br J Ind Med* 40: 145–152.

23. Suzuki, Y., Selikoff, I.J. (1992). Pathologic characterization of malignant mesothelioma among asbestos insulation workers. *Proc 8th Int Conf Occup Lung Disease* 1: 296–313.

24. McLemore, T.L., Roggli, V., Marshall, M.V., Lawrence, E.C., Greenbert, S.D., Stevens, P.M. (1981). Comparison of phagocytosis of uncoated versus coated asbestos fibers by cultural human pulmonary alveolar macrophages. *Chest* 80: (Suppl): 39–41.

25. Vorwald, A.J., Durkan, T.M., Pratt, P.C. (1951). Experimental studies of asbestosis. *Arch Ind Hyg Occup Med* 3:1–43.

26. Leigh, J., Hull, B., Ruck, E., Mandryk, J., Rogers, A.J. (1992). Lung asbestos fibre content by type and length and mesothelioma site and cell type. *Proc 8th Int Conf Occup Lung Dis* 1: 351–356.

27. Adams, V.I., Unni, K.K., Muhm, J.R., Jett, J.R., Ilstrup, D.M., Bernatz, P.E. (1986). Diffuse malignant mesothelioma of pleura. Diagnosis and survival in 92 cases. *Cancer* 58: 1540–1551.

28. Chahinian, A.P., Pajak, T.F., Holland, J.F., Norton, L., Ambinder, R.M., Mandel, E.M. (1982). Diffuse malignant mesothelioma: prospective evaluation of 69 patients. *Ann Intern Med* **96**: 746–755.

29. Brenner, J., Sordillo, P.P., Magill, G.B., Golbey, R.B. (1982). Malignant mesothelioma of the pleura: review of 123 patients. *Cancer* **49**: 2431–2435.

30. Kannerstein, M.D., Churg, J. (1977). Peritoneal mesothelioma. *Hum Pathol* **8**: 83-94.

31. Rogers, A.J., Leigh, J., Berry, G., Ferguson, D.A., Mulder, H.B., Ackad, M. (1991). Relationship between lung asbestos fiber type and concentration and relative risk of mesothelioma – A case-control study. *Cancer* **67**: 1912–1920.

32. McDonald, J.C., Armstrong, B., Case, B., *et al.* (1989). Mesothelioma and asbestos fiber type: evidence from lung tissue analysis. *Cancer* **63**: 1544–1547.

33. McDonald, A.D., McDonald, J.C., Pooley, F.D. (1982). Mineral fibre content of lungs in mesothelioma cases in North America. *Ann Occup Hyg* **26**: 417–422.

34. Wagner, J.C., Pooley, F.D., Berry, G., *et al.* (1982). A pathological and minerological study of asbestos-related deaths in the United Kingdom in 1977. *Ann Occup Hyg* **26**: 423–431.

35. Mowé, G., Gylseth, B., Hartveit, F., Skang, V. (1985). Fiber concentration in lung tissue of patients with malignant mesothelioma. *Cancer* **56**: 1089–1093.

36. Gaudichet, A., Janson, X., Monchaux, G., *et al.* (1988). Assessment by analytical microscopy of the total lung fibre burden in mesothelioma patients matched with four other pathological series. *Ann Occup Hyg* (Suppl) **32**: 213–223.

37. Tuomi, T., Huuskonen, M.S., Virtamo, M., Tossavainen, A., Tammilehto, L., Mattson, K., Lahdensuo, A., Mattila, J., Karhunen, P., Liippo, K., Tala, E. (1991). Relative risk of mesothelioma associated with different levels of exposure to asbestos. *Scand J Work Environ Health* **17**: 404–408.

38. Roggli, V.L., Pratt, P.C., Brody, A.R. (1993). Asbestos fiber type in malignant mesothelioma: analytical scanning electron microscopic study of 94 cases. *Am J Ind Med* **23**: 605–614.

39. Rom, W.N., Travis, W.D., Brody, A.R. (1991). Cellular and molecular basis of the asbestos related diseases. *Am Res Respir Dis* **143**: 408–422.

40. Rogers, A., Leigh, J., Berry, G., Ferguson, D., Mulder, H., Ackad, M., Morgan, G.G. (1994). Dose-response relationship between airborne and lung asbestos fibre type, length and concentration and the relative risk of mesothelioma. *Ann Occup Hyg* **38**: (Suppl. 1): 631–638.

41. Muhle, H., Bellmann, B., Pott, F. (1994). Comparative investigations of the biodurability of mineral fibres in the rat lung. *Environ Health Perspect* **102**: (Suppl. 5): 163–168.

42. Oberdörster, G. (1994). Macrophage-associated responses to chrysotile. *Ann Occup Hyg* **38**: 601–615.

43. Wagner, J.C., Berry, G., Skidmore, J.W., Timbrell, V. (1974). The effects of the inhalation of asbestos in rats. *Br J Cancer* **29**: 252–269.

44. de Klerk, N.H., Musk, A.W., Williams, V., Filion, P.R., Whitaker, D., Shilkin, K.B. (1996). Comparison of measures of exposure to asbestos in former crocidolite workers fron Wittenoom gorge, W. Australia. *Am J Ind Med* **30**: 579–587.

45. Churg, A., Wright, J., Gilks, B., Depaoli, L. (1989). Rapid short-term clearance of chrysotile compared with amosite asbestos in the guinea pig. *Am Rev Respir Dis* **139**: 885–890.

46. Churg, A. (1994). Deposition and clearance of chrysotile asbestos. *Ann Occup Hyg* **38**: 424–425.

47. Doll, R., Peto, J. (1985). *Effects on Health of Exposure to Asbestos*. HSC, London, HMSO.

48. Doll, R. (1989). Mineral fibres in the non-occupational environment: concluding remarks. In: Bignon, J., Peto, J., Saracci, R. (eds). *Non-occupational expsoure to mineral fibres*. IARC, Scientific Publications, Lyon, France **90**: 486-496.

49. Musk, A.W., de Klerk, N.H., Eccles, J.L., Hobbs, M.S.T., Armstrong, B.K., Layman, L., McNulty, J.C. (1992). Wittenoom, Western Australia: a modern industrial disaster. *Am J Ind Med* **21**: 735–747.
50. Armstrong, B.K., Musk, A.W., Baker, J.E., Hunt, J.M., Newall, C.C., Henzell, H.R., Blunsdon, B.S., Clarke-Hundley, D., Woodward, S.D., Hobbs, M.S.T. (1984). Epidemiology of malignant mesothelioma in Western Australia. *Med J Aust* **141**: 86–88.
51. Armstrong, B.K., de Klerk, N.H., Musk, A.W., Hobbs, M.S.T. (1988). Mortality in miners and millers of crocidolite in Western Australia. *Br J Ind Med* **45**: 5–13.
52. Cookson, W.O., de Klerk, N.H., Musk, A.W., Glancy, J.J., Armstrong, B., Hobbs, M. (1986). The natural history of asbestosis in former crocidolite workers of Wittenoom Gorge. *Am Rev Respir Dis* **133**: 994–998.
53. de Klerk, N.H., Armstrong, B.K., Musk, A.W., Hobbs, M.S.T. (1989). Cancer mortality in relation to measures of occupational exposure to crocidolite at Wittenoom Gorge in Western Australia. *Br J Ind Med* **46**: 529–536.
54. Scott, B., Mukherjee, S., Lake, R., Robinson, B.W.S. (2000). Malignant mesothelioma. In: *Textbook of Lung Cancer.* Hansen H., ed. London, Martin Dunitz, 273–293.
55. Berry, G. (1991). Prediction of mesothelioma, lung cancer, and asbestosis in former Wittenoom asbestos workers. *Br J Ind Med* **48**: 793–802.
56. de Klerk, N.H., Armstrong, B.K., Musk, A.W., Hobbs, M.S.T. (1989). Prediction of future cases of asbestos-related disease among former miners and millers of crocidolite in Western Australia. *Med J Aust* **151**: 616–620.
57. Hansen, J., de Klerk, N.H., Musk, A.W., Hobbs, S.T. Environmental exposure to crocidolite and mesothelioma. *Am J Respir Crit Care Med* 1998; **157**: 69–75.

=4=

Mesothelioma and Exposure to Asbestos in South Africa: 1956–62

†J. Chris Wagner

Asbestos

South Africa has deposits of three types of asbestos of value and in certain regions these ore bodies can be exploited commercially. It is important to note that at certain times the amount of the three types of asbestos produced has been comparable, and so have the workforces. By far the most mined asbestos fibre in the world (accounting for 95%) is the white, chrysotile, found in serpentine rock, the ore of which can be mined in the Eastern Transvaal and Swaziland. Amosite (accounting for 1% of the world market) occurs in the Northern Transvaal, is greyish-brown in colour, is an amphibole and is found in banded ironstone. Crocidolite, or blue asbestos (accounting for 2% of the worlds market), at one stage was colour graded, the lavender-blue being the most valuable. It is also an amphibole occurring in banded ironstone. It is found in the north-west Cape (Griqualand West). It is also found in the Northern Transvaal, where in some situations, amosite and crocidolite occur in the same seam. Exploitation of the Transvaal deposits of crocidolite peaked during the Second World War and then declined.

The mining of crocidolite in Griqualand West (north-west Cape) was begun south of Prieska, the southern most town in these asbestos fields, in 1893. In that year 100 tons of crude ore was produced. The early method of mining was open-cast quarrying.[1] In the Cape, the black workers (unlike elsewhere in South Africa) carried out the blasting. They also did the quarrying, whilst their women cobbed the fibre, and their children recovered any asbestos fibres that had been discarded. Cobbing, or knapping as it was originally called, consists in separating the rock from the fibre by striking the fragments with a square faced hammer. The women then sorted the fibre into different lengths. The work was supervised by the whites. The fibre was bought by companies on the tribute system.

Gradually, as the overseas market for crocidolite increased, underground mining started at the richer strikes, so that by 1918[2] there were mines in the south near Prieska and 150 miles to the north at Kuruman. In 1930 Hall listed 104 sites in the asbestos mountains, but there were only 12 actual mines.[3] Most of these mines were worked by black workers, but white farmers were working outcrops, especially during times of drought.

There was a greatly increased demand for crocidolite immediately before and during the First World War, with mills being built in the towns of Prieska and Kuruman. Following a lull, the industry revived in the late 1930s, increasing further during the Second World War. Then came another major increase between 1950 and 1960, production rising from 40 000 tons to 100 000 tons. By this time, the mills were modernised and mining occurred on a large scale with underground shafts. Only in Prieska did the tribute system continue and there was an active mill in the town. In other areas the mill was attached to the mine.

By 1962 as the mills became larger the amount of dust increased, as did the size of the tailings dumps, which released more dust during dry and windy conditions. Furthermore, the demand from the manufacturing industry for fine crocidolite fibre increased the amount of dust. The large tailings dumps contained about 20% fibre in the vicinity of active and previous sites of mills.

Mesotheliomas

During the Second World War, a Royal Air Force hospital was built in Kimberly, which is in the northern part of the Cape Province. After the war, this hospital was presented to the South African government, which decided it should be used for the treatment of tuberculosis. Dr C. A. Sleggs was appointed as Superintendent. The area covered by the hospital stretched from the Orange Free State in the east, to what is now Namibia in the west. Before 1950, tuberculosis was endemic in the whole of this area. In the next few years, with the advent of specific anti-tuberculous treatment, Sleggs noticed that there was a difference in the response to treatment of those with tuberculous pleurisy.[4] Patients from the eastern part of the area showed a good response, whilst there was a poor response from some of the cases from the west. Twelve of these latter were seen by thoracic surgeons in Capetown, Pretoria or Johannesburg. In all cases a diagnosis of metastatic carcinoma from an unknown primary site was made. By February 1956, there were a further 6 cases in this (west-end) hospital.

In February 1956 in Johannesburg, a black male patient came to necropsy examination. He was thought to have had tuberculous pleurisy and had been treated in the main mine hospital in Johannesburg but did not respond to treatment. Aspiration of his pleural cavity had failed, as the fluid was thick and sticky. A diagnosis of empyema was made and subsequently given as the cause of death. However, at postmortem examination the findings were different with the presence of a huge gelatinous tumour filling the right thoracic cavity, completely surrounding and compressing the right lung, infiltrating the pericardium and displacing the mediastinum. Mesothelioma was a rare tumour. At this time most pathologists agreed with R. A. Willis[5] that these tumours did not exist and that any tumour found in the pleural cavity was a metastasis from a primary site elsewhere.[6] Wagner carried out the postmortem, and he consulted the professor of pathology at Witwatersrand University (B. J. P. Becker). Becker suggested that a detailed examination should be made to eliminate any other primary tumour. None was found and the diagnosis of mesothelioma was agreed. As part of the histological investigation, clumps of asbestos bodies were observed in the lung tissue, but no evidence of asbestosis.

This case was presented to the local thoracic society group by Olaf Martiny[7] and Chris Wagner about 2 months later. In the meantime, Dr Sleggs was still perturbed over his cases, and consulted L. Fatti, senior thoracic surgeon, and his partner, P. Marchand, both of whom visited Kimberly. The marked similarity of clinical and radiological findings of Dr Sleggs' cases and the case that Wagner and Martiny had presented was noted by both these surgeons. Dr Sleggs sent 2 needle biopsies from his other cases, but the material was insufficient for a definite diagnosis. Marchand carried out open biopsies on the cases in the West-End hospital. By the end of 1956 pathology had been seen from 10 large pleural biopsies and 2 post-mortem examinations. Obviously, a definite diagnosis could only be given after death, followed by a full post-mortem examination. All material was shown to Professor P. Steiner from Chicago, who had seen a number of mesotheliomas previously, and he agreed with the diagnosis that had been made. He asked why there were so many of these rare tumours.

An association with asbestos was considered at an early stage, partly because asbestos bodies had been found in the first case and the range of the asbestos mountains was 90 miles west of Kimberly. Other possible aetiologies were suggested. Was there a virus implicated, the situation being similar to that in East Africa, with the Epstein-Barr virus? Could radioactivity play a part as monazite, the ore of thorium was known to occur in the region? Was there a local genetic disposition, associated with tuberculosis?

Of the first 16 cases collected only 4 had worked in the asbestos industry. The biopsies from these cases were mainly from the parietal pleura, but from 3 there were fragments of lung tissue that contained a few asbestos bodies. The majority of these 16 people had lived in the Kuruman district.

Evidence against the implication that asbestos was responsible for the development of these tumours was that only a quarter of the cases had admitted working with asbestos. Secondly, since asbestos mining had been in progress for more than 50 years in this region, it would be expected that the tumours could have been recognised at an earlier date. Later it was discovered from the records that a pleural endothelioma was first reported in 1917 and that several other tumours had been notified but always considered to be from a primary site elsewhere. Thirdly, none of these tumours had been observed where other types of asbestos were produced. Fourthly, Doll had shown a dose response associated with other asbestos diseases, occurring in heavily exposed (for more that 20 years) individuals.[8] The majority of the mesothelioma cases denied having worked with asbestos at all. Their occupations were diverse, including housewives, domestic servants, cattle herders, farmers, a water-bailiff, an accountant and later an international goal-keeper.

It was not until the middle of 1958 when Paul Marchand interviewed two brothers that it was realised that a different question must be asked. One brother had a mesothelioma, while the other had a suspicious x-ray. Marchand asked the latter whether either of them had worked in the asbestos industry, to which he replied that his father had owned a small asbestos mine and that they used to play on the dumps as children. All the cases were then re-interviewed (or the relatives), mainly by Dr Sleggs. From this information, it was clear that the majority had had exposure to blue asbestos. They had lived in the vicinity of either the mills or the tailings dumps. Exposure could be as little as 6 months even 40 years before. Some were exposed as infants and others at school where the neighbouring dumps made excellent play slides. The first patient diagnosed with mesothelioma whose occupation was given as a bath attendant was found to have herded sheep in the Kuruman area when young.

Could these tumours have occurred in those countries where the Cape blue had been exported? Preliminary enquiries in Europe during 1957–58 by Wagner[9] elicited evidence of one tumour in the Midlands, United Kingdom, and also one in Turin, Italy. E. McCaughey reported 15 cases,[10] which he had seen in Belfast, Northern Ireland, but no association with asbestos was considered. (Webster in 1959 stated that he had seen two further cases at the London Hospital, United Kingdom; personal communication).

In 1958 Dr Harold S. Stewart, Head of Cancer Research at the National Institutes of Health, Washington, DC, and an authority on geographical distribution of cancer, was keenly interested in these findings and he persuaded Dr A. J. Orenstein, Director of the South African Pneumoconiosis Unit, that Wagner and Sleggs should present papers at the International Pneumoconiosis Conference, to be held in Johannesburg in 1959. These papers were 'The pathological aspects of asbestosis in South Africa'[6] and 'Clinical aspects of asbestosis in the Northern Cape'.[4] The main topics of this conference were the diseases associated with the major industries of gold and coal mining. On the whole, no one appeared strongly interested in the mesothelioma problem, except for Dr J. C. Gilson, Director of the British Pneumoconiosis Unit.

It was decided to publish two further papers. The first had to concentrate on the precise nature of the pathology, as there was still doubt, internationally, about the existence of mesothelioma. The second paper would concentrate on the epidemiological, clinical and radiological findings, confirming the increased incidence. The first paper was submitted to the *British Journal of Industrial Medicine* in 1960.[11] According to Professor J. Gough of Cardiff, UK, who had seen the pathological material, the editorial board were about to reject the paper, as their senior pathologist did not accept the existence of mesotheliomas, but Gough persuaded them otherwise (personal communication). The clinical paper gave evidence of even further tumours associated with exposure to blue asbestos, in the Cape area and elsewhere in South Africa. By the end of 1961, 67 mesotheliomas had been diagnosed, 30 having occupational exposure, and 8 further cases having worked with crocidolite in other industries. Of the other 29, 22 had been born on the Cape asbestos fields. At this stage, there were only 2 people for whom no evidence of occupational or environmental history could be obtained.

At the Pneumoconiosis Conference in 1959, the question was again raised as to why there were no tumours found with the other types of asbestos. All had been active for at least 30 years. It is a legal requirement that respiratory organs of miners who died should be submitted to the Pneumoconiosis Bureau, in Johannesburg. Other than those submitted from the Cape, no mesotheliomas had been received. In 1959, Drs G. K. Sluis-Cremer (Director of Research from the Pneumoconiosis Bureau), J. C. Gilson and J. C. Wagner undertook a visit to the mines and hospital in the Transvaal and Swaziland. Evidence of several carcinomas of the lung were seen in the amosite area and several cases of pulmonary fibrosis among the chrysotile workers. No mesotheliomas were seen. Later, Sluis-Cremer and Wagner accompanied Sleggs to the Prieska district, where several mesotheliomas were seen.[12]

Officially, even in 1962, there was not sufficient evidence to implicate crocidolite as a major factor in the development of mesotheliomas. It was puzzling that unlike other industrial hazards, even the environmental exposure could be extremely short, in some cases only a few months. Then there was a long latent period, as with exposure to radio-active substances, but there was no evidence of radioactivity in this situation. The majority of patients with mesothelioma had worked or lived in the northwest Cape, but a few people, working elsewhere with the Cape blue, had also developed the tumour. Experimental work with rats[13] given various types of dust had produced a few pleural tumours, but most of the animals had died too early from rat bronchiectasis. Further evidence was required that this was an occupational hazard, and most worrying of all was the evidence of environmental exposure, which differed so much from carcinoma in asbestos workers. The answer was to undertake an investigation in Britain, a country with a major crocidolite industry. If positive evidence was obtained it would be important to compare these findings with the situation in Canada, a major producer of chrysotile. Further work with suitable animals was also essential.

References

1. Wagner PA. Asbestos. Mineral deposits of South Africa. In: PA Wagner (ed.), *Third Mining and Metallurgical Conference.* Johannesburg, 1929; 272–277.
2. Wagner PA. Asbestos. *South African Journal of Industries* 1917; 1–22.
3. Hall AL. Asbestos in the Union of South Africa. *Mem. No. 12 Geological Survey of South Africa,* 1930.
4. Sleggs CA. Clinical aspects of asbestosis in the Northern Cape. In: AJ Orenstein (ed.), *Proceedings of the Pneumoconiosis Conference, Johannesburg.* London: J&A Churchill, 1959.
5. Willis RA. *Pathology of tumours.* London: Butterworth, 1948.
6. Wagner JC. Some pathological aspects of asbestosis in the Union of South Africa. In: AJ Orenstein (ed.), *Proceedings of the Pneumoconiosis Conference, Johannesburg.* London: J&A Churchill, 1959; 376–381.
7. Martiny O. Report of a case of mesothelioma. *Proceedings of the Transvaal Medical Officers Association* 1956; **35**: 355–363.
8. Doll R. Mortality from lung cancer in asbestos workers. *Br J Ind Med* 1955; **12**: 81–86.
9. Wagner JC. Memo on pneumoconiosis research in Europe. Submitted to the *C.S.I.R.*, 1958.
10. McCaughey WTE. Mesotheliomas of the pleura. *J Patho Bact* 1958; **76**: 517.
11. Wagner JC, Sleggs CA, Marchand P. Diffuse pleural mesotheliomas and asbestos exposure in the North-West Cape Province. *Br J Ind Med* 1960; **17**: 260–271.
12. Sleggs CA, Marchand P, Wagner JC. Diffuse pleural mesotheliomas in South Africa. *S Afr Med J* 1961; **35**: 29–34.
13. Wagner JC. Experimental productions of mesothelial tumours of the pleura by implantation of dusts in laboratory animals. *Nature* 1962; **96**: 180–181.

=5=

Mesothelioma and Exposure to Asbestos in South Africa: 1962–2000

Neil White and Eric Bateman

As described in the previous chapter, South Africa features strongly in the modern story of mesothelioma. However, from promising beginnings the record is a trail of missed opportunities to prevent the disease and avert the medical disaster and human tragedy that resulted. Involved are more than 2700 South Africans who are reported to have died from mesothelioma and possibly thousands more who may die from this condition; government officials who failed in their duty to protect citizens from preventable harm; profit-orientated mine owners; a medical scientific community that for a variety of reasons had minimal discernible impact on policy or practice that might have prevented mesothelioma; a dysfunctional state compensation system for exposed workers and a legal system that offered no practical means of redress for people who develop mesothelioma consequent upon environmental exposures. It is not a happy story nor one of which the medical scientific communities or public at large can feel proud! But the story must be told if only for the sake of those that have suffered, and for its value as a cameo of life in South Africa during the middle and latter half of the twentieth century.

This chapter provides a brief review of the mineralogy, mining and use of asbestos in South Africa, an analysis of the not very extensive body of literature on mesothelioma in South Africa and the sometimes tortuous route of asbestos research. Environmental and occupational exposures related to mesothelioma are reviewed, as are current important preventive strategies. Future prospects for mesothelioma prevention, while they do not seem bright, are not without some hope.

Three minerals, three epidemics

All three of the major commercial forms of asbestos – Cape crocidolite (blue asbestos), amosite (brown asbestos) and chrysotile (white asbestos) occur in South Africa. Amosite, together with Cape and Transvaal crocidolite, belongs to the amphibole family of asbestos minerals, whereas chrysotile is a serpentine asbestos.

In their monograph on asbestos mining and disease in South Africa, Felix *et al.*[1] have traced the history of the mining of each of the these forms of asbestos, and demonstrated their links with local epidemics of asbestos-related diseases, and through exportation of massive amounts of these minerals, with disease in workers and communities around the globe.

The South African asbestos trade began in the early nineteenth century following the discovery and mining of crocidolite near Prieska in the Northern Cape in 1806. This town is at the southern end of a region with numerous asbestos occurrences, extending some 50 km in width and 400 km in length northwards to South Africa's border with Botswana, where the now defunct Pomfret, the largest of the crocidolite mines, is situated.

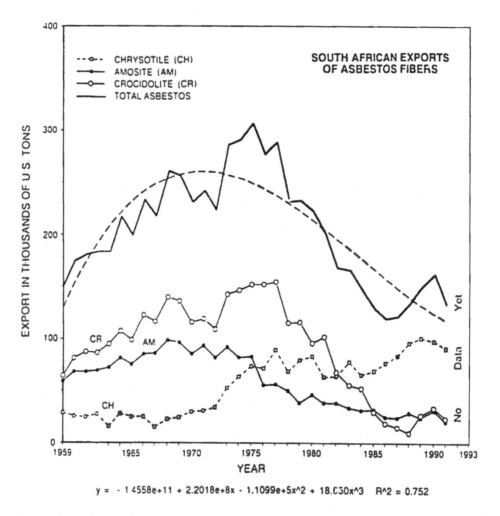

$$y = \cdot 14558e+11 + 2.2018e+8x \cdot 1.1099e+5x^2 + 18.030x^3 \quad R^2 = 0.752$$

Figure 5.1. *South African exports of chrysotile, amosite and crocidolite, 1959–91.*

Initially, and well into the first half of the twentieth century, crocidolite mining was outcrop and small digging operations run by tributers and farmers. Mining and milling were highly labour-intensive. Fibre was cobbed from rock by hand-held hammers, sieved by hand, sorted by a combination of a hand and mechanised method, and transported in Hessian sacks to its destination. Women and child labour was extensively employed in sorting and cobbing.

Trans-national companies became predominant in the mining of asbestos for international markets, a process that began with the establishment of the United Kingdom based Cape Asbestos Company that began mining and milling operations at Prieska in 1893. By 1919 more than 3000 tons of Cape crocidolite fibre were being produced per year. By the 1930s trans-national corporations dominated the asbestos mining scene in South Africa.

Amosite – a name derived from the acronym for Asbestos Mines of South Africa – occurs in the Lydenburg district, with the major deposit being at Penge where mining was carried out from 1914 to 1992. Numerous deposits occur north-west of Penge in a 45 km arc and during the mid-twentieth century were mined for amosite and Transvaal crocidolite in numerous small operations using crude technologies that caused extensive environmental pollution and exposed the labour force to high levels of asbestos dust.

Chrysotile mining in the Barberton district of Mpumalanga Province began at a number of sites after 1915. Exploitation of the major deposit at Msauli began in 1937. Msauli is currently South Africa's only operational asbestos mine, now employing less than 350 people.

A recent review of South African asbestos production, exports and destinations from 1959–93[2] confirms that sales of crocidolite and amosite reached their peaks in 1977 when South Africa exported a total of 380 000 tons of asbestos (Fig. 5.1), making it the third biggest supplier in the world in that year.

In the early 1960s Europe and North America were the major purchasers of South African asbestos, but sales of amphiboles to these countries declined steeply after 1980 as the dangers of this fibre type became known. By 1989–91, supply to these regions was surpassed by the Far East, which took over 90% of chrysotile, and 70% of amosite produced. Crocidolite sales in 1992 were only 5% of their former peak and amosite sales ceased following the ban on its importation into Japan. In that year an additional 21 countries continued to import crocidolite although in reduced quantities and South Africa remained the seventh largest world supplier of asbestos, providing 4.1% of global production (3 million tons). In 1992 the Middle Eastern countries took nearly 40%, Europe 28% and Africa 21% of crocidolite produced. In Africa, only Zimbabwe (152 561 tons in 1992) and Swaziland (32, 818 tons) mine asbestos, both of which produced chrysotile exclusively, destined for the export market.

At its height in the 1970s, the South African asbestos mining industry employed about 20 000 asbestos miners, but by 1986 this figure had declined to 6000.[3] In 1999, the only remaining functioning mine is the chrysotile mine at Msauli, which, it is estimated, will be exhausted within 3 years. Its closure may signal the end of the mine production of asbestos, but is not the finale to two aspects of the asbestos exposure hazard – exposure in industry, and environmental exposure, which in South Africa are each responsible for approximately as many mesotheliomas as occur in miners.

Twenty thousand tons of chrysotile are still used in the country annually. Its chief use is in the manufacture of asbestos-containing cement building materials and pipes, an industry which currently employs more than 3000 workers. A variety of other smaller industries remain important sources of exposure. Levels of environmental pollution in some regions remain huge. In the Northern Cape alone there are 82 asbestos dumps scattered about the countryside at or near the sites of defunct mines. It is in this region that the lethal association was first made.

Mesothelioma and asbestos – the beginnings

The association between asbestos and mesothelioma was first correctly made in people from the Northern Cape Province crocidolite fields, an association that was subsequently confirmed and accepted worldwide.[4,5] Considering that crocidolite had already been exploited for 150 years and that thousands of people had been exposed, many at an early age and under crude conditions, it is perhaps surprising that it had not been considered earlier. It appears that there were sufficient cases for Sleggs, Wagner and Marchand to assemble their series of 33 cases of this usually rare tumour in only four years!

In reviewing developments subsequent to the discovery of this association, Felix *et al.* recount that at the 1959 Pneumoconiosis Conference held in Johannesburg a resolution was adopted to further investigate the relationship between asbestos exposure and mesothelioma, and in 1961 the Pneumoconiosis Research Unit (PRU) of the government-sponsored Council for Scientific and Industrial Research (CSIR) embarked on a field survey in the northern Cape and at Penge. The first year of the study cost 12 000 rand. Asbestos mining companies contributed 8000 rand and the South African Cancer Association contributed 4000. It must have soon been clear to the researchers that they were dealing with a serious instance of environmental pollution. Flynn[6] recounts that Webster was charged with the unpleasant task of informing the asbestos industry of the environmental disaster in the Northern Cape and that crocidolite was the carcinogenic factor. This information apparently evoked a negative response which included a campaign to denigrate the scientists involved, accusing them of "trying to destroy a valuable export industry for self-aggrandisement".[6] Funding of the project by the industry and the Cancer Association was not renewed for a second year of the study, and consequently the field-work was never completed. However, the CSIR contributed 10 000 rand to finalise the research report on the work completed, but subject to an undertaking by the Research Advisory Committee of the PRU that "such a 'report' would not be published or made available outside the unit [PRU], other than to sponsors and the various members of the working committees that had been concerned with the conduct of the 'survey' ".[6]

The 1960 survey comprised a random sample of the inhabitants over the age of 20 years of every tenth house in three towns in the north-western Cape Province and one town in the north-eastern Transvaal.[7] Among the 1341 examinees, 4.8% of people not industrially exposed had asbestos bodies in their sputum and/or lung or pleural changes suggestive of asbestos exposure evident on x-ray examination. At that time fibre concentrations in the general ambient atmosphere were measured at 0.09 fibres per mL.[7]

The most notable conclusions were, first, that dust levels in the region were so high that "people who live or have lived in proximity to asbestos mines or mills are in danger of contracting asbestosis, even though they have had no industrial exposure to asbestos dust inhalation". . . and, second, that "an alarmingly high number of cases with mesothelioma of the pleura have been discovered and there is evidence to suggest that mesothelioma is associated with an exposure to asbestos dust inhalation which need not be industrial".[7]

Most of the data in the PRU report was subsequently published,[8] but the initial suppression of the results may be considered as the first symptom of an unhealthy relationship between parties who as a consequence failed to act in the public interest. It signalled the beginning of a process of acquiescence by various state agencies to the asbestos industry's demand for continued exploitation of crocidolite and amosite, despite the evidence of their potent carcinogenicity. This in turn resulted in a period of little epidemiological and field research in relation to mesothelioma in South Africa. It was not until the mid-1980s that substantial new epidemiology on mesothelioma in South Africa was published. Instead, such asbestos-related research as was carried out was either not specifically directed at mesothelioma or was based on pathology series. However, the most important consequence of the suppressed report is that control of atmospheric pollution caused by asbestos mining operations was not scheduled and controlled by the Atmospheric Pollution Prevention Act of 1965, administered by the Department of Health. Control of occupational and environmental asbestos exposure in relation to mining remained the sole responsibility of the Department of Minerals. Finally, it would appear that there was no intention at the time nor attempt to inform the residents of Prieska and the other affected towns investigated of the conclusions from the study.

Mesothelioma: reporting of cases and trends, 1955–92

After the 1959 Pneumoconiosis Conference in Johannesburg, the National Research Institute of Occupational Diseases (NIROD – subsequently the National Centre for Occupational Health [NCOH]) in association with the Asbestos Tumour Reference Panel – a panel of expert histopathologists established in 1965 – continued to record and check each diagnosis of mesothelioma reported to it. In 1973 Webster published the group's experience of the first 232 cases.[9] Later, Zwi *et al.* released results of a case series of mesothelioma compiled from a variety of sources, provided an estimate of mesothelioma incidence and described characteristics of 1347 cases identified in South Africa between 1976 and 1984.[10] Other case series have also been reported.[11–13]

In 1986, a South African National Cancer Registry (SANCR) was established within the South African Institute for Medical Research (SAIMR). The SANCR essentially incorporated the work of the Asbestos Tumour Reference Panel (ATRP) and centralised reporting of cancer diagnoses made by pathologists at all major public and private institutions in South Africa.[14] Between 1986 and 1992, 1158 cases were reported to the SANCR.

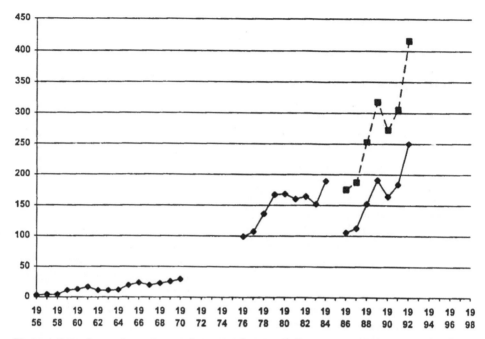

Figure 5.2. *Annual numbers of cases of mesothelioma occurring in South Africa, 1955–92. (Data sources: 1955–70, Webster[9]; 1976–86, Zwi et al.[10]: 1986–92 NCR.[14] Dotted line 1986–92 is an extrapolation of NCR data – see text.)*

The 2737 biopsy-confirmed cases of mesothelioma recorded in these three reports (Fig. 5.2) permit some conclusions concerning mesothelioma incidence and trends. Of these reports, the article by Zwi *et al.* is likely to provide the best estimates as the authors actively sought cases from sources not accessed by the SANCR's passive reporting system.

Together these series allow us to conclude that there has been and remains significant under-detection and under-reporting of mesothelioma, particularly in blacks in South Africa; that the incidence of malignant mesothelioma in South Africa is comparable with the highest figures found anywhere else in the world, with indications that it is probably higher; and that the country is still on the upward slope of the 'epidemic'.

In the nine-year study period covered by Zwi *et al.*,[10] only 796 (59%) of their 1347 cases were known to the ATRP. When the SANCR began reporting in 1986, the 105 cases detected that year represented only 55.6% of the number reported by Zwi *et al.* for 1984. Moreover, of the 408 deaths due to mesothelioma that had been entered into the death registers at Central Statistical Services, only 47 cases (11.5%) had been notified to the Department of Health (which made the disease a notifiable condition in 1979).

As further evidence of under-diagnosis, there are marked racial differences in mesothelioma rates, those in whites being considerably higher than in the other population groups. In fact, the majority of cases occurred in whites, despite the fact that they make up only about one-fifth of the total population, and represented only one-twentieth of the asbestos mining workforce.

Zwi *et al.* speculated that several factors might account for this. Whites have better access to health services than people of other races in South Africa, increasing the possibility of diagnosis. He also considered that under-diagnosis was prevalent in areas of highest incidence because experienced doctors were reluctant to subject people to invasive procedures for untreatable conditions, whilst inexperienced doctors would treat all pleural effusions as tuberculosis. Differing intensities and duration of exposure to asbestos, and different life expectancy between the races could result in real differences in the incidence of this tumour. Whites tended to be more permanently settled in mining areas and had longer duration of exposure, but generally occupied less dusty categories of employment. Shorter life expectancy in blacks and coloureds might mean that "members of these populations do not live long enough to develop mesothelioma...".[10] In a study of mortality in amphibole miners in South Africa, Sluis-Cremer *et al.* showed that miners have a higher risk of dying at an earlier age than the general population for many reasons, but principally tuberculosis and accidents. In the same study they showed that 4.7% of deaths in crocidolite miners and 0.6% in amosite miners were due to mesothelioma.

A third possibility, supported by recent follow-up data on the mining workforce is that subjects at risk were lost to surveillance and that the earlier studies are a serious underestimate. The infamous migrant labour system resulted in many (black) people returning not only to rural areas within the Republic of South Africa, but also to other southern African countries, thus escaping detection. In a 1997 study of gold miners from the Eastern Cape, Trapido found that, of the men in a cohort who worked in mining between 1969 and 1980, 55% of the cohort had already died.[15] If we conservatively estimate that there was a cohort of 40 000 crocidolite miners during the same period and 55% of them have died with 4.7% of the deaths due to mesothelioma, there should have been 1034 cases, or approximately double the total number of cases in black males reported by Zwi *et al.* and the NCR over an eighteen year period.

These studies strongly suggest that under-diagnosis rather than lower risk explains the racial differences in incidence. This has important implications for the future planning of surveillance and provision of compensation to the former asbestos workforce. At present it is clear why cases did not simply appear by themselves. Medical care is limited in rural areas, doctors have little to offer most people in whom mesothelioma is

Table 5.1. *Standardised incidence rates per million population aged 15 years and over for mesothelioma in the Republic of South Africa (1976–84) by race and sex.*[10,14]

	White		Coloured		Black	
	Male	*Female*	*Male*	*Female*	*Male*	*Female*
1976–84						
Overall	32.9	8.9	7.6	3.0	24.8	13.9
95% C.I.	22.7–46.4	2.5–15.8	3.5–15.8	0.6–8.8	16.2–36.9	7.7–23.5
1992	54.0	20.8	5.2	2.4	6.4	6.0

diagnosed, and the cumbersome compensation system calls for great patience and persistence, and at best provides late relief for the bereaved.

Zwi *et al.* estimated mesothelioma incidence rates, especially for whites, that were among the highest ever reported, being almost four to six times higher than those in England and Wales, and at least as high in white males as had been reported from Western Australia[16] – the only other place in the world where significant amounts of crocidoilite were mined. Age-standardised incidence rates (ASIR) per million in those aged 15 years and over are shown in Table 5.1. During the 9-year study period the ASIR in white males rose from 23.6 per million in 1976 to 40.5 per million in 1984. A comparable figure from the 1992 NCR report is 54 per million, giving an indication of a steady increase in mesothelioma incidence over the years.

When ASIR from the SANCR in 1992 are compared to those of Zwi *et al.* it is notable that there has been a significant increase in the ASIR for mesothelioma in the white population, particularly in white women. There has been no significant change in the black population. The rates in the coloured population were particularly low in 1992 – double the number of cases in this group were reported in 1990 and 1991.

Based on Zwi *et al.*'s estimate it seems reasonable to assume that cases registered annually by the NCR represent 60% of all biopsy-proven cases. In Figure 5.2, the NCR statistics are inflated based on this assumption. Based on this assumption the total number of biopsy-proven mesothelioma cases in 1992 would have been 416, giving an ASIR for the whole South African population over age 15 of 16.6 per million.

The SANCR does make some interesting comparisons possible. From the 1992 report it is obvious that mesothelioma does not warrant the epithet 'rare' tumour. If basal and squamous skin cancers are excluded, mesothelioma is the twentieth most common cancer diagnosis in the general male population, being more common than cancers such as pancreatic or thyroid cancer, myeloma or Hodgkin's lymphoma. If the skin cancers are not included, in 1992 mesothelioma was the fifteenth most common cancer in both men and women over the age of 70.

Asbestos exposure and mesothelioma

Four case series have been published that detail the source of exposure in 505 cases of histologically proven mesothelioma in South Africa (Table 5.2).[9,11-13] Most of the cases where exposure was not known or where it was believed that there was no exposure are from the first case series. If these 61 cases are excluded, of the remaining 444, in 118 or 26.6% the exposure was confirmed as being environmental only, whilst in the remainder a source of occupational exposure was identified with a slight majority of cases being reported from secondary industry.

Occupational mesothelioma

Mining-related exposures in asbestos mines or mills contribute the largest proportion of cases (145 cases or 44.5%) of those mesotheliomas where exposure is known. Mesothelioma has been described in relation to both crocidolite and amosite exposure, but given

Table 5.2. *Reported sources of occupational or environmental asbestos exposure in 505 histologically proven cases of mesothelioma in South Africa.*

	Webster 1973[9]	Cochrane 1978[11]	Solomons 1984[12]	Rees 1988[13]	Total
Mining					
mining	64	7	9	14	94
processing	14	4	4	18	40
transport	1	5	2	3	11
Railways					
maintenance	8	16	11	1	36
transport	—	3	4	—	7
Marine engineering	1	2	6	1	10
Asbestos cement					
manufacture	—	10	5	6	21
Construction					
asbestos cement	—	3	—	—	3
insulation	—	—	1	—	1
other	3	—	7	—	10
Boilermaker/artisan	6	2	4	15	27
Motor workshop	1	—	1	1	3
Miscellaneous	4	3	14	38	59
Environmental					
exposure only	76	13	7	22	118
No exposure	32	1	5	3	41
Exposure not known	22	—	—	1	23
Total cases	232	69	80	123	504

the relative paucity of cases in relation to amosite it seems that crocidolite is more carcinogenic than amosite.[17] A study of the causes of death in a cohort of South African amphibole miners has shown that 4.7% of the crocidolite miners in the study had died from mesothelioma – the proportional mortality ratio.[17] This is substantially higher than the same proportion in amosite miners (0.6%) and in Quebec chrysotile miners (0.4%).[17]

No cases of mesothelioma have been described where exposure has been to South African chrysotile alone. Caution is necessary before suggesting that it is safe, as South African health effects data in relation to chrysotile mining are unreliable. One case of mesothelioma has been described from Swaziland where the chrysotile ore body is an extension of that found in neighbouring South Africa.[18]

The South African chrysotile mining labour force has been conspicuously under-investigated, compared to miners in Zimbabwe[19] or Swaziland.[20] A pre-radiographic survey of the health of chrysotile miners was conducted in 1931.[21] There is no further published record on South African chrysotile mines until 1997 when in abstract form a report describes a substantial prevalence of asbestos-related diseases in Msauli miners being made redundant.[22] These workers were medically examined at the request of the National Union of Mineworkers.

In an interesting parallel, for many years Zimbabwean chrysotile was held to be non-mesotheliomagenic[23] because of an absence of reported cases of mesothelioma in Zimbabweans other than those exposed to crocidolite in non-mining occupations. Zimbabwean chrysotile is reportedly not contaminated by tremolite.[24] Formal review of the Zimbabwean National Cancer Registry and other sources in 1991 revealed two cases of mesothelioma in former chrysotile miners.[19]

Most mesothelioma cases result from exposures to asbestos in its many and varied uses in secondary industry. During the 1960s and 1970s, as South Africa became industrialised a substantial and diversified asbestos industry developed.[25] Formal control and limitation of asbestos exposure was only regulated in 1987 in terms of the Occupational Health and Safety Act.

This diversity of use made of asbestos in secondary industry is reflected by the wide range of occupations, particularly in the most recent series on cases in South Africa reported by Rees et al.[13] Three major occupations stand out: the maintenance of steam locomotive and other railways-related exposures; the asbestos cement industry, including the use of asbestos cement products in construction; and boiler makers and other artisans who use asbestos for lagging and similar insulation applications.

Compensation for patients with occupational mesothelioma

Prior to 1993, compensation for miners developing occupational diseases, including mesothelioma, was racially discriminatory. The Occupational Diseases in Mines and Works Amendment Act of 1993 abolished racial discrimination in the amounts paid, but awards are modest – usually about 70 000 rand given as a lump sum. The funding of future awards is of some concern as payments are made from the miners' Compensation Fund, maintained by current mining employers pro rata for the number of miners that they employ and their level of risk. If a mine has ceased operation the Act can require the state to make up the cost to the Fund of that mine's compensation. Since the asbestos mining industry is essentially defunct, all compensation costs of former miners in South Africa have come either from general revenues or from current mining employers.

Outside of the mining industry, compensation for occupational diseases, including mesothelioma, is governed by the Compensation for Occupational Injuries and Diseases Act (1993)[COIDA]. A striking feature in the past has been the low rate of claims. A recent analysis of numbers of mesothelioma cases compensated in South Africa has been reported by Rees et al.[26] (Table 5.3). They note that of the 242 cases reported to the

Table 5.3. Mesothelioma cases compensated in South Africa 1992–97.

	Number of cases compensated						
	1992	1993	1994	1995	1996	1997	Total
COID Act	12	—	15	57	52	54	178
ODMW Act	—	—	19	21	29	15	84
Total	12	—	34	78	81	69	262

NCR in 1992, probably 180 were occupational. Although data are incomplete it seems that the numbers of cases being reported, particularly from secondary industry (COID Act), are increasing. Nevertheless in 1997 only approximately a third of the expected number of cases were being accepted for compensation (69 of 180). Civil court actions claiming damages for personal injury caused by asbestos-related diseases have not been a feature in South Africa until very recently, as is detailed below.

Environmental mesothelioma

Evidence from mesothelioma case studies

In the vast majority of the cases of mesothelioma in South Africa where there was known to have only been environmental exposure to asbestos, this exposure has occurred in the Northern Cape in proximity to mines, mills and dumps.

A high proportion of cases of environmental origin (26.6%) is unique to South Africa. The only comparable example is Australia, the only other country to have mined crocidolite in significant amounts. Ferguson *et al.*[27] found that in 726 cases of mesothelioma registered in Western Australia during 1980–85, 43 cases or 6% had environmental exposure only, and only in six cases (<1%) was environmental asbestos exposure due to residence in an asbestos mining region (Wittenoom).

Webster[9] and Solomons[12] do not detail the source of environmental exposure to asbestos of the patients in their series but in a later series that included these and other environmental cases totalling 100, Webster[28] gave the following distribution: 93 cases originated from exposures in relation to mining in the Northern Cape; 3 in relation to amosite and Transvaal crocidolite in the Northern Province; and in the balance there was some uncertainty about the exact source of exposure. Cochrane[12] and Rees *et al.*[13] have detailed environmental exposure in a further 25 cases, 23 from the Northern Cape, and most could recall some asbestos exposure. In Rees' series one case was in a teacher who had worked in asbestos cement classrooms in 1934–75. Another was a policeman in the Northern Province who made regular trips to asbestos mines. The authors are aware of a medical colleague who died of mesothelioma in his mid-40s whose exposure was a childhood in the Northern Cape as a son of a local general practitioner. In summary, 93% of all environmental mesothelioma cases in South Africa originate from exposures in relation to crocidolite mining activities in the Northern Cape.

Zwi *et al.* were able to characterise exposure in 759 of their cases of mesothelioma, but did not provide many details. They do, however, state that in 30.3% of their cases there was environmental exposure and in a further 12.3% of cases both environmental and occupational exposure, again mainly in the Northern Cape. They provide the additional detail that in men only 16.8% of cases were environmental, whereas in women 124 out of 176 cases (70.5%) were solely due to environmental exposure.

Evidence from epidemiological surveys

In a survey carried out during the late 1970s, Talent *et al.*[29] investigated the health status of 1185 former crocidolite miners in the area around Kuruman, Northern Cape. A substantial prevalence of asbestos-related disease (ARD) was detected among the surviving miners who could be traced and examined. There were an unprecedented six incident cases of mesothelioma in the cohort. In addition, during the time that the research clinic operated near Kuruman (1974–79) 61 cases of mesothelioma were identified among patients attending the local hospital. Thirty-seven had some asbestos or cobbing exposure, and the remaining 24 only environmental exposure.

The findings of Talent *et al.* were part of a growing awareness in the South African medical community in the late 1970s and early 1980s of the extent of the mesothelioma problem growing in the country. This awareness spawned a number of insightful epidemiological studies quoted in this text. It also resulted in a number of publications by concerned scientists, calling for better control of South Africa's asbestos hazard.[3,25,30]

Sources of meaningful epidemiological data are limited in South Africa, as is research funding. In the late 1970s, Botha *et al.* set out to establish standardised mortality ratios for mesothelioma and other cancers for crocidolite mining districts in the Northern Cape, based on one of the few such sources – official death records kept by the Department of Statistics. The study was partly funded by the asbestos industry. In a well documented story of scientific suppression Cape Asbestos Company's health consultant was able to delay publication of Botha's paper for several years.

Investigative journalist Laurie Flynn[6] established that Botha's research findings had been leaked before publication to the South African Asbestos Producers Advisory Committee (SAAPAC), who then engaged a firm of consulting actuaries to critique the analysis. SAAPAC was represented on the advisory panel of the NIROD's Asbestos Research Project during this time – a position they occupied by virtue of their partial funding of the project. For years asbestos producers in South Africa were in the enviable position of being able to influence asbestos research at source.

The Directorship at the National Centre for Occupational Health changed in 1982. When finally published in 1986, Botha *et al.*'s study[31] showed that in the crocidolite mining districts of Kuruman, Hay and Prieska, the average annual crude death rates from asbestosis and/or mesothelioma in the age group 35–74 years were 30–100 times higher than in the rest of South Africa. The SMRs for these conditions compared to control districts ranged from 7.86 to 10.30.

Zwi *et al.*[10] clearly showed that mesothelioma deaths are under-registered in South African death statistics but nevertheless Botha *et al.*'s study had amply demonstrated the concentration of mesothelioma risk in these districts, even though it may have been underestimated.

A better estimate of the impact of asbestos exposure and mesothelioma in the Prieska district (population 14 000) comes from the study by Reid *et al.*[32] In a record linkage study of a birth cohort (1932–36) in this district it only proved possible to calculate mortality rates for whites. The cumulative mortality rate for mesothelioma in the cohort did not differ between men and women, nor was there much difference in rates for mesothelioma – 15 per 1000 (95% C.I. 5.5–24.5) – and respiratory neoplasm – 25.1 per 1000 (95% C.I. 12.2–38.0). Thus for the residents of Prieska, there is no significant difference in their risk of lung cancer and mesothelioma.

Compensation for patients with environmental mesothelioma

There is currently no form of financial compensation in South Africa for people who develop mesothelioma from environmental exposure. It has at various times in the past been mooted that the Department of Health should establish such a fund, but nothing has been forthcoming. It also appears that there has been no successful civil legal action for personal injury damages in this context. As we discuss below, this situation may be changing.

Preventing occupational mesothelioma

Since 1987 the use of asbestos in South African secondary industry has followed Asbestos Regulations framed in terms of the Occupational Health and Safety Act.[27] Among the provisions are a Permissible Exposure Limit (PEL) of 1 f/mL and an Action Exposure Limit (AEL) of 0.5 f/mL for all types of asbestos. More importantly and in line with trends elsewhere, there has been major substitution of most of the former uses of asbestos, particularly amphibole asbestos.

Most of the occupations listed in Table 5.2 are of historical interest only and are of little importance as current prevention strategies. For example, steam locomotives are being replaced. The asbestos cement industry used significant amounts of crocidolite in its products until the mid-1980s when substitution with chrysotile began.

In the future the main occupational asbestos hazard in industry will be the removal of asbestos, particularly in situations where it has been used as insulation on boilers, steam pipes and in buildings. It is not clear that this risk is adequately controlled by the current Asbestos Regulations and it is important that contractors are monitored to prevent unacceptable practices and methods of removal such as using untrained, daily paid workers to do this kind of work.

Although amphibole asbestos is no longer mined in South Africa, it is sobering to read Felix *et al.*'s account[1] of regulation of the health effects of asbestos mining by the Department of Minerals. Standards applied in South Africa have lagged behind those applied in Europe and North America. Sluis-Cremer[17] estimated that in surface workings in 1945, dust counts at crocidolite mines were 30–160 f/mL, and were 8–30 f/mL in 1970. In the 1970s, at a time when European countries were beginning to ban the importation of crocidolite, the PEL for asbestos surface workings was 10 f/mL. In 1984 the current uniform surface and underground mining standard of 2 f/mL was introduced.[1] In 2001 the Department is proposing that this limit be reduced to 1 f/mL for all types of asbestos.[33]

For many years asbestos producers strongly resisted the scientific evidence that asbestos was linked to cancer. Kuyper of Cape Asbestos argued at the 1969 Pneumoconiosis Conference that "the industry's engineers are still reluctant to agree with the alleged relationship between asbestos dust (principally crocidolite dust) and mesothelioma or that a transient encounter with the dust could lead to the development of the disease 20–30 years later; or that in consequence there is likely to be an increase in the number of cases of mesothelioma in the foreseeable future".[1]

This was a debate that the engineers clearly won because preventing mesothelioma was never a serious consideration in the setting of South Africa's PEL for asbestos. Felix *et al.* characterise state controls of the mining industry as reflecting more of an interest in encouraging mining and the use of asbestos products than an effort to protect miners and their communities from harm. This certainly rings true for crocidolite mining. Despite all that has been said, written and suffered for mesothelioma, state agencies in South Africa were prepared to countenance the continued mining of crocidolite well into the 1990s,[34] with operations presumably ceasing only because there was no longer anyone prepared to buy the product.

Preventing environmental mesothelioma

The focus for the prevention of environmental mesothelioma has to be twofold: the rehabilitation of the areas polluted by asbestos during mining and milling of the mineral and the education of the affected communities about the asbestos hazard. The extent of the problem of environmental pollution by asbestos in the affected regions is enormous. Living for the most part in complete ignorance of the health threat posed by asbestos, many communities have been seriously polluted with asbestos. Although initial remedial efforts by local and Provincial governments were slow and sporadic, a more concerted effort has been made by the Department of Minerals in recent years. The government has spent 44 million rand on this process, and estimates that a further 52 million is needed to complete this task. Companies have contributed less than 5% of the rehabilitation costs.

Felix[35] has documented the asbestos pollution of communities in the Northern Province asbestos fields in the proximity of Penge, together with community-based efforts to ameliorate the problem. Mills in the Pietersburg asbestos fields were originally situated in valleys near mines, often alongside streams and what later became the major roads of the area. African miners settled close to the mills. Over the years these remote, rural settlements grew into well established villages. In common with the conditions under apartheid, they had no piped water, no electricity, impoverished schools and health care facilities, and were served by rutted gravel roads.

Mafefe is the most densely populated (12 000 inhabitants) district in these asbestos fields. At least nine mills operated in the Mafefe district, each creating a large asbestos tailings waste dump. Apparently, the communities in the valley were never informed of the hazards of asbestos. After the mills closed, the abandoned dumps provided building material for the local people. Asbestos tailings were either mixed with clay to plaster mud homes or mixed with cement to make bricks. In 1987, half of all public buildings and 36% of 644 homes in Mafefe had been constructed with asbestos tailings. The grounds surrounding these homes were inadvertently contaminated with asbestos fibers during construction. In a random radiological survey of 389 residents performed in 1987, 34% had pleural changes.

Pollution conditions similar to Mafefe are to be found in the Kuruman district where many people live in proximity to mine dumps and crocidolite tailings have been used in brick making for homes. Most of the dumps and the areas around the mills in the crocidolite fields were not rehabilitated when the workings were abandoned. During the heyday of crocidolite mining, levels of environmental pollution were astounding. Personal accounts of this period include a blue haze that was usually visible over towns such as Prieska and Kuruman. In Prieska the mill was situated in the centre of the town. Balls of asbestos fluff would collect in homes and settle as dense mats in the ceiling boards. Immense dumps of asbestos tailings were left open to the climate. In this arid countryside fibre could be carried great distances on the wind. The industry used Hessian sacks and only changed to impermeable sacks in the 1980s. This meant that transporting the fibre was always a messy business. Asbestos tailings were used as gravel surfacing for roads. At one time rolled blue asbestos fibre was used to make up the greens at the Prieska golf course. In another instance, blue asbestos was used for a softer landing in the long jump pit at the Prieska school athletics field.

Some of the larger abandoned mines and dumps are no longer close to human settlement and have largely been forgotten. An example of this is Koegas, at the southern end of the Cape crocidolite belt. Like Prieska, Koegas is on the Orange River and its massive dumps stand astride the river open to climate and at risk of wind and water erosion into the river. Pomfret at the other end of the asbestos fields is also remote, but because it is close to the Botswana border, when the mine closed, its land, all the buildings and its immense dumps were bought by the state Public Works Department and up until 1998 used to house military personnel and their families. Although Pomfret's dumps were rehabilitated by contouring, soil coverage and planting of indigenous vegetation, heavy traffic in this arid area is again exposing the underlying asbestos tailings.

Treating mesothelioma

People who develop this cancer have a poor prognosis and, internationally, experience with treating mesothelioma has been discouraging. It is not clear that any treatment available to us confers benefit above that provided by simple palliation. This grim outlook seems to have discouraged clinical interest in this condition in South Africa. Specialised oncology therapies are only available in major centres and none of these are particularly close to the asbestos fields. Individual clinicians have over time developed considerable experience in the palliation of this cancer, but little of this experience has been published.[36]

The nihilism that surrounds the clinical management of mesothelioma has other consequences. In high-prevalence areas a typical case of mesothelioma (a painful pleural effusion that does not respond to anti-tuberculous therapy) is often not subjected to pleural biopsy unless drainage and pleurodesis becomes nescessary. Pleural biopsy is viewed as conferring no benefit other than confirming the diagnosis and carries a not insubstantial risk of tumour recurrence at the biopsy site – a troublesome complication that requires radiotherapy and distant referral.

Future prospects for mesothelioma

The future prospects for mesothelioma in South Africa are not encouraging. It could be expected that the occurrence of mesothelioma will peak some 20 to 30 years after the peak of crocidolite exploitation. This peak production was in 1977 and we may well be approaching this point in the epidemic. It can be expected that the epidemic will continue at least for the lifetime of those large numbers of people exposed to crocidolite in mining and industry up until the late 1980s. In view of the lack of timely, effective environmental rehabilitation in most affected communities it can be expected that mesothelioma will still be a spectre in the lives of children being born into these communities even today.

The asbestos tragedy has been described as "one of the most colossal blunders of the twentieth century" by Bill Sells,[2] a former executive of Johns-Manville, once a major US manufacturer of asbestos products. Sells wrote in 1994, "In my opinion the blunder that cost thousands of lives and destroyed an industry was a management blunder, and the blunder was denial," instead of the "responsibility . . . and product stewardship" demanded of so serious a situation.

Although asbestos in other countries could be considered a colossal blunder of management denial it is perhaps easier to understand the South African citizenry as the naive victims of a superbly conducted confidence trick carried out in the names of jobs, development and prosperity. Even now the con victim is scratching his head, looking at the dud cheque and saying to himself, "How did they do it?"

The only new developments in South Africa's asbestos tragedy have followed the advent of democratic government in 1994. For the first time asbestos polluted communities and workers are fully represented in the country's legislature. For the first time there has been a concerted, concerned focus by the legislature on asbestos-related matters through the Portfolio Committee for the Environment and Tourism. As part of this process a National Asbestos Summit was held in November 1998 to develop action-oriented strategies to address the main areas of current concern related to asbestos. The Summit was the culmination of a consultative process that sought to involve all interested and affected parties, including ex-mining communities, trade unions, scientists, government officials and industrialists. The declaration adopted at the summit expressed the intention, within "reasonable time"' to review compensation and other remedial systems; to strengthen the establishment of a "comprehensive health-care system", a Presidential Asbestos fund, and a Parliamentary Commission of Inquiry; to intensify inclusive processes of rehabilitation and sustainable development of communities in former asbestos mining areas; and to establish research towards the phasing out of chrysotile and ensure appropriate legislation for the above.

A second new development is the court actions for personal injury being brought against Cape Plc in the UK courts by former employees in South Africa. On 14 December 1998, the House of Lords agreed that the cases could be heard and possible compensation awarded in Britain. If successful, many more cases are likely to follow, not only from South Africa, but from the many countries that received the deadly ore.

For South Africa the outline of the last chapters of the asbestos story has been written by the Asbestos Summit. Researchers and clinicians will be in demand to ensure that the process is informed by sound decisions and realistic assessments of risk. Prevention of further exposure must be the over-riding priority.

References

1. Felix, M.A., Leger, J.P., Ehrlich, R.I. Three minerals, three epidemics – asbestos mining and disease in South Africa. In: *The Identification and Control of Environmental Diseases*, Princeton, NJ: Princeton Scientific, 1994.
2. Harington, J.S., McGlashan, N.D. South African asbestos: production, exports and destinations, 1959–1993. *Am J Ind Med* 1998; **33**: 321–326
3. Becklake, M.R. Control of asbestos-related disease in the RSA [opinion]. *S Afr Med J* 1987; **71**: 208–210.
4. Marchand, P.E. The discovery of mesothelioma in the North-Western Cape Province in the Republic of South Africa. *Am J Ind Med* 1991; **19**: 241–246.
5. Wagner, J.C. The discovery of the association between blue asbestos and mesothelioma and the aftermath. *Br J Ind Med* 1991; **48**: 399–403.
6. Flynn, L. South Africa blacks out blue asbestos risk. *New Scientist* 1982; **22**: 237–239.
7. South African Council for Scientific and Industrial Research. Pneumoconiosis Research Unit (1964). *Field Survey in the North Western Cape and at Penge in the Transvaal (Asbestosis and Mesothelioma)*. Report No. 1164, PRU Johannesburg SAIMR.
8. Sluis-Cremer, G.K. Asbestosis in South Africa – certain geographical and environmental considerations. *Ann N Y Acad Sci* 1965; **132**: 215–234.
9. Webster, I. Asbestosis and malignancy. *S Afr Med J* 1973; **47**: 165–171.
10. Zwi, A.B., Reid, G., London, S.P., Kieklkowski, D., Sitas, F., Becklake, M.R. Mesothelioma in South Africa – 1976–84: incidence and case characteristics. *Int J Epidemiol* 1989; **18**: 320–329.
11. Cochrane, J.C., Webster, I. Mesothelioma in relation to asbestos fibre exposure. *S Afr Med J* 1978; **54**: 279–281.
12. Solomons, K. Malignant mesothelioma – clinical and epidemiological features – a report of 80 cases. *S Afr Med J* 1984; **866**: 407–412.
13. Rees, D., Goodman, K., Fourie, E., Chapman, R., Blignaut, C., Bachman, M., Myers, J. Asbestos exposure and mesothelioma in South Africa. *S Afr Med J* 1999; **89**: 627–34.
14. Cancer in South Africa. *Annual Reports of the National Cancer Registry (NCR) of South Africa.* SAIMR, Johannesburg, 1986–92.
15. Trapido, A.S., Mqoqi, N.P., Williams, B.G., White, N.W., Solomon, A., Goode, R.H., Macheke, C.M., Davies, A.J., Panter, C. Prevalence of occupational lung disease in a random sample of former mineworkers, Libode District, Eastern Cape Province, South Africa. *Am J Ind Med* 1998; **34**: 305 – 313.
16. Armstrong, B.K., Musk, A.W., Baker, J.E. Epidemiology of mesothelioma in Western Australia. *Med J Aust* 1984; **141**: 86–88.
17. Sluis Cremer, G.K., Liddell, F.D.K., Logan, W.P.D., Bezuidenhout, B.N. The mortality of amphibole miners in South Africa 1946–80. *Br J Ind Med* 1992; **49**: 566–575.
18. Stayner, L.T., Dankovic, D.A., Lemen, R.A. Occupational exposure to chrysotile asbestos and lung cancer risk: a review of the amphibole hypothesis. *Am J Public Health* 1996; **86**: 179–186.
19. Cullen, M.R., Baloyi, R.S. Chrysotile asbestos and health in Zimbabwe. I. Analysis of miners and millers compensated for asbestos-related diseases since independence (1980). *Am J Ind Med* 1991; **29**: 161 – 169.
20. McDermott, M., Bevan, M.N., Elmes, P.C., Allardice, J.T., Bradley, A.C. Lung function and radiographic change in chrysotile mines in Zimbabwe. *Br J Ind Med* 1982; **39**: 338–343.
21. Slade, G.F. *The Incidence of Respiratory Disability in Workers Employed in Asbestos Mining.* (1931) MD Thesis. University of the Witwatersrand, Johannesburg.

22. Kisting, S.K. Respiratory health surveillance program on asbestos mines in South Africa – findings of medical audits over a five year period. (1997) Abstract. ICOH / ISEOH: 12th International Symposium: *Epidemiology in Occupational Health*. Harare, Zimbabwe.
23. Davies, J.C.A. Mesothelioma is a fibre-specific tumour [opinion]. *S Afr Med J* 1988; **73**: 327–328.
24. Baloyi, R. *Exposure to Asbestos among Chrysotile Miners, Millers and Mine Residents and Asbestosis in Zimbabwe*. Helsinki, Finland: University of Kuopio (1989). Dissertation.
25. Myers, J.E., Aron, J., Macun, I.A. Asbestos and asbestos-related disease: the South African case. *Int J Health Serv* 1987; **17**: 651–666.
26. Rees, D., Keilkowski, D., Lowe, R., Nokwe, N., Lobidu, K. A report on occupational health indicators for South Africa. NCOH Report No. 1/99. NationalCentre for Occupational Health. Johannesburg.
27. Ferguson, D.A., Berry, A., Jelihovsky, T., Andreas, S.B., Rogers, A,J., Fung, S.C., Grimwood, A., Thompson, R. The Australian mesothelioma surveillance program, 1979–1985. *Med J Aust* 1985; **147**: 166–172.
28. Webster, I. Discussion: In: Glen W.H., ed. *Proceedings of Asbestosis Symposium*, National Institute for Metallurgy. Johannesburg, South Africa: National Institute for Metallurgy; 1979, p 79.
29. Talent, J.M., Harrison, W.O., Solomon, A., *et al*. A survey of black mineworkers of the Cape crocidolite mines. In: Wagner J.C., ed. *Biological Effects of Mineral Fibres*. Lyon: International Agency for Research on Cancer. Vol 2, 1980.
30. Benatar, S.R., Bateman, E.D. The asbestos hazard (Editorial). *S Afr Med J* 1982; **6**: 881–882.
31. Botha, J.L., Irwig, L.M., Strebel, P. Excess mortality from stomach cancer, lung cancer and asbestosis and/or mesothelioma in crocidolite mining districts in South Africa. *Am J Epidemiol* 1986; **123**: 30–40.
32. Reid, A., Keilkowski, D., Steyn, S.D., Botha, K. Mortality of an asbestos exposed birth cohort. *S Afr Med J* 1990; **78**: 584–586.
33. Department of Mineral and Energy. Mine Health and Safety Inspectorate. Proposed Regulations for Occupational Hygiene. DME, Pretoria, 3 April 2000.
34. Harrington, J.S. McGilashan, ND. The South African asbestos trade 1994 – 1999 [letter]. *Am J Ind Med* 2000; **37**: 229.
35. Felix, M.A. *Environmental Asbestos and Respiratory Disease in South Africa*. PhD thesis. Faculty of Medicine, University of Witwatersrand, Johannesburg, 1998.
36. Lerner, H.J., Schoenfeld, D.A., Martin, A., Falkson, G., Barden, E. Malignant mesothelioma. The Eastern co-operative Oncology Group Experience. *Cancer* 1983; **52**: 1981–5.

= 6 =

Clinical and Palliative Care Aspects of Malignant Mesothelioma

Y. C. (Gary) Lee, Richard I. Thompson, Andrew Dean and
Bruce W. S. Robinson

Malignant mesothelioma has a number of characteristics with respect to its diagnosis, natural history and management that separates it from other malignancies. Over the past half-century, its diagnosis has frequently been difficult to establish in individual cases. This is because the disease usually already involves the pleural or peritoneal cavity extensively when it presents and clinically mimics secondary cancer; because the diagnosis ultimately depends on cytological or histological appearances, which are difficult to differentiate from reactive pleural diseases on the one hand and secondary cancers (especially adenocarcinoma) on the other; because for many years the sheer existence of the tumour was denied by the world's most eminent pathologists; and because there are no unique tumour markers, in serum or effusion, to identify it and follow its course.

Often it is the clinical and radiological appearances as well as the behaviour of malignant mesothelioma that are as helpful for diagnosis as cytology or histopathology. In particular, malignant mesothelioma tends to extend locally within and around the cavity of its origin and patients uncommonly exhibit clinical features of metastatic malignancy.

The relationship of asbestos exposure to the development of malignant mesothelioma has been well established and accepted since the seminal report by Wagner et al. in 1960.[1] Minor degrees of exposure, such as washing of asbestos-contaminated work clothes by workers' wives, have increasingly been recognised as potential sources of significant exposure. Despite that, in 20% or more of the patients no history of definite exposure to asbestos can be identified. Unlike the instance of lung cancer, smoking does not increase the risk of mesothelioma in asbestos-exposed individuals.[2,3] Irradiation has been reported as an uncommon cause of mesothelioma.[4]

Patient profile

Malignant mesothelioma is 2–6 times more common in males as a result of patterns of workplace exposure in the past. Because of the exponential shape of the relationship between risk and time since asbestos exposure and the ages at which most patients have been exposed in the past, the incidence of mesothelioma increases with age, with two-thirds of the patients presenting between 50 and 70 years of age. It was previously estimated that up to 10% of asbestos workers may develop the disease with an average latency of more than 30 years.[2] However, this type of calculation is not particularly meaningful as the risk of disease is determined by the type of asbestos, duration and intensity of exposure, timing of exposure in a person's life and time since exposure. For example, individuals exposed to asbestos as children may have a risk which increases over their lifetime.

The pleura is the most common site of malignant mesothelioma with a slight predominance to the right pleural cavity (60% of cases). Peritoneal mesothelioma can account for up to 25% of all cases of malignant mesothelioma.[5,6]

Clinical presentation

Symptoms

Symptoms of malignant mesothelioma may be non-specific and of insidious onset resulting in delay in presentation and diagnosis. The average time between onset of symptoms and diagnosis is 2–3 months with 25% of the patients presenting more than 6 months after development of symptoms.[7] Symptoms and clinical signs can arise from constitutional complaints, unilateral pleural disease, local invasion or distant spread. The most frequent presenting symptoms are those related to the local effects of the tumour.

Constitutional symptoms

Weight loss (30%), cough (10%) and fatigue are not common in the early presentation.[8] Hypertrophic pulmonary osteoarthropathy and intermittent hypoglycaemia are unusual and far more common with the rare localised fibrous mesothelioma than with malignant mesothelioma. Constitutional symptoms resulting from the medications, especially narcotic analgesics, necessary for management of pain and dyspnoea can be major problems as the disease advances.

Serous effusions

Effusion is the most common presentation and will occur at some stage of the disease course in most (95%) patients, especially those with epithelioid tumour. Blood-staining of the effusion is very common. Dyspnoea (40–70%) and non-pleuritic chest pain (60%) are common.[9] Clinical signs of pleural effusion are often the only abnormal findings on physical examination of patients with pleural mesothelioma. Ascites, on the other hand, is the most common presentation of peritoneal mesothelioma. When an asbestos-exposed patient presents with a pleural effusion and chest wall pain in the absence of other clinical features, mesothelioma is always suspected.

Local invasion

Direct invasion of adjacent structures is characteristic of malignant mesothelioma. Symptoms can therefore occur as a result of superior vena cava obstruction, spinal cord compression, Horner's syndrome, oesophageal compression, chest wall masses and malignant pericardial disease. Metastasis along tracks of previous invasive procedures (e.g. thoraco-centesis) is a feature of malignant mesothelioma with reported incidences between 2 and 51% (mean 19%) of cases, although not all of them require intervention and they rarely break through the subcutaneous tissue.[10] Chest wall, rib or intercostal nerve involvement are common causes of pain. Pericardial invasion may lead to pericardial effusion, cardiac tamponade and/or arrhythmias, resulting in chest pain and dyspnoea. Invasion into the contralateral hemithorax or the peritoneal cavity can occur as the disease progresses, leading to worsening breathlessness.

Distant spread

Extrathoracic spread was found in 54–82% of cases on post-mortem examination, but is often clinically silent and rarely the cause of death.[9] Intra-abdominal involvement of liver, adrenals and kidneys can also occur. Of cases undergoing autopsy, 44% had hilar or mediastinal lymph node metastasis.[11] Intracranial metastases were seen in 3% of the cases and were more likely from sarcomatous mesothelioma. 'Miliary mesothelioma' has been described,[12] but is rare.

Peritoneal mesothelioma

Abdominal distension with ascites and, in advanced disease, palpable abdominal masses (due mainly to omental tumour deposits) and small-bowel obstruction are frequent. This can be a result of primary peritoneal mesothelioma or trans-diaphragmatic spread of tumour from pleural mesothelioma.

Localised fibrous mesothelioma

This is a rare form of disease accounting for less than 5% of all pleural tumours.[13] It is different from malignant mesothelioma in that symptoms and effusions are uncommon. There is no established relationship between this form of tumour and asbestos exposure. Hypertrophic pulmonary osteoarthropathy is relatively common[14] and intermittent hypoglycaemia has been reported (4–5%).[15] It is usually amendable to surgery with good long-term prognosis after resection.

Physical signs

The physical signs of malignant pleural mesothelioma are usually those of a pleural effusion or pleural mass (reduced chest expansion, stony dullness to percussion, reduced intensity or absence of breath sounds, etc.). Large effusions or tumour masses can cause mediastinal displacement. The tumour may erode through the chest wall and cause localised tenderness and/or palpable masses (Figure 6.1). When the tumour has spread within the pleural cavity it is common to see a 'fixed' hemithorax, with reduced chest expansion. Mesothelioma masses alone cause dullness to percussion and reduced breath sounds, but occasionally breath sounds are harsh, almost bronchial in the absence of effusions. Signs of compression or invasion of mediastinal struc-

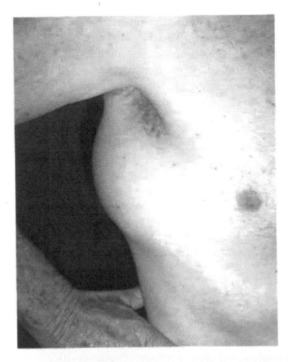

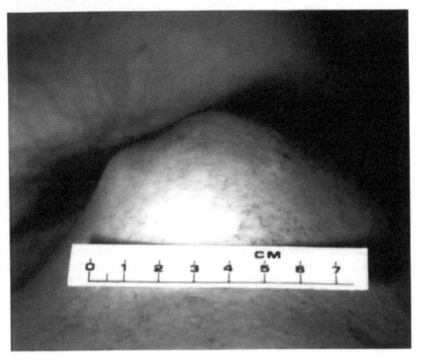

Figure 6.1. *Subcutaneous meso-thelioma lumps in the axillae of two patients. In both cases the tumour spread through the chest wall via a previous thoracentesis site.*

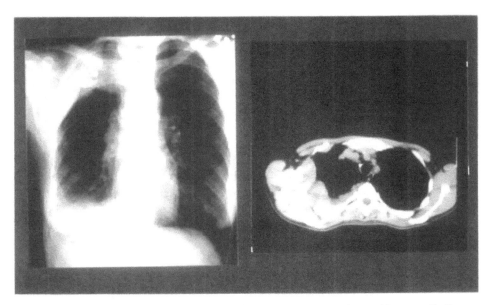

Figure 6.2. Radiological appearance of a patient presenting with mesothelioma. Shown are the chest x-ray (left) and thoracic CT scan (right), clearly demonstrating a large mass in the right upper zone with some pleural fluid on that side.

tures, particularly the superior vena cava or the phrenic or cervical nerves, may be present. Signs of extrathoracic involvement are uncommon on presentation, occurring in only 11% of patients in one large series.[16] Clubbing of the fingers is not a feature of malignant mesothelioma and when present may indicate co-existing pulmonary fibrosis from asbestosis.

Signs of ascites, abdominal tenderness or palpable abdominal masses are common with peritoneal mesothelioma.

Investigations

Occupational history

A detailed occupational and environmental/residential history is an important part of the investigation of suspected mesothelioma. Malignant mesothelioma should be considered in any patient with a history of asbestos exposure presenting with pleural effusion or ascites. A competent occupational history is also vital for the patient to pursue workers' compensation issues promptly following diagnosis.

Imaging (see also Chapter 10)

A chest x-ray commonly reveals a unilateral pleural effusion with or without evidence of pleural thickening. Occasionally patients have a large visible mass at presentation (Figure 6.2). Pleural thickening and encasement of the underlying lung may neutralise the mediastinal shift caused by the effusion or even result in contracture of the affected hemithorax. Other signs of asbestos exposure, particularly pleural plaques (especially pleural calcification) and asbestosis (20%), may be present.[17] Patients with pleural plaques are not at higher risk of developing mesothelioma if the influence of the degree of their exposure on risk can be accounted for as in the Wittenoom cohort of Western Australia.[18]

Computed tomography (CT) commonly shows nothing other than the pleural fluid, but may demonstrate lobulated or non-lobulated pleural thickening (92%), thickening of interlobular fissure (86%), effusion (74%), areas of pleural calcification (20%) or chest wall invasion (18%).[19] Changes of asbestosis (subpleural lines, parenchymal bands, reticular changes and honeycombing) and the occasional findings of pericardial or lymph node involvement are far better demonstrated by CT than by plain x-ray. CT is unable to differentiate between malignant mesothelioma and benign pleural changes (sensitivity 72%; specificity 83%),[20] nor can it aid in the differentiation between mesothelioma and metastatic adenocarcinoma. Therefore imaging cannot be regarded as a substitute for cytology or biopsy in establishing the diagnosis.

Magnetic resonance imaging (MRI) and positron emission tomography (PET) scanning can better define the extent of tumour extension and chest wall invasion, especially on coronal images, but are expensive and not readily available in many centres.

As the ultimate diagnosis of mesothelioma rests upon cytology or histology, the diagnosis is dependent, in most cases, on material obtained by thoracocentesis or pleural biopsy. CT and MRI are not routinely indicated in the diagnosis or management of pleural mesothelioma. In cases where repeated pleural aspiration ± biopsies failed to yield the diagnosis, CT scan may help to locate and guide fine needle aspiration of any pleural mass for diagnostic material. Although CT and MRI can aid in the staging process, they have no definite role in the practical management of the patient unless there is a specific clinical indication, e.g. localising direct spinal cord invasion to aid in radiotherapy planning. In our unit, they are only employed if the patient is enrolled in clinical trials of novel therapies where accurate measurement of the tumour size is important to judge therapeutic response. This can be done accurately (Nowak *et al.*, unpublished observations).

PET with 2-fluoro-2-deoxy-D-glucose (FDG) holds promise in aiding the detection of mesothelioma and its differentiation from benign pleural diseases and has been shown to be useful in the evaluation of malignant mesothelioma in a small series achieving a sensitivity of 91% and a specificity of 100% in a highly selected population.[21]

Blood tests

There is no specific haematological or biochemical test for the diagnosis of mesothelioma. Non-specific abnormalities including anaemia, thrombocytosis and hypergammaglobulinaemia occur often but are seldom of clinical significance. The erythrocyte sedimentation rate is often very high. Results of liver function tests are often mildly abnormal in the absence of liver metastases, and include hypoalbuminaemia.

Thoracocentesis and biopsy

A definitive diagnosis of mesothelioma can only be established with cytological or histological confirmation. The usefulness of thoracocentesis depends in part on the experience of the cytologist as it is often difficult to distinguish between reactive mesothelial cells and malignant ones with certainty on cytology. The yield of aspirate cytology of pleural or peritoneal effusions varies from 33% to 84%.[8,22]

Closed pleural biopsies at the time of pleural aspiration can improve the diagnostic yield of the procedure by 30–50%.[9] Accuracy of diagnosis depends on the morphologic appearance and results of tumour marker staining using light microscopy (see Chapter 8) and can be improved with the use of electron microscopy. In suitable cases where a pleural-based tumour can be identified on imaging, CT-guided percutaneous biopsy has a high success rate for establishing the diagnosis. Bronchoscopy, bronchoalveolar washings or lavage and gallium lung scanning have no useful role in the diagnosis of mesothelioma and are not routinely employed. The usual appearance at bronchoscopy is that of extrinsic compression of the central airways related to the amount of fluid or tumour bulk. Bronchial washings and bronchoalveolar lavage may show asbestos bodies and provide evidence of asbestos exposure.

Medical thoracoscopy is valuable in the diagnosis of mesothelioma. Performed under sedation with adequate analgesia, this procedure allows extensive inspection of the pleural cavity and multiple biopsies under direct vision. In experienced hands, the diagnosis can be established in up to 98% of cases by medical thoracoscopy with good patient tolerance and very few complications, as was shown in one prospective study of 188 mesothelioma patients.[23] The direct examination of the pleura can aid in staging, and the presence of tumour on the visceral surface is reported to carry prognostic implications.

If the diagnosis can be established (e.g., with cytologist on-site) at the time of the thoracoscopy, chemical pleurodesis can be performed during the same procedure. An intercostal chest tube is usually left in situ for 24 to 36 hours after the procedure and can be used to administer chemical pleurodesis if the diagnosis from the aspirate cytology becomes available during that time. Talc offers the best rate of successful pleurodesis amongst commonly used agents. It can cause pain and, occasionally, acute respiratory distress syndrome,[24] but these are easily controlled and rare, respectively. The use of cytokines, especially transforming growth factor beta, as a novel pleurodesis agent has shown promise as a possible alternative in the future.[25]

Medical thoracoscopy can only be performed if there is free pleural space and should be avoided if the pleural space has been obliterated by tumour or adhesions. Video-assisted thoracoscopy (VATS) under general anaesthesia is an alternative to medical thoracoscopy. In cases where there are dense adhesions precluding thoracoscopy, an open biopsy may be necessary. This procedure is more invasive and carries a higher morbidity, especially regarding implantation of tumours in the wound, and requires a longer hospital stay. It should only be performed if medical thoracoscopy is contraindicated or failed to produce a diagnosis.

Due to the high likelihood of needle track metastasis in mesothelioma patients, prophylactic radiotherapy to sites of instrumentation after any invasive procedure to the pleura has been advocated – 21 Gy over 3 days was shown to be adequate to prevent needle tract spread in 20 consecutive patients who received thoracoscopy in a randomised trial. In contrast, 8 out of 20 subjects in the control group who received no prophylactic radiotherapy developed at least one chest wall metastasis at the site of instrumentation.[10]

Differential diagnosis

Distinguishing between reactive mesothelial cells and malignant mesotheliomas is not always easy. Differentiation between mesothelioma and metastatic malignancies, especially adenocarcinoma, can also be difficult (See Chapter 8). Localised fibrous mesothelioma, pleural lipoma, liposarcoma and primary pleural thymoma are rare alternative causes of pleural tumours.

Clinical staging

Butchart's ongoing clinical staging protocol for malignant mesothelioma has recently been superseded by the International Mesothelioma Interest Group's revised staging of mesothelioma,[26] including the notion of an early stage with involvement of parietal

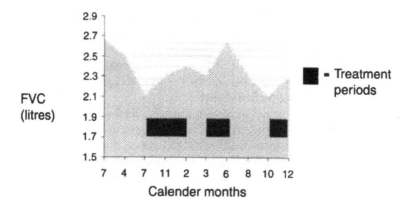

Figure 6.3. Monitoring vital capacity (VC) or forced VC is one way of monitoring response to therapy, provided the values are not complicated by pleural effusion or the presence of other active pulmonary disease. Shown are the FVC measurements (litres) over time (expressed as calendar months) in a patient whose condition responded to several cycles of gemicitabine plus cisplatin chemotherapy with reduction in tumour size and contemporaneous increase in FVC.

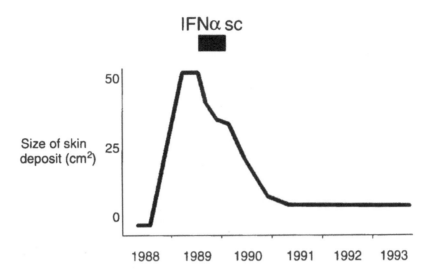

Figure 6.4. *Monitoring the size of subcutaneous lumps is one way of monitoring response to therapy. Shown is the area of such a lump measured over time in a patient who showed a prolonged response to a short period of therapy with subcutaneous recombinant human interferon alpha 2a.*

but not visceral pleura associated with a better prognosis.[27] Staging is not always easy to carry out and necessitates additional investigations which do not relate to determining treatment. Hence, staging is not routinely carried out in day-to-day practice. It may be useful in the future when more promising treatments become available.

The concept of 'mesothelioma in situ' has been reported[28] but is not yet widely accepted. It is likely that early detection techniques will require the use of molecular probes.

Prognostic factors

The average survival of mesothelioma patients in Western Australia is in the order of nine months. Age, performance status, sarcomatoid histology, weight loss and duration of symptoms before diagnosis are recognised prognostic factors.[2,29] The clinical staging (using the Butchart classification) is correlated with survival, and visceral pleural involvement by mesothelioma during thoracosopy carries a poorer prognosis than for patients with disease limited to the parietal pleura.[27] Histologically, epithelioid mesothelioma predicts better survival than the sarcomatous tumours.

Monitoring of disease progress

Clinical progress

Clinical assessment of advancing malignancy or possible response to any form of intervention may be made simply by measures of body weight, spirometry (FEV1, FVC)

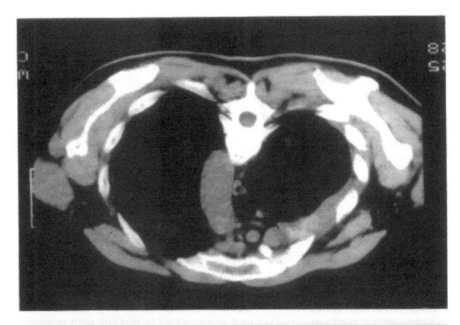

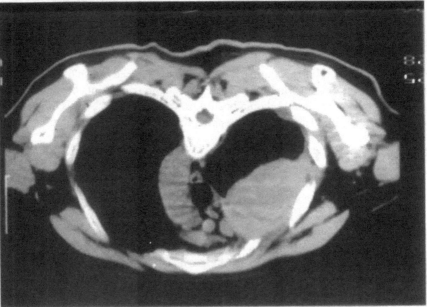

Figure 6.5. Monitoring mesothelioma responses using serial thoracic CT scans. Shown are two scans of the same patient taken before (top) and three months after (bottom) therapy with recombinant interferon alpha 2a. A partial response (greater than 50% reduction in tumour area) is obvious.

(Figure 6.3). Skin lump size can be a good gauge to treatment response (Figure 6.4). Quality of life assessment may be made using existing validated tools. Radiology, especially CT and MRI, may be useful depending on the research question being asked (e.g., response to chemotherapy in clinical trials).

Radiological progression

Monitoring of the clinical course of mesothelioma can be achieved with imaging. Routine chest x-rays are useful in the monitoring of the overall bulk of disease, but the distinction between pleural fluid and solid tissue is not always possible. The plain x-ray may also be helpful in the assessment of superimposed conditions such as cardiac failure or pulmonary consolidation.

Although CT scanning can provide good overall assessment of the extent of disease process,[30] it does not necessarily contribute to diagnosis or clinical management in most cases and should only be employed if there is a specific indication. It can accurately assess the overall thickness of the pleural disease as well as the dimensions of more specific nodules. This rarely influences medical management but is most useful in clinical trials to assess treatment response (Figure 6.5). Consistency of technique over a series of scans is necessary if accurate assessment of nodular progression or resolution is required. Scans should be performed according to an established protocol, so that continuity is achieved between one examination and the next. Helical and non-helical techniques can be used. Follow-up scans can be performed without intravenous contrast, assuming a baseline scan is obtained. If there is disease closely adherent to the mediastinum, it may be necessary to perform contrast enhanced scans, particularly if there is clinical evidence of superior vena cava obstruction. In cases of local spread of tumour that require intervention, e.g., spinal cord invasion or superior vena cava obstruction, CT scanning may be useful, especially in the planning for palliative radiotherapy. Area determination software is available on newer CT scanners, allowing tumour volume and 3-D reconstructions to be undertaken

Techniques have been developed for serial measurement of mesothelioma volume on CT scans that have been performed on machines without area-determination software. This involves tracing the tumour outline onto transparent sheets and then digitally determining its volume using dedicated software (Nowak *et al.*, unpublished observations).

Pleural fluid is usually clearly detectable using CT scanning. However, when there is increased density within the pleural fluid (e.g., following repeated pleural aspiration with associated haemorrhage), it can be difficult to distinguish the fluid from solid components. In those cases, ultrasound can provide better information. Reports have indicated that CT scanning, whilst it can detect gross chest wall invasion, is less sensitive than MRI. The ability of MRI to provide superior soft tissue contrast and multiplanar scanning facilitates the early detection of chest wall invasion.[31]

Ultrasound also has a role in the follow-up management of mesothelioma. Pleural effusions resulting from mesothelioma rapidly become multi-loculated as a result of the disease process. Thickened septations, sometimes nodular, can be readily seen with ultrasound. Repeated pleural aspirations, with presumably some haemorrhage, may also contribute to multi-loculation of effusions. Such effusions are then difficult to aspirate and ultrasound may be helpful in guiding pleural biopsy or aspiration of the largest loculations for relief of breathlessness. Almost invariably, ultrasound will demonstrate the characteristics of pleural effusion more accurately than CT. An example of mesothelioma progression monitored by CT series scanning is included (Figure 6.5).

Palliative and supportive care

From a practical perspective, patients with malignant mesothelioma develop a number of prominent symptoms, the management of which can be difficult even for those with experience in palliative care.

The anatomical site of disease can cause a variety of different pain types, e.g., lung invasion causing diffuse visceral pain, chest wall invasion causing well localised somatic pain and intercostal nerve invasion or vertebral invasion giving neuropathic pain. Dyspnoea is also exceptionally common and usually progressive in tandem with the disease process. Breathlessness associated with pleural effusion may be relieved by aspiration. Talc pleurodesis may delay the recurrence of breathlessness if the effusion reaccumulates rapidly and requires repeated aspiration.[32] Ultimately the enlarging pleural tumour results in reduced ventilatory capacity and leads to more breathlessness. There is no need for patients with malignant mesothelioma to put up with distressing symptoms. If visceral pain is the problem, titrated doses of opioids with regular laxative prescription together with anti-emetics if necessary should control the problem. The same is also true of the symptom of dyspnoea.

There is no ceiling dose of opioid for symptom relief. The dose reached should give adequate analgesia for the duration of action of the drug (e.g., 4 hours for liquid morphine, 12 hours for controlled/slow release morphine) without causing unnecessary side effects. If people are unable to tolerate a specific opioid, substitution with a different opioid such as methadone or fentanyl should be considered.

Somatic pain will often respond to the addition of paracetamol together with a non-steroidal anti-inflammatory medication, such as naprosyn. We find that neuropathic pain responds best to opioid together with an anticonvulsant such as carbamezapine or sodium valporate. If pain relief is achieved effectively and early in the disease, few patients ultimately require procedural pain relief such as intrathecal analgesia or regional nerve blockade. Early effective pain management helps prevent the wind-up phenomenon with its consequent escalation in opioid dosage.

As most currently available treatment for mesothelioma is essentially palliative and standard treatment must still be 'best supportive care', patients must be made aware of the ultimately terminal nature of their disease at the time of diagnosis. This can lead to a number of existential issues. Many patients still fear poor symptom control and misunderstand the use of analgesics. Patient education is therefore paramount and all patients should know that the ideal treatment is to maintain symptom relief with minimal unpleasant side effects. As debility progresses and other problems arise we strongly recommend the use of multidisciplinary teams to address all the issues. No one person is able to provide all aspects of palliative care and the use of a team will ensure optimal medical, nursing, spiritual, social and psychological management together with provision of the necessary physical aids.

Screening studies in at-risk individuals

There is little clinical role for screening of asbestos-exposed subjects for 'early mesothelioma' even though 'mesothelioma in situ' has been described.[28] This is because:

(i) There is no simple or effective screening procedure available. The pleural cavity is inaccessible for exfoliative cytology and routine thoracoscopy cannot be justified. Asbestos-related benign pleural disease is known to be a separate and frequent response of the pleural cavity to exposure and the recognition of either circumscribed plaques or diffuse pleural fibrosis would not be helpful in predicting mesothelioma. Pleural effusion in an asbestos-exposed individual should always be investigated with aspiration and pleural biopsy but when malignancy is identified the disease is almost always extensive.

(ii) There is no effective treatment of the disease. Screening cannot be justified, however easy or difficult it might be, until effective therapies for early disease become available.

The recent description of anti-mesothelioma antibodies in the serum of patients at presentation raises the possibility that, if these mesothelioma antigens can be identified, early antibody responses would be able to be detected.[33]

Psychosocial aspects

The psychosocial consequences of malignant mesothelioma are very important considerations in the management of patients and their families. Several features of mesothelioma set it aside from other incurable malignancies: (i) its known aetiology and long latency period that often create prolonged anxiety in 'at-risk' individuals; (ii) its tendency to occur within groups of workers who know each other as a result of previous employment; (iii) its reputation of being a particularly unpleasant terminal illness associated with significant suffering from pain, breathlessness and cachexia; and (iv) the issue of compensation and its legal consequences.

If patients are still working at the time of diagnosis, the timing of retirement requires careful consideration. Many decide to retire at the time of diagnosis irrespective of their symptoms, based on the fact that the median survival is about 9 months. However, we have managed cases with prolonged survivals of up to 10 years. Patients (and their family) may fare better emotionally and financially if they remain employed until symptoms prevent adequate performance at work.

After diagnosis, issues of compensation and litigation frequently arise. These may be complex because of local workers' compensation provisions and difficulties in assigning legal responsibility in cases where there may have been multiple employers during periods of exposure, often many decades ago. In some workforces, friendships and associations continue long afterwards and provide important sources of information and support for mesothelioma patients and their families. However, these groups can also have undesirable effects as those recently diagnosed often know of others whose experience with the disease has been especially unpleasant. The reputation of mesothelioma may induce profound fear and apprehension in patients, making the usually difficult task of symptom control even more so for the attending physician. Local cancer support groups or pneumoconiosis societies can be valuable in providing psychosocial support and assistance on legal matters.

The terminal care of a patient with mesothelioma should be carried out jointly by the physician who has been responsible for care of the patient throughout his illness, the family practitioner and an experienced palliative care team. It is important that advice on prognosis is consistent and management plans are carried out in a coordinated fashion, thus maintaining trust and confidence between the patient, family and physicians.

Conclusion

The worldwide incidence of malignant mesothelioma is currently calculated to be approaching its peak. However, as a result of ongoing exposure to amphiboles, it can be expected that there will be an ongoing need to care for patients well into the century. Until the biology of cancer is better understood (which may result in a generic anti-cancer treatment evolving) and unless a significant improvement in existing empirical anti-cancer modalities takes place, all forms of anti-cancer treatment for malignant mesothelioma should be part of clinical trials. There remains a need for better palliative measures for this unpleasant malignancy.

There is now a lot more research into mesothelioma than was previously the case, no doubt stimulated in part by the increasing numbers of cases presenting and the lack of effective therapies. It is to be hoped this will translate into early diagnosis and better treatment regimens in years to come.

References

1. Wagner, J.C., Sleggs, C.A., Marchand, P. Diffuse pleural mesothelioma and asbestos exposure in the North Western Cape Province. *Br J Ind Med* 1960; **17**: 260–271.
2. Pisani, R.J., Colby, T.V., Williams, D.E. Malignant mesothelioma of the pleura. *Mayo Clin Proc* 1988; **63**: 1234–1244.
3. De Klerk, N.H., Musk, A.W., Eccles, J.L., Hobbs, M.S.T. Contribution of asbestos, alcohol and smoking to deaths in subjects occupationally exposed to crocidolite at Wittenoom Gorge. In: Hurych, J., Lesage, M., David, A. eds. Proceedings of the 8th International Conference on Occupational Lung Diseases; 1992: Prague, Czech Republic: Czech Medical Society, 1993: 329–333.
4. Stock, R.J., Fu, Y.S., Carter, J.R. Malignant peritoneal mesothelioma following radiotherapy for seminoma of the testis. *Cancer* 1979; **44**: 914–919.
5. Antman, K.H. Current concepts: malignant mesothelioma. *N Engl J Med* 1980; **303**: 200–202.
6. De Klerk, N.H., Armstrong, B.K. The Epidemiology of asbestos and mesothelioma. In: Henderson, D.W., Shilkin, K.B., Langlois, S.L., Whitaker, D., eds. *Malignant Mesothelioma.* New York: Hemisphere Publishing Corporation, 1992: 223–250.

7. Chahinian, A.P., Pajak, T.F., Holland, J.F., Norton, L., Ambinder, R.M., Mandel, E.M. Diffuse malignant mesothelioma: prospective evaluation of 69 patients. *Ann Intern Med* 1982; **96**: 746–755.
8. Rusch, V.W. Diagnosis and treatment of pleural mesothelioma. *Semin Surg Oncol* 1990; **6**: 279–284.
9. Pass, H.I., Pogrebniak, H.W. Malignant pleural mesothelioma. *Curr Prob Surg* 1993; **30**: 921–1012
10. Boutin, C., Rey, F., Viallat, J.R. Prevention of malignant seeding after invasive diagnostic procedures in patients with pleural mesothelioma. *Chest* 1995; **108**: 754–758.
11. Kim, S.B., Varkey, B., Choi, H. Diagnosis of malignant pleural mesothelioma by axillary lymph node biopsy. *Chest* 1987; **91**: 279–282.
12. Musk, A.W., Dewar, J., Shilkin, K.B., Whitaker, D. Miliary spread of malignant pleural mesothelioma without a clinically identifiable pleural tumour. *Aust N Z J Med* 1991; **21**: 460–462.
13. Theros, E.G., Feigin, D.S. Pleural tumours and pulmonary tumours: differential diagnosis. *Semin Roentgenol* 1977; **12**: 239–247.
14. Fraser, R.G., Pare, J.A.P., Pare, R.D., Fraser, R.S., Genereux, G.P. *Diagnosis of Diseases of the Chest*. 3rd ed. Philadelphia: Saunders, 1991; 2712–2793.
15. Briselli, M., Mark, E.J., Dickersin, G.R. Solitary fibrous tumours of the pleura: eight new cases and review of 360 cases in the literature. *Cancer* 1981; **47**: 2678–2689.
16. Chailleux, E., Dabouir, G., Pioche, D. Prognostic factors in diffuse malignant mesothelioma. *Chest* 1988; **93**: 159–162.
17. Antman, K.H. Natural history and epidemiology of malignant mesothelioma. *Chest* 1993; **103**(4): 373S–376S.
18. De Klerk, N.H., Musk, A.W., Eccles, J.L., Glancy, J.J., Pang, S.C., Hobbs, M.S.T. Non-malignant pleuro-pulmonary disease and the development of malignant mesothelioma in Western Australia crocidolite workers. Proceedings of International Symposium in Epidemiology in Occupational Health; Sept. 23–25 1992: Cincinnati, Ohio: International Commission of Occupational Health, 1992; 161–166.
19. Muller, N.L. Imaging of the pleura. *Radiology* 1993; **186**: 297–309.
20. Leung, A.N., Muller, N.L., Miller, R.R. CT in differential diagnosis of diffuse pleural disease. *AJR Am J Roentgenol* 1990; **154**: 487–492.
21. Benard, F., Sterman, D., Smith, R.J., Kaiser, L.R., Albelda, S.M., Alavi, A. Metabolic imaging of malignant pleural mesothelioma with fluorodeoxyglucose positron emission tomography. *Chest* 1998; **114**(3): 713–722.
22. Whitaker, D., Sterrett, G., Shilkin, K. Early diagnosis of malignant mesothelioma: the contribution of effusion and fine needle aspiration cytology and ancillary techniques. In: Peters, G.A., Peters, B.J., eds. *Asbestos Disease Update, March 1989*. New York: Garland Law Publishing, 1989: 73–112.
23. Boutin, C., Rey, F. Thoracoscopy in pleural malignant mesothelioma: a prospective study of 188 consecutive patients. Part 1: Diagnosis. *Cancer* 1993; **72**: 389–393.
24. Milanez Campos, J.R., Werebe, E.C., Vargas, F.S., Jatene, F.B., Light, R.W. Respiratory failure due to insufflated talc. *Lancet* 1997; **349**: 251–252.
25. Lane, K., Cheng, D., Rogers, J., Blackwell, T., Davidson, J., Light, R.W. An innovative method by which pleurodesis can be produced in rabbits. *Chest* 1998; **114**(4): 364S.
26. Rusch, V.W. A proposed new international TNM staging system for malignant mesothelioma. From the International Mesothelioma Interest Group. *Chest* 1995; **108**(4): 1122–1128.

27. Boutin, C., Rey, F., Gouvernet, J., Viallat, J.R., Astoul, P.H., Ledoray, V. Thoracoscopy in pleural malignant mesothelioma: a prospective study of 188 consecutive patients. Part 2: Prognosis and staging. *Cancer* 1993; **72**: 394–404.
28. Whitaker, D., Henderson, D.W., Shilkin, K.B. The concept of mesothelioma in situ: implications for diagnosis and histogenesis. *Semin Diagn Pathol* 1992; **9**: 151–161.
29. Musk, A.W., Woodward, S.D. Conventional treatment and its effect on survival of malignant pleural mesothelioma in Western Australia. *Aust N Z J Med* 1982; **12**: 229–232.
30. Miller, B.H., Rosado-de-Christenson, M.L., Mason, A.C., Fleming, M.V., White, C.C., Krasna, M.J. Malignant pleural mesothelioma: radiologic-pathologic correlation. *Radiographics* 1996; **16**: 613–644.
31. Piwnica-Worms, D.R., Jochelson, M., Sarin, M., Sugarbaker, D.J., Pugatch, R.D. Malignant pleural mesothelioma: value of CT and MR imaging in predicting resectability. *AJR Am J Roentgenol* 1992; **159**: 961–966.
32. Kennedy, L., Sahn, S.A. Talc pleurodesis for the treatment of pneumothorax and pleural effusion. *Chest* 1994; **106**(4): 1215–1222.
33. Robinson, C., Callow, M., Lake, R.A. *et al*. Serologic responses in patients with malignant mesothelioma: evidence for both public and private specificities. *Am J Respir Cell Mol Biol* 2000; **22**: 550–556.

=7=

Pleuroscopy in the Management of Malignant Pleural Mesothelioma

Philippe Astoul and Christian Boutin

Pleural mesothelioma is more frequent than peritoneal mesothelioma, possibly because inhalation is the usual route of entry of the pathogenic fibres[1,2] and the incidence has risen in recent years[3] and is expected to peak sometime between 1990 and 2010.[4]

This disease is refractory to the standard therapeutic options since chemotherapy is only partially effective, radiation therapy simply provides palliation against pain, and surgery, even when performed at a relatively early stage, is controversial.[3-5] Perhaps because of this poor prognosis, early screening has not elicited great interest. However, this pessimism belies the fact that certain forms have a better prognosis when diagnosed early.[2,5-7] To better ascertain prognostic factors, multifactorial studies using the Cox model have been performed.[1,3,4,8-12] The most favorable factors are age less than 50 years, epithelial histopathological type, good general condition, and stage I disease (Table 7.1).

Pleuroscopy is an essential procedure for the management of malignant pleural mesothelioma (MPM) for several reasons:

- It provides insight into the pathogenesis of this disease in showing carcinogenetic asbestos fibres accumulating in black anthracotic zones of the parietal pleura.[13] Further study suggests that these zones could be the equivalent of the milky spots that have been observed in animals.[14]
- It allows clinical approach in the following aspects: i) *diagnosis* – the sensitivity and specificity of thoracoscopy is higher than any other method.[5,8,9,15,16] In addition, thoracoscopic biopsy is considerably more cost-effective than surgical biopsy. ii) *prognosis* – thoracoscopy allows division of stage I Butchart mesothelioma into two subgroups, Ia, which is an early stage with only parietal pleura involvement, and Ib, which is characterised by the invasion of visceral pleura. iii) *therapy* – in patients with early-stage disease pleuroscopy allows placement of an implantable port for local immunotherapy, which is a reasonable therapeutic approach.[17,18]

Symptoms and signs

The mean age at diagnosis of mesothelioma is 60 years. However, onset as early as the fourth decade can be observed in subjects with exposure to asbestos as children. The

Table 7.1. Multifactorial analysis of prognostic factors for mesothelioma: literature data.

Authors	Chahinian[1]	Alberts[11]	Antman[2]	Calavrezos[37]	Spirtas[36]	Ruffie[58]	Rusch[7]	Boutin[8]
Year	1982	1988	1988	1988	1988	1989	1991	1990
N° of patients	57	262	136	93	1197	170	83	188
Overall MS (months)	13	9.6	15	7	7	9	10	12
Classified favorable prognostic factors*	Epithelial type	PS	PS	PS	Age<50	Stage I	None	Epithelial type / Stage IA
	Age < 65	Medical treatment	Epithelial type	Epithelial type	Stage I	Platelets <400000		
	PS	White race	Absence of chest pain	Age*50	Treatment	No weight loss		No weight loss
	Surgery	S. Dg > 6 months	S. Dg > 6 months	No chest pain	Geographic origin			
	Response To CT	Stage I	Surgery	Stage I + II multimodal	Treatment			

*Favourable prognostic factors are listed in each column according to their statistical significance in each study.
MS : median survival.
S. Dg : interval between first symptom to diagnosis.
CT : chemotherapy.
PS : performance status.

incidence of mesothelioma is much higher in males. This is probably because occupational exposure to asbestos is less common in females.

Asbestos exposure has been reported in 20% to 90% of cases (mean 70%). This wide variation is due to differences in the occupational or environmental criteria used in various studies and to the importance of industrial use of asbestos in the regions where these studies were conducted. Previous radiotherapy has sometimes been noted.[19]

Functional or general manifestations are non-specific at the onset of the disease. Of 65 stage I patients in our department, the initial symptoms were cough and shortness of breath related to pleurisy. As shown in Table 7.2, pain and other changes such as weight loss were observed significantly less frequently in stage IA than IB. Interestingly, 5 symptomless stage IA patients were diagnosed incidentally. Pleural effusion is not especially large or painful at the beginning and in many cases x-ray fails to detect any mass. In non-pleural tumoural forms, localised pain, which is often moderate, is the most frequent first sign. Since mesothelioma has no characteristic clinical manifestations, this diagnosis should always be considered in any patient with pleural symptoms, especially in towns, harbours and geographic areas where the asbestos industry formerly developed. Systematic screening allowed detection of 3% of the patients in Ruffie's series.[10]

CT-scan images are variable. When pleural fluid is present at onset, the specificity of CT scan is limited. CT scanning is more precise if the fluid is removed, but it is most useful for follow-up. In our series, 20% of patients had lesions visible on CT scan, whereas 40% had fibrohyaline or calcified pleural plaques seen at thoracoscopy. Thoracoscopy allows excellent visualisation and diagnosis of these plaques. A decrease in the diameter of the affected hemithorax is frequent with mesothelioma, but this finding is also associated with infectious pleurisy. Mediastinal changes are more specific: uneven, nodular thickening of the mediastinal pleura, pericardium, hilus, and its lymph nodes. As will be discussed further on, mediastinal status is an important factor in staging the disease. Mediastinal changes develop at an advanced stage of mesothelioma and are a highly unfavourable prognostic feature.

Thoracoscopy technique

The rigid thoracoscopic system and cold light source that we use is manufactured by the Wolf Company (Knittlingen, Germany). Except for a few minor improvements in design and optics, this instrumentation is the same as previously described.[5,8,9] We use

Table 7.2. *Symptoms at the time of diagnosis.*

	Stage		
	IA (26 patients)	IB (39 patients)	
Cough/dyspnoea	10 (38.5%)	17 (43.6%)	NS
Pain	7 (27%)	21 (53.8%)	p<0.05
Altered general condition	4 (15.4%)	1 (2.6%)	
Weight loss	4 (15.4%)	25 (55.6%)	p<0.002
Routine x-ray examinaton/PNO	5 (1932%)	0	

direct (0°) and lateral (50°) viewing Panoview telescopes 35 cm in length and 7 mm in diameter and optical forceps for biopsy of the parietal and visceral pleura. Used in conjunction with modern video technology, this system provides excellent resolution and allows detailed inspection of the pleural cavity.

This procedure can be performed under local or general anaesthesia depending on the facilities. No tracheal intubation is required. During the procedure, 10 to 20 large biopsy samples from various sites in the diaphragm, parietal pleura, costovertebral gutter, posterior costophrenic angle and any suspicious zones of the visceral pleura are taken. At the end of the examination, a chest tube is inserted, which, in cases of parietal pleural biopsies, can be removed early, i.e. as soon as clinical examination shows that the lung is fully re-expanded.

Tolerance to thoracoscopy is good. Chest tube placement after diagnostic thoracoscopy lasted from a few minutes to a few hours. By contrast, the average duration of drainage in the 31 patients who had a talc poudrage at the end of thoracoscopy is 5 ± 0.5 days. [5]

The following complications were observed: extensive subcutaneous emphysema in 1 patient, localised pleural infection in 4 patients, haemorrhage less than 100 ml after injury of an intercostal vessel during biopsy in 3 patients, and fever ranging from 38° to 38.5°C for 24 to 48 hours in 26 cases. Fever was treated with paracetamol. Thoracoscopy appears to be a safe procedure with very few complications, only minor risks and no mortality.

Since 1986, when we started performing diagnostic thoracoscopy as an outpatient procedure, discharge of patients has never been delayed because of thoracoscopy-related complications. Seven patients died within 1 month of thoracoscopy, but the procedure was never the cause of death.

One potential complication that can arise at any time if the thoracic wall is trangressed, regardless of the device used, i.e. a scalpel, a trocar, a biopsy needle, or even a simple thoracentesis catheter, is the development of subcutaneous tumour masses in the wound. Such nodules ultimately develop in up to 80% of mesothelioma patients after pleural biopsy or thoracotomy and are usually quite painful. Elmes and Simpson[20] observed 34 cases in which tumour extended into the chest wall in a total of 237 patients with mesothelioma (4 after thoracentesis, 9 after needle biopsy, and 21 after thoracotomy). Although Law et al.[21] reported that these lesions were not particularly painful in their patients, we have developed a preventive technique for this frequent and often unpleasant complication.

Between 1973 and 1979, we observed seeding of the thoracic wall along the pathway of the trocar or drain in 12 patients in our series. Since 1979, to avoid this complication, we have been performing preventive radiation therapy at all points of entry. As

Table 7.3. Sensitivity of diagnostic methods for diffuse malignant mesothelioma.

Method	Number/total	Per cent
Fluid cytology	49/175	28%
Abrams needle biopsy	33/135	24%
Thoracoscopy	185/188	98%
Surgery	9/9	100%

previously described,[22] we wait 10 to 12 days to allow the incisions to heal and then perform radiotherapy of 12.5 to 15 MeV on the chest wall, applying 21 Gy over a 48-hour period in 3 sessions. The average penetration is 3 cm and the sides of the field are 4 to 12 cm at the site of the drain and puncture.

We assessed this preventive treatment in a series of 40 patients with mesothelioma who were randomly distributed into two equal groups. One group underwent radiotherapy after thoracoscopy and the other did not. None of the 20 treated patients developed nodules along the pathway of the drain or trocar. In contrast, 9 of the 20 untreated patients developed such nodules. In view of these results, we have been performing preventive radiotherapy systematically after diagnostic thoracoscopy in mesothelioma patients since 1982 and have not observed this complication since then.

Value of diagnostic thoracoscopy

Indications

The reported sensitivity of pleural fluid cytology ranges from 0% to 64%. Likewise, the sensitivity of needle biopsy varies from 6% to 38%. Herbert and Gallapher[23] claimed that the value of both these methods was limited and advocated surgical biopsy. With thoracoscopy the results achieved are similar in comparison to the surgery and better than fluid cytology or Abrams biopsy (Table 7.3). Cope or Abrams needle biopsy under CT-scan control is of limited sensitivity since sample volume is usually too small for histology and negative findings do not rule out mesothelioma.

Thoracoscopy is indicated in practically all cases of suspected mesothelioma. In a series of 188 patients,[24] the indications were chronic pleurisy in 88% of cases, empyema in 2%, chronic spontaneous pneumothorax in 1%, and radiographically documented pleural nodules without effusion in 9%. Of these patients, 80% recalled previous exposure to asbestos.

Thoracoscopic biopsy was positive in every case in which it was feasible. Thus sensitivity was 100% in 185 patients. Thoracoscopy was unfeasible in 9 cases and 'extended thoracoscopy'[25] was required in 5 patients with an achieved diagnosis (Table 7.4).

Thoracoscopic findings

In 137 of the previous 188 patients, the pleural cavity was completely free or displayed only loose or fibrinous adhesions that did not impede thoracoscopic examination. In the other 51 patients, the procedure was hindered by adhesions, and electrocoagulation was required for severe adhesions and to obtain a cavity of at least 10 cm³. Although complete examination was not possible in these cases, biopsy samples were almost always obtained from malignant lesions on the parietal and, if necessary, visceral pleura.

The following lesions were observed in the parietal pleura or diaphragm.

· Nodules or masses ranging from 5 mm to 10 cm in 92 patients (49%). In 25 - patients (13%), a grape-like aspect[9] characteristic of mesothelioma was noted.

Table 7.4. Diagnostic yield and complications of thoracoscopic pulmonary biopsy.

	Diagnostic yield (%)	No. of patients	Haemor-rhage	Pneumo-thorax	Infection	Death
Brandt[59]	87	457	1	–	–	–
Dijkman[31]	98	65	1	10	2	1
Faurschou[60]	100	7	–	–	–	–
Guy et al.[61]	100	14	6	3	–	–
Janik et al.[62]	100	17	–	–	–	–
Kapsenberg[63]	95	116	–	6	–	–
Rodgers[64]	94	81	3	4	–	–
Voellmy[65]	75	32	–	–	–	–
Wetzer et al.[66]	89	63	–	–	–	–
Boutin[5]	96	170	–	7	1	–
Total	**93**	**1031**	**5**	**30**	**3**	**1**

- Thickening of the pleura in 21 patients (11%). This thickening was more or less regular with elevated, pale, hard, poorly vascularised tissue suggesting malignancy.
- Malignant-looking pachypleuritis in association with nodules or masses in 63 patients (33.5%).
- Non-specific inflammatory aspect with fine granulations (1–2 mm in diameter), lymphangitis, congestion, hypervascularisation or local thickening of the pleura in 12 patients (6.5%).

The sensitivity of thoracoscopic biopsy was 98% (185 positive biopsies including 'extended thoracoscopy' out of 188 patients). In the 3 cases where this examination failed, thick adhesions prevented specimen collection and the diagnosis was only mesothelial hyperplasia. Conclusive biopsy samples were obtained by Abrams needle biopsy (1 patient), repeat thoracoscopy (1 patient) and surgical biopsy (1 patient). The histologic type of mesothelioma was epithelial in 135 cases (72%), mixed in 38 (20%), and fibrosarcomatous in 15 (8%).

In contrast with the almost perfect sensitivity of thoracoscopy, the cumulative sensitivity of fluid cytology and needle biopsy was only 38.2%. The sensitivity of these conventional procedures in our patients with previously negative results was necessarily lower than in other series reporting initial plus repeat results. However, Herbert and Gallagher[23] concluded that the overall sensitivity of these techniques was poor and most investigators prefer open surgical biopsy.

We prefer thoracoscopy to thoracotomy because it is far less painful and safer for the patient. Although Ratzer et al.[26] were unable to achieve diagnosis twice and Law et al.[21] were successful in only 13 of 23 cases, thoracoscopy seems to be a highly reliable method. Martensson et al.[15] achieved diagnosis of mesothelioma in 23 of 24 thoracoscopies, Hirsch et al.[27] in 9 of 9 and Lewis et al.[28] in 28 of 28.

Detection of asbestos in the lung

In a mineralogic study carried out in collaboration with Sebastien[29] from the LEPI and CERCHAR laboratories in Paris, thoracoscopic lung biopsy proved to be highly useful in detecting asbestos fibres. Similarly, thoracoscopic lung biopsies carried out first in animals and then in man[30] demonstrate a high diagnostic yield with low morbidity. The technique is the same as published by Dijkman.[31] Biopsies are obtained using coagulating forceps introduced through a second point of entry under direct vision. One to eight specimens may be taken in each session. The high frequency allows perfect haemostasis and air-tightness. The pleural drainage usually lasts for 48 hours.

A 1989 review of 10 different series covering a total of 1031 patients revealed very few complications following thoracoscopic lung biopsy (Table 7.4). Only one death was attributed to the procedure. Although larger specimens may be taken using the new EndoGIA stapler, this device is not absolutely necessary to achieve asbestos fibre counts.

In a group of 25 'control' patients who had not been in known contact with asbestos, thoracoscopy carried out for reasons unrelated to asbestos exposure revealed the following fibre counts (Table 7.5):

$1.4 \pm 0.3 \times 10^6$ chrysotile fibres/g dry tissue;
$1.0 \pm 0.4 \times 10^6$ amphibole fibres/g dry tissue.

These figures contrast sharply with the following values obtained in subjects with known asbestos exposure:

$19.5 \pm 11.5 \times 10^6$ chrysotile fibres/g dry tissue;
$10.8 \pm 2.6 \times 10^6$ amphibole fibres/g dry tissue.

These findings confirm that the pulmonary asbestos burden is correlated with asbestos exposure and suggest that thoracoscopy allows differentiation of occupational or environmental mesothelioma. Contrary to the opinion of Churg and Wood,[32] thoracoscopic pulmonary biopsy seems to be an excellent method for mineralogic studies of the peripheral lung.

Detection of asbestos in the parietal pleura

Benign and malignant pleural plaques, the most frequent manifestation of occupational or environmental exposure to asbestos fibre, develop more often on the parietal pleura or the diaphragm than on the visceral pleura. Surprisingly few asbestos fibres have been found in the parietal pleura. An explanation for this paradox would be that the distribu-

Table 7.5 *Assessment of asbestos burden by thoracoscopic lung biopsy – mean asbestos fibre counts (x 10⁶/g dried lung tissue) ± SEM.*

	Control patients (n=25)	Occupational exposure (n=30)	Environmental exposure (n=8)
Chrysotile	1.4 ± 0.3	19.5 ± 11.5 (NS)*	2.7 ± 1.5 (NS)*
Amphiboles	1 ± 0.4	10.8 ± 2.6 (p<0.01)*	20.1 ± 8.1 (p<0.01)*

Biopsy samples were analysed by electron microscopy according to the Sebastien technique.[28] Pulmonary asbestos burden correlates with known asbestos exposure whether occupational or environmental (patients from north Corsica).
* Student's t test *versus* mean fibre counts in control (unexposed) patients.

tion of fibres in the parietal pleura is heterogeneous. If samples were taken from pleural plaques or tumours,[33] more fibres might be found. Dodson *et al.*[34] were the first to detect substantial numbers of Stanton fibres (10% of the total fibre burden).

In mice subcutaneously injected fibres are known to concentrate in the milky white spots of the parietal pleura of mice.[35] Animal studies have also shown that these milky spots trap soot particles and Indian ink. In man milky spots are not observed but black spots frequently occur on the parietal pleura near lymphatic vessels and cancer nodules in patients with anthracosis.[5] We speculate that asbestos fibres might concentrate in the same areas that trap visible substances such as coal particles and thus that anthracotic black spots could correspond to the milky spots described by Kanazawa.[35]

Samples were collected from 14 subjects including 8 with and 6 without a history of asbestos exposure. Amphibole fibres were more common than chrysotile in all samples. Nearly one-fourth of fibres in black spots (22.5%) and in the lung (21.7%) measured 5 μm or more in length. In 3 patients with mesothelioma, the concentration of fibres was higher in black spots than in the lung. Like milky spots in the parietal pleura, black spots are characterised by the presence of macrophages, lymphocytes and mesothelial cells. This histological similarity was confirmed by scanning electron microscopy.

The findings indicate that black spots concentrate particles and asbestos fibres that may lead to inflammation and/or cancer. Thus black spots allow correlation of experimental data and clinical observations. These areas may be the starting points for asbestos pleural plaques on the parietal pleura. They could also account for the finding that early-stage mesothelioma is more often observed on the parietal and diaphragmatic pleura than on the visceral pleura.

Prognosis of mesothelioma

Prognosis depends on numerous factors which have been studied separately or in multiple correlation studies (Cox model). Despite their methodological interest, multivariate studies (Table 7.1) have been somewhat disappointing. As previously stated, good overall condition, no weight loss and a good performance status are favourable prognostic factors. Common sense would warrant the same conclusions without complex calculations. The value and significance of age, sex, and symptom-to-diagnosis interval have varied widely from one study to another. Treatment was cited as a favourable factor in 5 out of 7 series,[1,2,11,36,37] but none of these studies was randomised, and no definite conclusions can be drawn, especially with regard to surgery.[7]

Histological type

The histological type appears to be important. Epithelial or mixed forms have a better prognosis than fibrosarcomatous forms. Mean survival is 10 to 17 months for the former patients and 4 to 7 months for the latter. In our series, the fibrosarcomatous type had the most unfavourable prognosis, with a mean survival of 5.25 months.

Disease stage

Disease staging is useful not only to establish prognosis but also to allow evaluation of the effectiveness of treatment. The most widely used and first classification is that of Butchart,[6] which includes 4 stages (Table 7.6). Only patients in the first 2 stages are eligible for curative treatment. In stage II, the chest wall and/or mediastinum is involved with or without mediastinal lymph nodes. In all classification systems, mesothelioma at stage III or IV is fatal in from a few weeks to 4 or 5 months.

Although cited as a good prognostic sign in 4 multivariate studies, stage I disease was a highly favourable factor in only 2. In the previous series, mean survival at stage I was 13.4 months. This was statistically different from the other stages but hardly exceeded overall average survival. These facts could mean either that stage is not an important prognostic factor or that the Butchart system is inadequate. In this regard it should be emphasised that the number of patients in stage I, which has ranged from 30%[11] to 77%,[38] tends to be overestimated.

Thoracoscopy

Thoracoscopic features seem to allow more accurate staging. In 50% of cases, patients with the longest survivals had tumours with an inflammatory or non-specific lymphangitic appearance.[39] The mean survival for these patients (12 in our series) was 28.3 months. In the other 50% of these cases, small nodules (less than 5 mm in diameter), fine granulations or slight pleural thickening were observed. In this early stage of the disease, the mediastinum as well as the visceral pleura appears normal through the thoracoscope as well as on CT scan. Unlike Canto *et al.*[40] no lesions exclusively on the visceral pleura

Table 7.6. *Survival as a function of Butchart classification.*

	Butchart[6] Survival (months)	Nb	Antman[1] Survival (months)	Nb	Brenner[10] Survival (months)	Nb	Alberts[11] Survival (months)	Nb
Stage I: localised tumour in homolateral pleura	13	17	31	16	62	13	202	11
Stage II: involvement of mediastinal organs or of the wall or of the contra-lateral pleura	4	11	4	9	52	11	35	8
Stage III: subdiaphrag-matic involvement	2	9	5	5	7	4	13	7
Stage IV: remote metastasis	0	–	2	4	0	–	12	2

Nb = number

were noted and it can be concluded that in most cases mesothelioma develops from the parietal or diaphragmatic pleura and invades the visceral and mediastinal pleura later. This is consistent with the location of benign asbestos plaques only on the parietal or diaphragmatic pleura. As reported by Adams *et al.*, in 19 of their 20 patients,[41] was observed in comparison to less involvement of the visceral pleura than the parietal pleura or diaphragm. If the visceral pleura was involved to any extent, mesothelioma had a very unfavourable prognosis with a median survival of 10 months. Conversely, the median survival for 48 patients with a normal visceral pleura was 22.4 months.

Staging of mesothelioma is an important but difficult problem that must be solved so that effective treatment when it becomes available can be applied at the earliest stage of the disease. Rusch and Ginsberg[42] listed the following requirements for validation of a classification system:

- confirmation of diagnoses by a panel of pathologists
- good prognostic value
- corroboration by a prospective study.

The Butchart system has been criticised because it overestimates the number of patients in stage I, and because assessment of tumour thickness by conventional x-ray and even CT scan is difficult in the case of ipsilateral effusion. This criticism is equally valid for all other classification systems. The Mattson system[43] differs from the Butchart system mainly with regard to pericardial involvement, which is included in stage II rather than in stage I. The Dimitrov system[44] is based on measurement of the largest diameter of the tumour by CT scan, and this would be much easier by thoracoscopy.

The TNM system proposed by Chahinian *et al.*[1] has the advantage of being based on an international system. A simpler TNM classification has been proposed by the UICC.[42]

In fact, thoracoscopy shows that patients with parietal pleura involvement, which often occurs at an early stage of the disease, should be classified separately, while patients with involvement of visceral pleura, which has, in our series, the same prognostic significance as mediastinal involvement, should be classified in another group. Based on this finding we divided stage I into two subcategories:

Stage IA. The parietal and/or diaphragmatic pleura are involved, but the visceral pleura appears disease-free by both thoracoscopy and CT scan (26 patients in our series). Median survival of stage IA patients is 28 months.

Stage IB. The features are the same as stage IA plus evident visceral pleura involvement (70 patients). Median survival is only 11 months at stage IB. Thus, as soon as the visceral pleura is invaded, the prognosis becomes much worse, whatever treatment is attempted.

In stage II, where the mediastinum is involved, survival is only 10 months, suggesting that mediastinal involvement may occur very soon after visceral pleura invasion, and in some cases may even be synchronous.

Recently, a group of investigators working under the direction of V. Rush agreed on a new TNM system that included stages IA and IB. [45]

Therapeutic thoracoscopy

Talc poudrage pleurodesis

In most cases, the goal of treatment of mesothelioma is simply to prevent recurrent effusions and obtain the longest possible survival with the best quality of life. As previously seen, the efficacy of chemotherapy and/or radiotherapy is controversial, and surgery is generally non-curative.

Thoracoscopy permits effective palliation with less morbidity than surgery or even chemotherapy or radiation therapy. Permanent pleurodesis may be achieved at the end of the thoracoscopic examination by spraying 6 to 10 mL (3–5 g) of talcum powder into the pleural space. A chest tube is inserted and all air is aspirated from the chest cavity. A final x-ray is taken to assess the position of the tube and to confirm full re-expansion of the lung. Drainage or aspiration under negative pressure (50–100 mmHg) is maintained for 4 to 6 days.

Talc poudrage prevented fluid reaccumulation in 81% of cases, versus 83% after surgery.[46] When effusions recurred despite poudrage, surgery was contraindicated by poor general condition. A second talc poudrage in 2 patients produced good results.

Complications included one case of empyema after poudrage which resolved after drainage and pleural lavage, and 4 deaths (3, 4, 7 and 10 days after talc poudrage) in patients in very poor general condition. Three perioperative deaths occurred, one 60 days after pleuropneumonectomy from a bronchial fistula and two 10 days after pleurectomy. The median survival in the three groups was 210 days after surgery, 330 days after talc poudrage, and 120 days for supportive care alone.

The decreased survival observed in the untreated group was most likely due to the advanced stage of the tumours. Conversely, there was no significant difference between the surgery and talc poudrage groups. These groups, however, were not randomised.

The proportion of survivors at 1 year for these 3 groups was 47% after talc poudrage, 28% after surgery, and 13% for supportive care.

Surgery did not prevent subsequent distant metastasis. Among patients surviving more than 3 months, metastasis developed in 8 of 12 patients after surgery as compared to 12 of 32 patients after talc poudrage.

Role of thoracoscopy in intrapleural treatment

Talc pleurodesis is a purely palliative procedure that enhances the functional and general status of the patient by eliminating the need for repeated puncture. A more active therapy is available to some patients. It is intrapleural chemotherapy using either a sclerosing agent (doxorubicin) or an antimitotic agent (5-fluorouracil, thiotepa, or bleomycin). Tolerance is proportional to the sclerosing effect, which itself depends on the cytotoxic effect. This is particularly true for bleomycin.[47] Patients with minimal peritoneal or pleural disease (<5 mm in depth) experience the best response rates to intracavitary chemotherapy.[48] The necessity of inserting a catheter or chest tube for the administration of intrapleural chemotherapy inevitably poses a high risk of infection.

Markman *et al.*[49,50] treated 8 patients with malignant mesothelioma with intrapleural cisplatin (100 μg/m^2 in 250 mL of saline). Only one patient showed a response, but these patients had more extensive disease, which severely limited the diffusion of drug throughout the pleural cavity. Two of 7 patients treated intrapleurally with cisplatin combined with cytarabine showed a response.[51] A Lung Cancer Study Group trial published by V. Rusch *et al.*[52] included 46 patients. The overall response rate was 49%. The outcome of this trial was encouraging enough to warrant inclusion of the regimen in subsequent trials for pleural mesothelioma.

The incidence of pleural adhesions and the heterogeneity of lesions in the pleural cavity led us to place the catheter near the lesions under visual control during endoscopy to obtain the best possible delivery of intrapleural chemotherapy. The incidence of pleural infection due to catheter handling led us to place a subcutaneous port-A-cath at the level of the 4th intercostal space in the anterior axillary region. The catheter is tunnelled for 6 to 8 cm under the skin and the tip is placed under visual control. Healing is obtained after 8 to 12 days and treatment can begin after two weeks. Limiting contact with ambient air has practically eliminated the problem of pleural infection. Our experience now includes 70 patients treated in the department plus over 100 patients from a multicentric study. Using interferon gamma[47,48] and interleukin-2,[53,54] we have obtained objective response with prolonged survival.

Another indication for thoracoscopy is assessment of tumour response. Follow-up can be accomplished using repeated pleural fluid cytology,[51] but when there is no more liquid, cytology is not feasible. Others judge response on the decrease in the amount of fluid.[50] It appears that a second thoracoscopy is the most effective means of visualising tumour response. In our patients we perform thoracoscopy and CT scan before treatment to achieve diagnosis and staging. Then 15 to 30 days after treatment we perform CT scan after fluid removal. If CT scan shows that the lesions have stabilised or regressed, we repeat thoracoscopy to confirm response.[51] In 8 cases[47] we observed complete regression with negative biopsies. Thus thoracoscopy appears to be an excellent method for evaluating tumour response.

Conclusion

As thoracoscopy is a simple and safe procedure, we recommend that it be used liberally for the following diagnostic indications.

Table 7.7. *Effectiveness of thoracoscopy and surgery in preventing fluid recurrence.*

	Thoracoscopy	**Surgery**
N° of patients with pleural fluid	32	12*
Results		
Good	26 (81%)	10 (83%)
Poor	6	2
Hospital mortality at 1 month	4	2

* Of patients who underwent surgery, only 12 had chronic pleural effusions.

- Patients with a history of previous asbestos exposure presenting chest pain, recent and untreatable cough, unexplained loss of weight, pleural effusion, empyema, or spontaneous pneumothorax. Thoracoscopy should be undertaken early. In our experience several patients developed mesothelioma after false-negative cytology. In these patients thoracoscopy was performed only after recurrence of fluid, and as a result diagnosis was delayed for several weeks or months.
- X-ray or CT scan documented changes in visible pleural plaques.
- Recent unexplainable pleurisy particularly in patients from areas liable to asbestos exposure.

In all these cases manifestations are very minor and most physicians are reluctant to recommend a highly invasive procedure like exploratory thoracotomy. For malignant mesothelioma this reluctance is detrimental to survival, since we observed complete responses to cytokines only in patients in the earliest stage of disease.

To allow more widespread use, thoracoscopy should not be restricted to the surgeon, and physicians should be trained to perform this procedure for diagnostic purposes. More and more groups, even in the USA or Canada, where resistance to thoracoscopy has traditionally been strong, are starting to report their experience.[55-57]

References

1. Chahinian, A.P., Pajak, T.F., Holland, J.F., Norton, L., Ambinder, R.M., Mandel, E.M. Diffuse malignant mesothelioma (prospective evaluation of 69 patients). *Ann Intern Med* 1982; **96**: 746–755.
2. Antman, K., Shemin, R., Ryan, L., *et al*. Malignant mesothelioma: prognostic variables in a registry of 180 patients, the Dana-Farber Cancer Institute and Brigham and Women's Hospital experience over two decades, 1965–1985. *J Clin Oncol* 1988; **6**: 147–153.
3. MacDonald, A.D., MacDonald, J.C. Epidemiology of malignant mesothelioma. In: Antman, K., Aisner, J. (ed.) Asbestos-related malignancy. Boston, Grune and Stratton Inc., 1986; 31–35.
4. Nicholson, W.J., Perkel, G., Selikoff, I.J. Occupational exposure to asbestos: population at risk and projected mortality – 1980–2030. *Am J Ind Med* 1982; **3**: 259–311.
5. Boutin, C., Viallat, J.R., Aelony, Y. Practical thoracoscopy. Berlin-Heidelberg: Springer-Verlag, 1991.
6. Butchart, E.G., Ashcroft, T., Barnsley, W.C., Holden, M.P. Pleuropneumonectomy in the management of diffuse malignant mesothelioma of the pleura (experience with 29 patients). *Thorax* 1976; **31**: 15–24.
7. Rusch, V.W., Figlin, R., Godwin, D., Piantadosi, S. Intrapleural cisplatin and cytarabine in the management of malignant pleural effusions: a lung cancer study group trial. *J Clin Oncol* 1991; **9**: 313–319.
8. Boutin, C., Viallat, J.R., Cargnino, P., Farisse, P. Thoracoscopy in malignant pleural effusions. *Am Rev Respir Dis* 1981; **124**: 588–592.
9. Boutin, C. Thoracoscopy in malignant mesothelioma. *Pneumologie* 1989; **43**: 61–65.

10. Brenner, J., Sordillo, P.P., Magill, G.B., Golbey, R.B. Malignant mesothelioma of the pleura. *Cancer* 1982; **49**: 2431–2435.

11. Alberts, A.S., Falkson, G., Goedhals, L., Vorobiof, D.A., van der Merwe, C.A. Malignant pleural mesothelioma: a disease unaffected by current therapeutic maneuvers. *J Clin Oncol* 1988; **6**: 527–535.

12. Delaria, G.A., Jensik, R., Faber, L.P., *et al.* Surgical management of malignant mesothelioma. *Ann Thorac Surg* 1978; **26**: 375–382.

13. Boutin, C., Dumortier, P., Rey, F., Viallat, J.R., De Vuyst, P. Black spots concentrate oncogenic asbestos fibres in the parietal pleura; thoracoscopic and mineralogic study. *Am J Respir Crit Care Med* 1996; **153**: 444–445.

14. Le Bouffant, L., Bruyere, S., Daniel, H., Tichoux, G. Etude expérimentale de devenir des fibres d'amiante dans l'appareil respiratoire. *Rev Fr Mal Respir* 1979; **7**: 707–716.

15. Martensson, G. Thoracoscopy in the diagnosis of malignant mesothelioma. *Poumon-Coeur* 1981; **37**: 249–251.

16. Martensson, G., Hagmar, B., Zettergren, L. Diagnosis and prognosis in malignant pleural mesothelioma: a prospective study. *Eur J Respir Dis* 1984; **65**: 169–178.

17. Boutin, C., Viallat, J.R., Astoul, P.H. Le traitement des mésothéliomes par interferon gamma et interleukine-2. *Rev Pneumol Clin* 1990; **46**: 211–215.

18. Driesen, P., Boutin, C., Viallat, J.R., Astoul, P.H. Implantable access system for prolonged intrapleural immunotherapy. *Eur Respir J* 1994; **7**: 1889–1892.

19. Antman, K.H., Corson, J.M., Li, F.P., *et al.* Malignant mesothelioma following radiation exposure. *J Clin Oncol* 1983; **1**:695–700.

20. Elmes, P.C., Simpson, J.J. The clinical aspects of mesothelioma. *Q J Med* 1976; **179**: 427–449.

21. Law, M.R., Hodson, M.E., Turner-Warwick, M. Malignant mesothelioma of the pleura: clinical aspects and symptomatic treatment. *Eur J Respir Dis* 1984; **65**: 162–168.

22. Boutin, C., Irisson, M., Rathelot, P., Petite, J.M. L'Extension pariétale des mésothéliomes pleuraux malins diffus après biopsies. Prévention par radiothérapie. *Presse Med* 1983; **33**: 1823.

23. Herbert, A., Gallagher, P.J. Pleural biopsy in the diagnosis of malignant mesothelioma. *Thorax* 1982; **37**: 816–821.

24. Boutin, C., Rey, F. Thoracoscopy in pleural malignant mesothelioma: a prospective study of 188 patients. Part 1: Diagnosis. *Cancer* 1993; **72**: 389–393.

24. Boutin, C., Rey, F., Gouvernet, J., Viallat, J.R., Astoul, P.H., Ledoray, V. Thoracoscopy in pleural malignant mesothelioma: a prospective study of 188 patients. Part 2: Prognosis and staging. *Cancer* 1993; **72**: 394–404.

25. Janssen, J., Boutin, C. Extended thoracoscopy: a method to be used in case of pleural adhesions. *Eur Respir J* 1992; **5**: 763–766.

26. Ratzer, E., Pool, J.L., Melamed, M.R. Pleural mesotheliomas: clinical experiences with thirty-seven patients. *Am J Roentgenol* 1967; **99**: 863–880.

27. Hirsch, A., Brochard, P., De Cremoux, H., *et al.* Features of asbestos-exposed and unexposed mesothelioma. *Am J Ind Med* 1982; **3**: 413–422.

28. Lewis, R.J., Sisler, G.E., Mackenzie, J.W. Diffuse, mixed malignant pleural mesothelioma. *Ann Thorac Surg* 1981; **31**: 53–60.

29. Sebastien, P. La biométrologie des fibres inhalées. Dissertation, University of Paris XII, 1982.
30. Boutin, C., Viallat, J.R., Cargnino, P., Rey, F. Thoracoscopic lung biopsy. Experimental and clinical preliminary study. *Chest* 1982; **82**: 44–48.
31. Dijkman, J.H. Thorakoskopie bei immunsupprimierten patienten. *Pneumologie* 1989; **43**: 116–118.
32. Churg, A., Wood, P. Observations on the distribution of asbestos fibres in human lungs. *Environ Res* 1983; **31**: 374–380.
33. Kohyama, N., Suzuki, Y. Analysis of asbestos fibers in lung parenchyma, pleural plaques, and mesothelioma tissues of North American insulation workers. *Ann N Y Acad Sci* 1991; **643**: 27–52.
34. Dodson, R.F., Williams, M.G., Corn, C.J., Brollo, A., Bianchi, C. Asbestos content of lung tissue, lymph nodes and pleural plaques from former shipyard workers. *Am Rev Respir Dis* 1990; **142**: 843–847.
35. Kanazawa, K., Birbeck, M.S.C., Carter, R.L., Roe, F.J.C. Migration of asbestos fibres from subcutaneous injection sites in mice. *Br J Cancer* 1970; **24**: 96–106.
36. Spirtas, R., Connelly, R., Tucker, M.A. Survival patterns for malignant mesothelioma: the SEER experience. *Int J Cancer* 1988; **41**: 525–530.
37. Calavrezos, A., Koschel, G., Husselmann, H., *et al*. Malignant mesothelioma of the pleura. *Klin Wochenschr* 1988; **66**: 607–613.
38. MacCornack, P., Nagasaki, F., Hilaris, B.S., *et al*. Surgical treatment of pleural mesothelioma. *J Thorac Cardiovasc Surg* 1982; **84**: 834–842.
39. Whitaker, D., Henderson, D.W., Shikin, K.B. The concept of mesothelioma in situ: implications for diagnosis and histogenesis. *Semin Diagn Pathol* 1992; **9**: 151–161.
40. Canto, A., Saumench, J., Moya, J. Points to consider when choosing a biopsy method in cases of pleuritis of unknown origin, with special reference to thoracoscopy. In: J. Deslauriers et L.K. Lacquet (eds), *Thoracic Surgery: Surgical Management of Pleural Diseases*. 6. St Louis, MO: CV Mosby, 1990; 49–53.
41. Adams, V.I., Unni, K.K., Muhm, J.R., Jett, J.R., Ilstrup, D.M., Bernatz, P.E. Diffuse malignant mesothelioma of pleura: diagnosis and survival in 92 cases. *Cancer* 1986; **58**: 1540–1551.
42. Rusch, V.W., Ginsberg, R.J. New concepts in the staging of mesothelioma. In: Deslauriers, J., Lacquet, L.K., (ed). *Thoracic Surgery: Surgical Management of Pleural Diseases*. 6. St Louis, MO, C.V. Mosby, 1990, 336–343.
43. Mattson, K. Natural history and clinical staging of malignant mesothelioma. *Environ J Respir Dis* 1982; **63**: 124:87.
44. Dimitrov, N.V., MacMahon, S. Presentation, diagnostic, methods, staging and natural history of malignant mesothelioma. In: Antman, K. Aisner, J., (eds), *Asbestos Related Malignancy*, Boston, Grune & Stratton Inc., 1986; 225–238.
45. International Mesothelioma Interest Group. A proposed new international TNM staging system for malignant pleural mesothelioma. *Chest* 1995; **108**: 1122–1128.
46. Viallat, J.R., Rey, F., Astoul, P.H., Boutin, C. Thoracoscopic talc poudrage pleurodesis for malignant effusions. Review of 360 cases. *Chest* 1996; **110**: 1387–1393.
47. Boutin, C., Viallat, J.R., Van Zandwijk, N., *et al*. Activity of intrapleural recombinant gamma-interferon in malignant mesothelioma. *Cancer* 1991; **67**: 2033–2037.

48. Boutin, C., Nussbaum, E., Monnet, I., *et al*. Intrapleural treatment with recombinant γ-interferon in early stage malignant pleural mesothelioma. *Cancer* 1994; **74**: 2460–7.
49. Markman, M., Cleary, S., Pfeifle, C., Howell, S.B. Cisplatin administered by the intracavitary route as treatment for malignant mesothelioma. *Cancer* 1986; **58**: 18.
50. Markman, M., Howell, S.B., Green, M.. Combination intracavitary chemotherapy for malignant pleural disease. *Cancer Drug Deliv* 1984; **1**: 333.
51. Rusch, V.W., Piantadosi, S., Holmes, C. The role of extrapleural pneumonectomy in malignant pleural mesothelioma. *J Thorac Cardiovasc Surg* 1991; **102**: 1–9.
52. Rusch, V.W. Intrapleural chemotherapy for malignant pleural effusion. In: Deslauriers, J., Lacquet, L.K. (ed.) *Thoracic Surgery: Surgical Management of Pleural Diseases*. 6. St Louis, MO, C.V. Mosby, 1990, 409–414.
53. Astoul, P.H., Viallat, J.R., Laurent, J.C., Brandely, M., Boutin, C. Intrapleural recombinant IL-2 in passive immunotherapy for malignant pleural effusions. *Chest* 1993; **103**: 209–213.
54. Astoul, P.H., Picat-Joossen, D., Viallat, J.R., Boutin, C. Intrapleural administration of interleukin-2 for the treatment of patients with malignant pleural mesothelioma, a phase II study. *Cancer* 1998; 15; **83**: 2099–2104.
55. Aelony, Y., King, R., Boutin, C. Thoracoscopic talc poudrage pleurodesis for chronic recurrent pleural effusions. *Ann Intern Med* 1991; **115**: 778–782.
56. Menzies, R., Charbonneau, M. Thoracoscopy for the diagnosis of pleural disease. *Ann Intern Med* 1991; **114**: 271–276.
57. Mathur, P., Martin, W.J. Clinical utility of thoracoscopy. *Chest* 1992; **102**: 3–4.
58. Ruffie, P., Feld, R., Minkin, S., *et al*. Diffuse malignant mesothelioma of the pleura in Ontario and Quebec: a retrospective study of 332 patients. *J Clin Oncol* 1989; **7**: 1157–1168.
59. Brandt, H.J. Biopsie pulmonaire sous contrôle visuel. *Poumon-Coeur* 1981; **37**: 307–311.
60. Faurschou, P. Diagnostic thoracoscopy in pleuro-pulmonary infiltrates without pleural effusion. *Endoscopy* 1985; **17**: 21-25.
61. Guy, P., Kasparian, P., Guibout, P. Biopsies pulmonaires par thoracoscopie. *Poumon-Coeur* 1983; **39**: 179–181.
62. Janik, J.S., Nagaraj, H.S., Groff, D.B. Thoracoscopic evaluation of intrathoracic lesions in children. *J Thorac Cardiovasc Surg* 1982; **83**: 408–413.
63. Kapsengerg, P.D. Thoracoscopic biopsy under visual control. *Poumon-Coeur* 1981; **37**: 313–316.
64. Rodgers, B.M. Thoracoscopy in children. *Poumon-Coeur* 1981; **37**: 301–306.
65. Voellmy, W. Résultats diagnostiques de la thoracoscopie dans les affections du poumon et de la plèvre. *Poumon-Coeur* 1981; **37**: 67–73.
66. Wetzer, K., Schilling, W., Wenzel, D., Scheuler, D. Die thorakoskopische Lungenbiopsie. *Z Erkrank Atem-Org* 1980; **155**: 82–88.

= 8 =

Pathology of Mesothelioma

Amanda Segal, Darrel Whitaker, Douglas Henderson and
Keith Shilkin

Since its first recognition over a century ago, malignant mesothelioma has been the subject of social, epidemiological, legal and scientific interest. From an epidemiological and social viewpoint, this interest has derived largely from the strong association between malignant mesothelioma and exposure to asbestos, often with implications for litigation. For the pathologist, the diagnosis of mesothelioma is challenging, not only because of the histological diversity of this tumour, but also because of the difficulty in distinguishing mesothelioma from both reactive serosal processes and from metastatic disease involving the serosa. There has been controversy in the past, as to whether a diagnosis of mesothelioma could be established reliably on cytological examination of serous effusions or fine needle aspiration (FNA) samples – or histological examination of small biopsy specimens – and there have been claims that the diagnosis should only be made after a full post-mortem examination or evaluation of substantive tissue derived at thoracotomy or laparotomy. More recently, however, there has been a gradual shift towards acceptance that the diagnosis can be confidently reached on cytological specimens or small tissue samples, given the support of ancillary studies – in particular immunohistochemical and ultrastructural assessment. The pathology of mesothelioma continues to stimulate interest, reflected in the relative explosion in the literature in the last few years in the form of papers dealing mainly with the differential diagnosis of malignant mesothelioma.

In this chapter we seek to give an overview of the pathology of mesothelioma. Emphasis has been placed on the more challenging and common diagnostic problems seen by the pathologist, in particular distinguishing reactive and reparative mesothelial processes from malignant mesothelioma in both effusion cytology and biopsy material.

Sample types in the diagnosis of mesothelioma

Depending on the type of mesothelioma and the clinical presentation, there are several samples that may independently or collectively be examined to establish a diagnosis of mesothelioma (Figure 8.1). By optimising sampling procedures, the clinician can greatly influence and enhance the pathologist's ability to offer a definitive diagnosis. Although

THE INVESTIGATION OF SUSPECTED MESOTHELIOMA

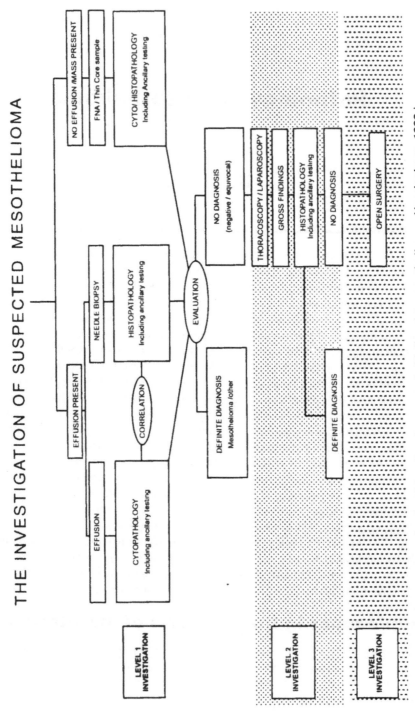

Figure 8.1. A diagnostic pathway. (After Henderson et al., Malignant mesothelioma, *Hemisphere, 1992.*)

thoracoscopic wedge biopsies – and even open biopsy via thoracotomy – are sometimes required to establish a diagnosis of mesothelioma, there are several less invasive forms of sampling which may be diagnostic in some settings. These latter sample types are discussed below.

Effusion fluid

When a serous effusion is present an adequate sample (preferably over 50 mL of fluid) should be collected and sent to the cytology laboratory; this will enable smears and a cell block to be prepared. In addition, some of the cell deposit can be set aside for ultrastructural examination.[1] In our hands a definite diagnosis of malignant mesothelioma can be made on cytology of effusions in the majority of cases.

Closed needle biopsy

Although taking a closed needle biopsy (of the Abrahams' type) at the time of tapping the effusion was the standard practice in the past, we have seen a reduction in this form of sampling related to a significant proportion of inadequate or inconclusive biopsies. The high diagnostic yield from effusion cytology has probably also influenced this decline.

Fine needle aspiration (FNA)

FNA has a role in sampling sites such as chest wall lesions or lymph nodes, and is also often used as a first line investigation of pleura-based lesions, when an effusion is absent. Such samples can be obtained under radiological guidance and at the same time as thin core biopsy samples.

Thin core biopsy samples

Over the last few years we have seen an increase in the use of thin core sampling for pleura-based lesions, especially when there is no accompanying serous effusion. This form of sampling is well tolerated by patients, who require only simple local anaesthesia with lignocaine. Thin core samples are obtained with the aid of a spring-loaded Temno biopsy sampler (Bauer Medical, Clearwater, Florida, USA), using a 16-gauge or occasionally 19-gauge, 9 cm long needle to collect one to three samples. The resultant specimens measure up to 12 mm in length and approximately 1 mm in diameter (Figure 8.2). Thin core samples are often taken immediately after an FNA sample; the cores can be used as a valuable adjunct by making 'roll smears', without damaging the specimen (Figure 8.3). The tissue cores can also be divided to collect a small sample for electron microscopy (EM). Tissue cores obtained in this manner are well preserved and suitable for histopathology and immunophenotyping. Limitations of thin core biopsy include sampling of areas of necrosis in some tumours, and sclerotic fibrous lesions such as desmoplastic mesothelioma. Thin core samples are rarely diagnostic in the setting of desmoplastic mesothelioma, where thoracoscopic wedge biopsies or open biopsies are usually required; these latter forms of biopsy allow inclusion of chest wall tissues – skeletal muscle and adipose tissue – important for the recognition of invasion.

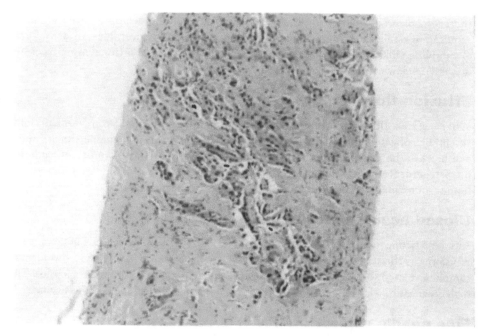

Figure 8.2. Core biopsy. Malignant mesothelioma. H&E stain.

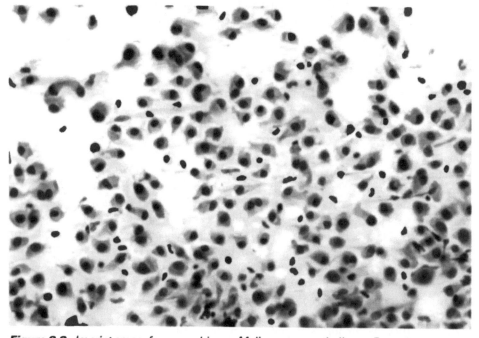

Figure 8.3. Imprint smear from core biopsy. Malignant mesothelioma. Papanicolaou stain.

In summary, thin core samples are a valuable diagnostic aid in our approach to the tissue diagnosis of malignant mesothelioma, particularly for the diagnosis of epithelioid (epithelial) or biphasic subtypes; the limitations of this form of biopsy for the diagnosis of desmoplastic mesothelioma must be recognised.

Serosal reactions

Serosal healing

Serosal surfaces are covered by a mesothelial membrane, consisting of a single cell layer of mesothelial cells resting on a basement membrane and with a further supporting and delicate layer of connective tissue. This gossamer-like covering provides an outer boundary to the parietal serosa and to the internal visceral organs. It is specialised in both form and function to provide a well lubricated surface that facilitates intra-thoracic and intra-abdominal movement, and also plays an important role in local fluid regulation. Because of its monolayer nature, tissue integrity is achieved by complex cell-to-cell interdigitation and the formation of abundant cell junctions which result in an interlocking structure. Damage to the serosa as a result of surgery or inflammation is generally followed by healing that is normally complete within 10 days. The nature of this healing may differ depending on the nature of the injury, i.e., whether a surface or deep wound occurs. There is good experimental evidence to show that simple denudation is followed by local healing with proliferation of surface mesothelial cells adjacent to the wound surface.[2] In deeper wounds involving the connective tissue of the serosa, a more complex process may occur. Whereas this repair is characterised chiefly by a predominance of proliferating fibroblasts, other spindled or elongate polygonal cells that have the ultrastructural and immunophenotypic characteristics of mesothelial cells also participate. In tissue culture it is recognised that mesothelial cells can modulate from a vimentin-positive, keratin-negative spindled form to a keratin-positive, vimentin-negative polygonal form.[3] There is some controversy as to whether these deeply located mesothelial cells arise from a subserosal stem cell,[4] or from proliferative surface mesothelial cells which – due to the injury or as part of the inflammatory process – migrate into the extracellular matrix of the wound. We will not speculate further here about the origin of the healing cell, but it must be borne in mind in the context of the differential diagnosis of serosal biopsies that a variable number of keratin-positive spindle cells will be present throughout the healing process, and morphological transition between spindled and epithelioid cells can be found in the superficial regions of the wound. In this context, the differential diagnosis between a serosal reparative process and sarcomatoid or desmoplastic mesothelioma requires caution and critical assessment.

Distinction between reactive serosal processes and mesothelioma

Reactive processes involving the mesothelium-lined serous cavities are common, are seen in a variety of clinical settings, and may result in proliferation of mesothelial cells, fibroblasts or both. Florid mesothelial or fibroblastic proliferation may be caused by processes as diverse as physical trauma, surgical procedures, pulmonary infarction, infection, recurrent pneumothoraces, collagen-vascular diseases, cirrhosis and the presence of adjacent tumour.[5-7] Obtaining adequate clinical information is an important step to avoid misinterpretation of florid reactive processes as neoplastic; conversely, a history of asbestos exposure is not required for the diagnosis of mesothelioma.

Difficulties in evaluating florid reactive processes can arise within both cytological and histological specimens.[8] Two significant areas of difficulty are:

· Distinguishing mesothelial hyperplasia from well differentiated epithelioid mesothelioma: this problem is mainly encountered with effusion cytology, but also arises in biopsy specimens.

· Distinguishing fibrous pleuritis from desmoplastic mesothelioma: this is generally a problem seen in biopsy material, and in particular with small specimens.

While immunohistochemistry plays an important and primary role in distinguishing mesothelial hyperplasia from epithelioid mesothelioma, at this time its usefulness – apart from cytokeratin immunohistochemistry to facilitate identification of invasion – is of little or no significant value for the distinction of fibrous pleuritis from desmoplastic mesothelioma, where clinical and radiological correlation, obtaining adequate biopsy material and careful attention to light microscopic appearances are essential.

Electron microscopy is of little value in either of these problem areas.

Distinction of mesothelial hyperplasia from epithelioid mesothelioma

Cytology

Cytological examination of effusion fluids plays a major role in the primary diagnosis of malignant mesothelioma. The sensitivity of this technique varies between institutions, with some reports indicating less than one-third of mesotheliomas are diagnosable by this technique.[9,10] Accurate diagnosis depends on many factors, and – given technically well prepared specimens and experience in this area of cytopathology – a sensitivity of approximately 90% can be achieved.[11]

In the setting of a formal national quality assurance programme in cytology coordinated by the Royal College of Pathologists of Australasia, a case of biopsy-proven mesothelioma was included for assessment in the 1997 survey. Papanicolaou and Diff-Quik stained smears and an H&E stained cell-block section of the effusion sample were sent to 176 respondent laboratories in Australia: 98.8% of respondents correctly called the case malignant. Of these, 73.8% indicated mesothelioma, either making a specific cytologic diagnosis (49.4%) or favouring mesothelioma (24.4%). Twenty-five per cent made a diagnosis of adenocarcinoma, 'definite' (18.37%) or 'favoured' (6.8%). Only two respondents called the case benign or favoured benign.

These findings reflect a single case only, and it is therefore not possible to draw conclusions regarding the general accuracy of cytological diagnosis; however, given well prepared material and familiarity with the cytological diagnostic criteria, a correct diagnosis of malignant mesothelioma could be made by most laboratories. It could also be presumed that in an appropriate clinical setting, with the additional support of ancillary tests, a higher degree of accuracy may have been achieved.

In effusion cytology, the diagnosis of mesothelioma is a two-stage process:

· establishing malignancy; and
· demonstrating mesothelial characteristics in the malignant cells.

Difficulty in diagnosis relates both to the distinction between benign and malignant mesothelial proliferations, and between mesothelioma and other malignancies, usually metastatic adenocarcinoma. In technically well prepared samples, the mesothelial nature of the cells is often obvious and the difficulty is more often in establishing the malignant nature of the cells. There are numerous references highlighting cytomorphological criteria which are useful for a diagnosis of mesothelioma.[12-15] Despite the validity of these criteria, in our experience supportive ancillary studies, usually immunohistochemistry, are invariably required for diagnosis (see Ancillary studies section).

Some of the cytological criteria used to establish a diagnosis of malignancy are site specific. For example, in malignant mesotheliomatous *pleural* effusions, the fluid generally contains numerous well formed cell aggregates, the large numbers of aggregates being an important factor in establishing a malignant diagnosis (Figure 8.4).[16]

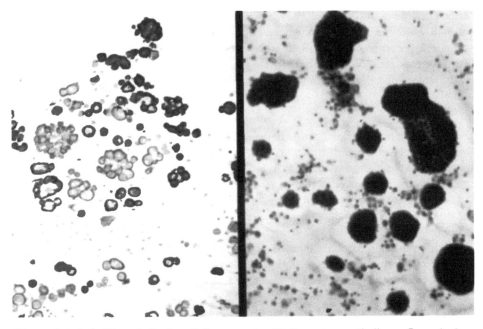

Figure 8.4. Left: *Pleural effusion. Cell aggregates. Malignant mesothelioma. Papanicolaou stain.* Right: *Pleural effusion. Malignant mesothelioma. EMA immunostain.*

However, aggregate cellularity is not such a reliable feature in pericardial and perito-neal specimens, where samples may contain moderate numbers of aggregates and still represent a benign process.[17,18] For example, we have seen a florid pericardial mesothelial reaction with numerous well formed papillary aggregates in a pericardial effusion three weeks after cardiac surgery. Recently, the term mesothelial/monocytic incidental cardiac excrescences (cardiac MICE) has been used to describe a reactive process occurring both within the pericardial cavity and within the heart, which is thought to represent a non-neoplastic accumulation of mesothelial and monocytic cells, sometimes related to previous cardiac catheterisation.[19,20]

Loosely cohesive aggregates of mesothelial cells may be seen in both reactive and neoplastic processes. However, tightly cohesive three-dimensional aggregates, often with a 'mulberry'-like external contour, and papillary arrangements, are generally indicative of mesothelioma, particularly in pleural fluid. Stromal cores within the aggregates are more commonly seen in malignant pleural effusions. Occasionally, mesothelioma presents as a single cell pattern, posing diagnostic difficulties both in detection and diagnosis.[21]

Nuclear atypia, generally the basis of establishing a malignant diagnosis in cy-tology, may sometimes be minimal in mesothelioma, probably reflecting that mesothe-lioma is often a diploid neoplasm.[14] Mitotic activity is likewise not a useful indicator of a malignant process. Other features therefore assume increased significance. Cell enlargement is an important finding, often with enlargement of the whole cell, rather than an increased nuclear:cytoplasmic ratio. Macronucleoli, while not a sole criterion of malignancy, should prompt careful evaluation, as this is a feature often seen in well differentiated mesothelioma.[12,22] Prominent cell engulfment as a feature of malignant mesotheliomatous effusions has been emphasised in some studies.[22]

The presence of any of the features cited above, especially with a history of past asbestos exposure, should initiate further studies, in particular immunohistochemical staining for epithelial membrane antigen (see Ancillary studies section).

Histology

In biopsy specimens the distinction between benign and malignant processes at the light microscopic level depends on the extent of the mesothelial proliferation, significant cytological atypia and invasion.[13,23] Again, there are potential problems, as malignant mesothelioma may be very well differentiated with bland and uniform cytomorphology, and conversely reactive processes may show atypia. Mitotic activity may be more promi-nent in reactive than malignant processes. Architectural complexity with formation of papillae is usually a feature associated with neoplasia, especially in a pleural location (well differentiated papillary mesothelioma is a distinct clinico-pathological entity, un-related to asbestos exposure; see below, section on Benign low grade mesothelial prolif-erations). Entrapment of reactive mesothelial cells in fibrinous exudates, and tangen-tial cutting may simulate invasion;[8,13,23] examination of multiple levels may demonstrate that the 'invasive' component represents in-foldings of mesothelium, with connection to the surface. Genuine invasion is usually more extensive, with a 'raining down' pattern over a broad front, and is often associated with insinuation of malignant cells into adjacent structures, such as subpleural adipose tissue.[13,23]

Occasionally, in cases of mesothelioma a small biopsy may reveal only a benign mesothelial proliferation: this may occur if the biopsy site includes only the mesothelial reaction adjacent to the tumour. The sampling problems associated with small biopsies highlight the invaluable role of effusion cytology.[24] Nance *et al.*[25] found that combined cytology and biopsy slightly improved the sensitivity for a diagnosis of pleural malignancy.

Although a very rare phenomenon, an unusual potential diagnostic pitfall in biopsy specimens is the spread of mesothelial cells to lymph nodes in reactive conditions, particularly in the setting of chronic effusion and serosal inflammation, thus mimicking metastatic disease and prompting a diagnosis of metastatic mesothelioma.[26,27] Conversely, mesothelioma can present with lymph node metastases on rare occasions.

Ancillary studies

Several types of ancillary studies have been reported to assist in the distinction between benign and malignant mesothelial proliferations, and these include immunohistochemistry, proliferation markers, ploidy and cytogenetics. Most attention has focused on immunohistochemical staining for epithelial membrane antigen (EMA), with some reports indicating that human milk fat globule (HMFG) can be used in a similar fashion.[28]

Our experience is almost entirely with EMA and we have found this marker to be very useful for this distinction. Most of the remaining ancillary studies are, as yet, of unproven value. While EM can play a vital role in distinguishing mesothelioma from other tumours, it cannot definitively distinguish between benign and malignant mesothelial cells.

Epithelial membrane antigen (EMA)

EMA expression has been described on the surface membranes of a wide variety of normal epithelia. The first report of EMA expression by malignant, but not benign mesothelial cells was in 1981.[29] Subsequent studies appeared to confirm the role of EMA in the distinction between benign and malignant mesothelial cells,[30,31] but there have also been studies questioning its value in this setting.[32] In our experience, and in studies from several other centres, EMA has been shown to play an important role in distinguishing between benign and malignant mesothelial cells. Immunohistochemical staining for EMA is particularly useful in effusion cytology, where strong, thick, linear membrane staining of both single cells and cell aggregates is a reliable pointer to neoplasia (Figure 8.4).[11,33,34] A negative EMA result, however, cannot be used to exclude the diagnosis of mesothelioma. There is also a role for the use of EMA as a screening test in effusions in patients with a known history of asbestos exposure, or in effusions which appear to contain reactive mesothelial cells, but in which there is evidence of cell aggregation. Strong EMA staining in this setting, especially with a 'thick membrane' distribution[34] warrants re-evaluation of the cytological and clinical findings. Some reactive effusions may show weak EMA positivity in a small proportion of cell aggregates and single cells; this form of staining does not imply malignancy and should not be confused with the typical thick membrane staining seen in the majority of cells in malignant mesothelioma.

Positive EMA staining may be seen in plasma cells, and it is therefore essential to ensure that the EMA-positive cell population is mesothelial in nature.

Interpretation of EMA staining in biopsy specimens may be more difficult than in effusion cytology. Biopsy samples may only show strong membrane staining along the luminal aspect of the tumour, while the deeper invasive portion shows weak or negative staining.[33] As in effusion samples, strong membrane staining with EMA in a biopsy should not be dismissed, even if present only on surface cells.

Other potential markers of malignancy

Discussion of all of these potential markers is beyond the scope of this chapter; however, a few brief comments will be made regarding some of the more important recent findings.

p53

Immunostaining for p53 protein accumulation has been claimed to be of value in distinguishing mesothelioma from reactive mesothelial proliferations. Esposito et al.[35] investigated 20 mesothelial hyperplasias and 35 mesotheliomas in formalin-fixed paraffin-embedded biopsy material and found positive staining in 85.7% of neoplasms and no staining in any case of hyperplasia. No difference was detected in p53 expression within the different sub-types of mesothelioma and over-expression did not correlate significantly with survival. They concluded that p53 over-expression is a frequent feature of pleural mesothelioma and useful in routine distinction between malignant and non-neoplastic mesothelial proliferations. Other studies have reported similar findings, but generally with lesser frequencies of p53 positivity in the mesotheliomas. [36-39]

In contrast to these findings, Walts et al.[40] in a study examining benign mesothelial cells and adenocarcinoma cells in effusions, found staining for p53 in 73% of benign fluids. Stoetzer et al.[41] found that the sensitivity and specificity of p53 staining in malignant (not necessarily mesothelioma) effusions depends on the antibody used.

Mayall et al.[42] concluded that the frequency of p53 gene mutation in mesothelioma is probably unrelated to the effects of asbestos, and that p53 mutations occur during tumour progression rather than as an initiation event.

Although not yet established for use in a routine diagnostic setting, some studies indicate that there may be a possible future role for p53 immunohistochemistry in distinguishing benign from reactive mesothelial proliferations, particularly in cases where EMA staining is equivocal. However, in view of the finding of high rates of p53 positivity in benign fluids in some series, and our own experience that p53 is of little value in this setting, further studies are required before its use can be advocated in a diagnostic setting.

Proliferating cell nuclear antigen (PCNA)

Esposito *et al.*[43] found statistically significant differences for PCNA expression between malignant mesothelioma and mesothelial hyperplasia. A positive relationship was also found between the level of PCNA expression and overall survival of those affected by malignant mesothelioma. Ramael *et al.*[44] found differences in the percentage of PCNA-reactive cells in mesothelioma, reactive mesothelial cells and normal mesothelium.

Further studies are required to assess the potential role of PCNA in distinguishing benign from malignant mesothelial proliferations.

AgNORs (silver-positive nucleolar organising regions)

Distinguishing mesothelioma from reactive mesothelial hyperplasia through analysis of AgNORs has been undertaken with some success in tissue biopsy samples,[45] but overlap has been found between benign and malignant reference ranges.[46] Wolanski *et al.*[47] found that the average count of AgNORs/cell in malignant mesothelioma was elevated compared with benign mesothelial proliferations, but there was considerable overlap, and this form of analysis was considered to be of little value in distinguishing benign from malignant mesothelial processes. However, AgNOR *area* – especially when considered in conjunction with EMA staining – increased the sensitivity for the diagnosis of mesothelioma.

The labour-intensive nature and specialised requirements of AgNOR studies render them of limited value in a routine diagnostic laboratory.

Ploidy

Many mesotheliomas (39–78%) are diploid with a low S-phase fraction. The diploid profile may explain the lack of malignant nuclear characteristics in cases of well differentiated mesothelioma. For this reason ploidy studies often fail to distinguish between benign and malignant mesothelial proliferations,[48-50] although one study concluded that flow cytometry may have a role in distinguishing benign effusions from mesothelioma.[51] Overall, the usefulness of flow cytometry and ploidy studies in the diagnosis of mesothelioma is limited.

Cytogenetics

As yet, no specific non-random chromosomal alterations have been found to be consistently associated with malignant mesothelioma. Lee and Testa[52] concluded that the complex profile of somatic genetic changes characteristic of m esothelioma implicates a multistep process of tumorigenesis. The presence of multiple recurrent cytogenetic deletions suggests that loss and/or inactivation of tumour suppressor genes are critical to the development and progression of these tumours. Deletions of 1p, 3p, 6q, 9p and 22q are relatively common and these are thought to be likely loci of tumour suppressor genes important in the transformation process. Popescu *et al.*[53] reported that deletions involving 3p are the most common and non-random chromosomal alterations in mesothelioma and are either spontaneous or asbestos-induced lesions at vulnerable genomic sites. They suggest that 3p abnormalities may be causally related to the development of mesothelioma. More recently, Balsara et al.[54] identified a novel recurrent site of chromosomal loss in mesothelioma. Using cell lines and comparative genomic hybridisation, they demonstrated frequent deletion of a discrete segment in 15q, suggesting that this region harbours a putative tumour suppressor gene whose loss or inactivation may contribute to the pathogenesis of many mesotheliomas.

At this stage cytogenetic studies do not play a major role in the routine diagnosis of mesothelioma. The lack of specific non-random alterations means that cytogenetic analysis would not be useful in distinguishing mesothelioma from other malignancies. It is potentially useful in confirming malignancy in cases where the differential diagnosis is between reactive and malignant mesothelial proliferation, but the specialised technical requirements limit its usefulness in routine diagnostic practice.

Recommended approach to the difficult case/clinical correlation
(reactive mesothelial proliferation versus epithelioid malignant mesothelioma)

- Clinical follow-up with treatment of any potentially reversible cause of effusion. Resolution of effusion favours a benign process; persistence or recurrence of effusion demands further samples be submitted for cytological assessment, i.e., larger volume of fluid (as much as possible); larger volumes usually yield better diagnostic material.
- Obtaining different sample types, e.g., radiologically directed core biopsies if there is a mass present or pleuroscopy with directed biopsy may be of value.
- Consider mesothelioma in situ/atypical mesothelial proliferation (see below) if effusion contains malignant cells, but there is no mass present, i.e. 'false' false positve.
- The term 'atypical mesothelial cells' is sometimes used in effusion cytology; such terminology should be qualified; e.g., 'Atypical mesothelial cells are favoured to be reactive; however, definitive diagnosis is not possible'. Sometimes the uncertainty reflects an insufficient sample on which to perform ancillary studies such as EMA, and in these cases it is preferable to give a recommendation; e.g., 'If the effusion is re-tapped, send further samples for cytological assessment'.

Distinction between fibrous pleuritis and desmoplastic mesothelioma

This distinction represents one of the most challenging areas in mesothelioma diagnosis.

Cytology

Effusion cytology has a minimal role in the differential diagnosis between fibrous pleuritis and desmoplastic mesothelioma. This reflects the minimal shedding of malignant cells from these fibrous lesions into effusions. In rare cases atypical spindle cells may be recognised in effusion fluids, although this recognition is often retrospective following diagnosis by another modality, such as core or open biopsy.

There may be an absence of mesothelial cells and lymphocytosis in the effusions associated with sarcomatoid/desmoplastic mesothelioma.

Histology

In biopsy material, the desmoplastic variant of mesothelioma may have large areas that are composed of paucicellular collagenous tissue containing bland spindle cells, which mimic either a pleural plaque or reactive process. Conversely, reactive processes may be highly cellular and mitotically active (Figure 8.5).

Mangano *et al.*[55] described useful light microscopic features in distinguishing desmoplastic mesothelioma from fibrous pleuritis. These features include storiform regions or a 'patternless pattern' (see below), plus one or more of the following:

- invasion of chest wall tissues;
- foci of bland necrosis (with storiform/micronodular architecture);
- frankly sarcomatoid foci; and
- distant metastasis.

These features would appear to be useful, although their identification requires an adequate sample.

Figure 8.5. *Pleural biopsy. Fibrous pleuritis with vigorous spindle cell reaction. Masson trichrome stain.*

The term 'patternless pattern'[56] refers to randomly arranged bundles of collagen fibres, in contrast to the organised appearance with zonation and perpendicularly oriented capillaries associated with reactive processes.

Invasion can be highlighted by cytokeratin staining, but cytokeratin positivity alone cannot be used to distinguish reliably between reactive and malignant processes, because proliferating deep serosal cells express cytokeratins, including high molecular weight forms. Demonstration of invasion into fat, skeletal muscle or lung parenchyma requires a sample in which these tissues are present, but the presence of subtle invasion by malignant cells can be dramatically highlighted with keratin stains. Keratin staining may also reveal underlying lung parenchyma which has been invaded and effaced by tumour cells and therefore overlooked on routine H&E stains. The distinctive pattern of alveolar septal invasion is a useful marker of malignancy.[57] Invasion of lung parenchyma by desmoplastic mesothelioma may also produce an organising pneumonia-like appearance.

Another useful feature characteristic of a reactive process is that most cellular areas tend to be orientated toward the luminal side of the pleura, whereas the deeper tissues tend to be less cellular; the reverse pattern is seen in malignant cases. Perpendicularly orientated capillaries, almost completely traversing the thickened pleura, favour a reactive process.[58]

In desmoplastic mesothelioma the collagen occurs as interweaving bands that may be branched, whorled, micronodular or storiform, usually different from the laminar or 'basket-weave' pattern of benign plaques, or the orderly stratified zonal pattern of organising pleuritis.

Foci of necrosis, a useful feature of malignancy if present, must be distinguished from the fibrinous surface exudate which can be seen in both benign and malignant processes. Caution is also needed as mesothelioma and fibrous pleuritis may co-exist in the same biopsy.

Ancillary studies

Ancillary studies have a limited role in the distinction between fibrous pleuritis and desmoplastic mesothelioma.

EMA

Unlike surface epithelial lesions, where EMA is of diagnostic value, the role of EMA in distinguishing reactive fibroblastic processes from desmoplastic mesothelioma is negligible, as desmoplastic/sarcomatoid mesothelioma is generally EMA negative; occasionally, subtle epithelioid foci which are EMA positive may be highlighted.

Cytokeratins

Cytokeratin stains play an important role both in confirming invasion (see above), and in distinguishing this form of mesothelioma from other sarcomas and melanoma (although there are several keratin-positive sarcomas, including synovial sarcoma, which is often both keratin and EMA positive); almost all desmoplastic mesotheliomas are cytokeratin positive.

At this time, the distinction between fibrous pleuritis and mesothelioma is not achieved by extensive immunohistochemical panels.

Other potential markers of malignancy

p53

The role of p53 in the setting of distinguishing between desmoplastic mesothelioma and fibrous pleuritis was examined by Mangano *et al.*[55] They found that although positive staining was more common in mesothelioma, the difference was not statistically significant.

Proliferation markers, flow cytometry/ploidy and cytogenetics

The role of these ancillary studies has not as yet been specifically addressed in the setting of desmoplastic mesothelioma versus fibrous pleuritis.

Markers of mesothelial differentiation

Some of the more recently described positive mesothelial markers may play a future role in this area. Calretinin, a marker of mesothelial cells, is positive in both epithelioid mesothelioma and in some cases of sarcomatoid mesothelioma, although the frequency with which sarcomatoid mesotheliomas are positive varies between different studies. Information regarding a possible role for calretinin in the setting of fibrous pleuritis versus sarcomatoid mesothelioma is not available at this time.

Cytokeratin 5/6 is another mesothelial marker which has recently become commercially available (see Cytology section), but there is little information available in the literature regarding CK5/6 staining in sarcomatoid mesothelioma.

Electron microscopy

Electron microscopy has a limited role in distinguishing desmoplastic/sarcomatoid mesothelioma from fibrous pleuritis. The cells of sarcomatoid mesothelioma usually display only fibroblastic or myofibroblastic features, and similar appearances will be present in fibrous pleuritis. Occasionally, mesothelial characteristics such as desmosomes, tonofilaments or microvilli may be present in sarcomatoid mesothelioma.

Recommended approach to the difficult case/clinical correlation
(fibrous pleuritis versus desmoplastic mesothelioma)

·   Clinical/radiological correlation: in the presence of a destructive/invasive lesion on radiology, a biopsy regarded as 'probable' or 'suspicious' for desmoplastic mesothelioma may sometimes be enough to establish a diagnosis for treatment/ medico-legal purposes. Assessment by a radiologist with expertise in the diagnosis of thoracic and asbestos-associated diseases is important; radiology may also be useful in guiding core biopsy or other forms of biopsy to areas most likely to yield diagnostic material. The role of core biopsies in an obviously malignant clinical/radiological setting is twofold: to establish the diagnosis of desmoplastic mesothelioma if possible and also to exclude other primary or metastatic malignancies.

· Obtaining multiple cores to improve sampling and increase the likelihood of detecting overtly sarcomatous areas or invasion may be of use in some cases.

· In cases where core biopsies have suggested desmoplastic mesothelioma, but a definitive diagnosis is not possible, thorascopic directed biopsy or open (decortication) biopsy may be undertaken. In view of the lack of established/effective therapy for desmoplastic mesothelioma, the reasons for proceeding to this invasive diagnostic procedure should be seriously considered, and in some cases a 'waiting' policy may be adopted. The circumstances requiring diagnosis may sometimes be legal rather than medical.

· In cases where it is not possible to establish a histological diagnosis, clinical/radiological follow-up to document progression of disease, and repeat biopsies may be useful in establishing a definitive diagnosis. Henderson *et al.*[59] have proposed a modification of criteria put forward by Lilis[60] for the clinicopathological recognition of mesothelioma:

1. A history of past asbestos exposure.
2. A prolonged lag time, usually >20 years, between the first exposure to asbestos and the subsequent pleural disease.
3. Development of clinical symptoms of chest pain or dyspnoea over a short time interval of weeks or months.
4. Nodular opacities projecting from the pleura, especially if there is rapid progression of the radiological abnormalities.
5. Usually no clinical evidence of extra-thoracic disease at the time of presentation.
6. Tissue diagnosis on an adequate specimen.

The probability of mesothelioma remains high when the first five criteria are met, but the biopsy is inadequate for definitive diagnosis, although it may militate against the other major diagnosis in this setting, namely pseudomesotheliomatous carcinoma.

Mesothelioma in situ (atypical mesothelial proliferation)

We and others have come to recognise what is believed to be a pre-invasive neoplastic mesothelial proliferation, which has the characteristics of an in situ lesion.[8,61] At this stage, the concept of mesothelioma in situ/atypical mesothelial proliferation has not advanced to a point at which surgical or chemotherapeutic intervention can be instituted on the basis of this diagnosis, unless there is also evidence of associated invasive mesothelioma.

Histologically, mesothelioma in situ is characterised by a solid, linear, or more often papillary, surface growth of atypical mesothelial cells, which are EMA positive

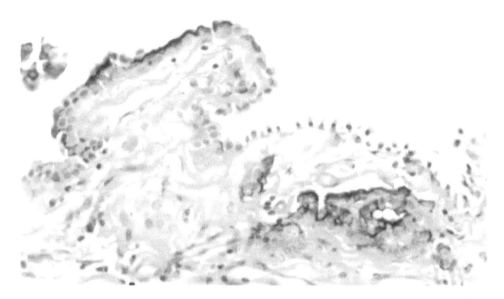

Figure 8.6. *Pleural biopsy. Transition between benign EMA-negative mesothelial cells and EMA-positive mesothelioma in situ, with a focus of invasive mesothelioma. H&E and EMA immunostain.*

(Figure 6). These lesions are often, although not always, found in patients with invasive disease and may be seen in close proximity to invasive malignant mesothelioma. This lesion can result in a 'false positive' diagnosis of mesothelioma; for example, there may be an effusion containing malignant cell clusters typical of mesothelioma, yet chest x-ray or CT scanning reveals no mass lesion. Mesothelioma in situ may have a characteristic pleuroscopic appearance of grains of sand. Distinction of mesothelioma in situ/atypical mesothelial proliferation from a hyperplastic lesion can be challenging. It has been shown that in contrast to benign proliferative mesothelial lesions these in situ/atypical lesions decorate strongly with EMA, as does invasive mesothelioma, thus helping to confirm the neoplastic nature of the cells (Figure 8.6).

Recommended approach/clinical correlation

- The importance of the recognition of this entity lies in the possible future development of interventional/'preventative' therapies, i.e. to allow treatment at the earliest detectable stage of disease; however, with our current knowledge there are insufficient data for treatment to be instituted on the basis of a diagnosis of mesothelioma in situ/atypical mesothelial proliferation.

- The existence of an in situ stage (stage 0) may provide a possible explanation for 'malignant cells' in effusions, where there is no clinical evidence of a tumour mass, i.e. no measurable disease; it may also explain long-term survival in such cases.

Malignant mesothelioma

Historically, it has been argued that accurate diagnosis of mesothelioma is possible only at post-mortem examination.[62] While this view now seems extreme, there are a number of potential pitfalls in the diagnosis of malignant mesothelioma, and studies have demonstrated poor interobserver agreement in mesothelioma diagnosis, particularly in small samples such as closed needle biopsies.[63]

Traditionally, invasive mesothelioma has been subclassified into the major categories of epithelioid (epithelial), biphasic and sarcomatoid, any of which may be desmoplastic. Epithelioid tumours account for approximately 60%, biphasic tumours approximately 30%, and sarcomatoid tumours approximately 10% of mesotheliomas.[33]

In addition, there are rare subtypes of mesothelioma including lymphohistiocytoid, small cell and deciduoid mesothelioma, as well as other mesothelial lesions which are generally benign and predominantly associated with the peritoneum.

There are a number of difficulties associated with the accurate subclassification of mesothelioma, although these are generally not of great clinical significance. Some of these difficulties include:

- Distinguishing poorly differentiated epithelioid mesothelioma from sarcomatoid mesothelioma.
- Distinguishing reactive from malignant spindle cells in the diagnosis of biphasic tumours; i.e., an epithelioid mesothelioma which has a florid fibroblastic stroma may mimic a biphasic tumour.
- When only small biopsy samples are obtained, the sample may not be representative of all areas, leading to differences in diagnosis between different sample types, e.g., thin core versus open biopsy.
- The nature of the specimen may determine how the tumour is subclassified, e.g., if the sample submitted is pleural fluid alone, biphasic tumours may be diagnosed as epithelioid, as the sarcomatoid component will generally shed minimal or no material and remain undetected.

The clinical value and significance of mesothelioma subclassification and grading is controversial due to the poor prognosis associated with all categories. Sarcomatoid mesothelioma appears to have a worse prognosis when compared with epithelioid mesothelioma (mean survival for epithelioid, mixed and sarcomatoid: 13, 10.2 and 5.8 months, respectively).[64] The majority of patients surviving more than 2 years have epithelioid or biphasic histology.[65] Beer et al.[66] found spindle versus epithelioid histology to be a useful prognostic marker, with significantly shorter survival for patients with the spindle cell (sarcomatoid) subtype of mesothelioma.

Recently, interest has focused on the potential for different responses to treatment by the different subtypes of mesothelioma; however, the difficulties associated with accurate subtyping discussed previously – limited sampling, different sample types and interobserver differences – should be recognised when such correlations are made, to avoid flawed conclusions.

Recognition of the various histological subtypes of mesothelioma is probably of greatest importance in avoiding potential errors in the differential diagnoses associated with the diverse growth patterns of mesothelioma; these are discussed in greater detail below.

Epithelioid mesothelioma

Distinction between epithelioid mesothelioma and adenocarcinoma has been, and remains, the subject of numerous publications dating back over several decades. The current approach, using histochemistry and immunohistochemical panels, facilitates the diagnosis in the vast majority of cases, although there is a subset of difficult cases, in which ultrastructural assessment may still be required.

Controversy remains as to which immunohistochemical markers are of greatest value[67] although there is general acceptance that distinction between mesothelioma and adenocarcinoma requires the use of a panel of antibodies rather than reliance on a single immunohistochemical result. The component antibodies included in these panels are undergoing change, with the recent commercial availability of several novel antibodies positive in mesothelioma (see below).

Effusion cytology

Approximately 60% of mesotheliomas can be diagnosed on morphological grounds in effusion specimens; 20% require additional ancillary studies (immunohistochemistry or EM) and 20% are undiagnosable by cytology, either due to inadequacy of the sample or the poorly differentiated nature of the tumour. We advocate the routine use of ancillary immunohistochemical studies in all cases.

The macroscopic appearance of the fluid sample (e.g., highly viscous) may reflect a high hyaluronic acid content and suggest mesothelioma even before microscopic assessment. Several studies have found quantifying hyaluronic acid levels to be of value in the diagnosis of mesothelioma, with high levels seen in mesotheliomatous effusions.[68-70]

In effusion specimens there are morphological (both architectural and cytological) features which may point to either adenocarcinoma or mesothelioma, some requiring assessment in cell-block preparations.[15]

Some of these useful microscopic features include:

·   The presence of a benign mesothelial population plus a 'foreign' population; this combination favours adenocarcinoma. In mesothelioma there may be a spectrum of mesothelial cells with transitional forms between bland and malignant.

·   The structure of the aggregates: smooth contoured aggregates are seen in adenocarcinoma while solid aggregates, with a 'mulberry'-like configuration and papillary architecture, characterise mesothelioma. These features are also reflected in cell-block preparations, in which hollow centres within aggregates favour adenocarcinoma, whereas collagen stromal cores are seen in mesothelioma.

- A columnar cell morphology favours adenocarcinoma.
- Eccentric nuclei favour adenocarcinoma.
- Dense cytoplasm with abundant peripheral glycogen favours mesothelioma.
- Cell-to-cell apposition with a window-like gap favours mesothelioma.
- Small squamous-like orangiophilic cells in the background favour mesothelioma over adenocarcinoma, although squamous cell carcinoma may need to be considered.
- Hyaluronic acid vacuoles are occasionally present and are strongly predictive of mesothelioma. Hyaluronic acid may also be seen in the background of smears.

Histology

Distinguishing between mesothelioma and adenocarcinoma in biopsy specimens presents similar problems to those encountered in cytological specimens. Often, the morphological clues present in a cytology specimen are not as easily recognised in biopsy material, particularly in small or distorted samples. The diagnostic sensitivity of a small biopsy is less than that of an effusion specimen, as the latter reflects cell shedding from a total serosal surface bathed in fluid. Classical features of well differentiated epithelial mesothelioma in biopsy material include tubulo-papillary or tubular configurations; papillary formations with connective tissue cores may project into large tubular structures. A microcystic architecture is sometimes present. Psammoma bodies are present in 5–10% of cases and represent a non-specific finding. The lining cells are usually cuboidal, and, as in effusion samples, the presence of cells with a columnar morphology is more suggestive of adenocarcinoma. Nuclei are often very bland. Less differentiated tumours may consist partly or wholly of sheets of cells without tubular or papillary patterns. These cells may show lack of cohesion, another useful discriminant from adenocarcinoma.[71]

Ancillary studies

Distinction between mesothelioma and adenocarcinoma is reliant on ancillary studies, with histochemical and immunohistochemical panels currently proving the most reliable and cost-effective approach. There is still a role for electron microscopy, but in a limited capacity and generally restricted to primary diagnosis in cases in which medico-legal issues arise or where there are atypical features or discrepant immunohistochemical findings, such as positivity for a glandular marker in a case which otherwise has mesothelial features. Ideally, cases included in clinical trials should be thoroughly assessed, including electron microscopy. Particular forms of adenocarcinomas may closely mimic mesothelioma in their clinical presentation, morphology and immunohistochemical profile, e.g., ovarian or primary peritoneal adenocarcinomas and metastatic renal carcinoma; EM has a diagnostic role in these settings (see below).

Histochemistry

Mucin histochemistry is routinely used to distinguish mesothelioma from adenocarcinoma, and when positive is very useful in establishing a diagnosis of adenocarcinoma (see also section on Uncommon/unusual diagnostic issues). The most reliable and commonly used stain for the demonstration of neutral mucin is PAS positive diastase. Approximately 60–75% of pulmonary adenocarcinomas produce mucin.

Some 20–55% of epithelial mesotheliomas contain hyaluronic acid. This can be demonstrated by performing Alcian blue or colloidal iron stains for acidic mucins. We do not routinely stain for acidic mucins as the water-solubility of hyaluronic acid means that it is often not found.

Immunohistochemistry

Markers negative in mesothelioma (exclusionary markers)

Since the value of carcinoembryonic antigen (CEA) as a negative marker of mesothelioma was first described in 1979,[72] the role of immunohistochemistry has expanded dramatically in this area of pathology. Most laboratories have devised a standard panel of immunohistochemical markers which aid in the differential diagnosis between mesothelioma and adenocarcinoma, and which ideally will have been technically optimised *within* that laboratory. The importance of close attention to methodology is highlighted by Wick,[73] who points out that discrepant results in the literature may be sometimes explained by methodological differences between laboratories.

Antibody panels can be applied to both cytological (usually cell-block) material and biopsy specimens. Until recently, such panels have tended to be based on antibodies which label membrane-related glycoproteins present in glandular epithelium, and generally absent in mesothelioma; these include CEA, Ber-EP4, B72.3, CD15, BG-8 and MOC-31. The literature contains numerous studies comparing the role and value of these markers, with various recommendations for different combinations as having greater specificity and sensitivity. The importance of using panels rather than single antibodies is recognised in most studies.[74–79]

Wick *et al.*[80] found that positive labelling with 2 out of 3 of the antibodies to CEA, CD15 (LeuM1) and B72.3 appears to exclude a diagnosis of mesothelioma.

MOC-31 is a monoclonal antibody which has recently become commercially available; there are studies indicating that it represents another valuable exclusionary marker,[81,82] but there are reports of low specificity in some studies.[83] In our experience this marker is of low specificity, with up to 39% of proven mesotheliomas staining positively; this appears to occur in the same group of mesotheliomas that demonstrate Ber-EP4 positivity (up to 28%).

Newer exclusionary antibodies such as thyroid transcription factor-1 (TTF-1)[84] and E-cadherin[85-87] are still undergoing assessment and are not yet utilised in most standard panels.

It is worth noting that some studies address only the differential diagnosis between mesothelioma and adenocarcinoma of *pulmonary* origin; the findings in such studies cannot be extrapolated to metastatic adenocarcinomas from other sites.

Our approach to diagnosis in cases that show equivocal results by immunohistochemistry is to proceed to electron microscopy. If there is no tissue specifically set aside for EM, material for analysis can be retrieved from paraffin blocks. In our experience ultrastructural assessment is of greater diagnostic value than performing additional immunohistochemical studies.

Markers positive in mesothelioma

Over recent years, antibodies have been produced which demonstrate positive staining in mesothelioma; however, most of these have not been commercially available.[88-91]

In the past, standard antibody panels have relied on an absence of staining for diagnosis, i.e., accumulation of negative immunostaining results to make the diagnosis of mesothelioma (diagnosis by exclusion); however, these newer antibodies are positive in mesothelioma. Antibodies effective in formalin-fixed, paraffin-embedded material, and which show positive staining in mesothelial cells are now available commercially; their potential role in clinical laboratories in a diagnostic setting is currently being more fully assessed. However, as with any new antibody, studies performed subsequent to initial enthusiastic reports have sometimes shown lower sensitivity and specificity than originally claimed. The ideal marker would label malignant mesothelial cells only; such a marker is not available and most of these newer antibodies will stain both benign and malignant mesothelial cells, and therefore cannot be used in isolation.

There is the potential for reducing the number of exclusionary antibodies included in standard panels, by the inclusion of one or more positive markers. Some of the more important newer antibodies, positive in mesothelioma, are briefly discussed below.

Positive markers which show promise (CK5/6 and calretinin)

CK5/6

Pulmonary adenocarcinomas exhibit a simple epithelial type of cytokeratin expression, characterised by cytokeratins 7, 8, 18 and 19 expression. Squamous carcinomas express cytokeratins 5 and 6 in addition to the simple epithelial-types of cytokeratin. Mesothelial cells (both normal and neoplastic) also express simple epithelial cytokeratins as well as cytokeratin 5, the latter not being expressed by pulmonary adenocarcinomas. This finding was first reported by Moll *et al.*[92] in 1989. They observed that cytokeratin 5 could be a useful marker to distinguish between these malignancies; however, the antibody used did not react in formalin-fixed, paraffin-embedded tissues. Recently, Clover *et al.*[93] used a commercially obtained monoclonal antibody to CK5/6 to demonstrate reactivity with all of the epithelial mesotheliomas examined (sarcomatoid or desmoplastic areas showed absent or weak staining). Only 5 out of 27 pulmonary adenocarcinomas showed any positivity (four of these cases showed weak or equivocal staining and one case showed focal staining only). Ordonez[94] reported 40 mesotheliomas positive and 30 pulmonary adenocarcinomas negative for CK5/6. Focal or weak positivity was seen in 14/93 non-pulmonary adenocarcinomas (10/30 ovarian, 2/10 endometrial, 1/18 breast, 0/10 kidney, 0/10 colonic and 0/87 prostatic). Fifteen out of fifteen lung squamous cell carcinomas were positive, as were 6/12 transitional cell carcinomas metastatic to lung, and 3/5 large cell undifferentiated carcinomas of lung.

Although only relatively few studies have been reported to date, CK5/6 appears to be a promising positive marker for mesothelioma, particularly useful in the distinction from pulmonary adenocarcinoma.

Calretinin

Calretinin is a calcium-binding protein of 29 kDa. The gene is expressed in central and peripheral neural tissues. In non-neural tissues strong and consistent immunoreactivity is seen in normal and reactive mesothelial cells, and calretinin is also expressed in eccrine glands, adipocytes, and keratinising thymic epithelial cells. In mesothelial cells there is both nuclear and cell membrane staining (Figure 8.7), although some studies describe only membrane and cytoplasmic staining.[95] Positivity for calretinin has been claimed to be a feature of the sarcomatoid component of biphasic and pure sarcomatoid mesothelioma by some authors,[96] but others have failed to confirm this observation.[97]

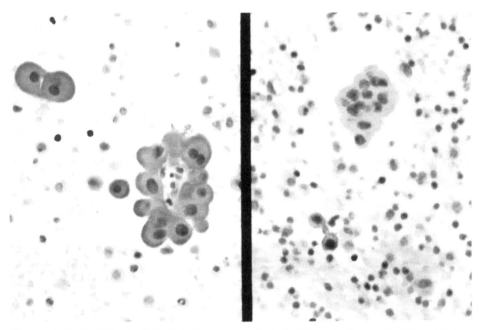

Figure 8.7. *Cell block. Calretinin immunostain.* Left: *Mesothelioma. Positive staining.* Right: *Adenocarcinoma. Negative staining in malignant cells. Positive staining in benign mesothelial cells.*

A study by Riera *et al.*[98] which showed reduced sensitivity and specificity for calretinin has been explained by Ordonez[67] as being attributable to differences in the antibodies used.

Calretinin has been described as the most sensitive and specific marker of mesothelial differentiation applicable to histologic and cytologic materials.[99]

In our experience in cell-block material from pleural effusion samples, both calretinin and CK5/6 show reliable positive staining in both benign and malignant mesothelial cells. The staining is generally strong with a clean background, and easily interpretable. Cases of metastatic breast, ovarian and lung carcinoma in pleural fluid were all negative for both of these markers in the malignant cell population; the background benign mesothelial cells provide a useful internal positive control (Figure 8.7).

Other positive mesothelial markers, probably of less value

HBME-1

HBME-1 is a mouse monoclonal antibody raised against a suspension of cells from a human mesothelioma cell line.[100] The antibody reacts with an epitope present in mesothelial microvilli in normal and malignant mesothelial cells. Reports of its value are somewhat conflicting, but several studies have concluded that due to overlapping staining patterns between mesotheliomas and adenocarcinomas, the specificity of HBME-1 is too low to be of practical value in this differential diagnosis.[101-103] In addition HBME-1 has been reported to react with some sarcomas and lymphomas.[104]

We have found that it is important to use HBME-1 at high dilution (in the range of about 1:5000 to 1:15 000); when used at too great a concentration (e.g., 1:50 to 1:100), it labels an unacceptably high proportion of carcinomas and it is desirable for laboratories using HBME-1 to carry out titration studies to ascertain the optimal dilution. In addition poorly differentiated mesotheliomas may be negative with HBME-1.

Thrombomodulin

Thrombomodulin is a transmembrane glycoprotein expressed by mesothelial cells, endothelial cells (preferentially by lymphatic endothelium), mesangial cells and placental syncytiotrophoblast. It exerts anticoagulant activity by activation of protein C. Its role in distinguishing adenocarcinoma from mesothelioma is controversial, with conflicting reports regarding its sensitivity and specificity;[74] however, some recent studies have concluded that thrombomodulin is sufficiently sensitive and specific to warrant inclusion in standard panels.[102-105] Difficulties in interpretation of staining can result from the positivity of endothelial cells for thrombomodulin.

Cadherins

Cadherins are a group of adhesion proteins that play an important role in the sorting of cells into specialised tissues during morphogenesis. There are several distinctive members of the cadherin family.[106] In the setting of distinction between mesothelioma and adenocarcinoma, N-(nerve) cadherin and E-(epithelial) cadherin are of importance, as N-cadherin is expressed in mesothelial cells and E-cadherin is expressed by epithelial cells of the lung. Preliminary studies appear to indicate a possible role for these antibodies in a diagnostic setting, although larger studies are needed.[86,87] We have not found this group of antibodies to be of diagnostic value, with E-cadherin staining all 29 mesotheliomas examined.

Of note, N-cadherin, which is positive in mesothelioma, is also positive in papillary serous and endometrioid carcinomas of the ovary, tumours which may enter the differential diagnosis of mesothelioma. However, the ovarian tumours are also positive for E-cadherin.[107]

CD44H

Malignant mesotheliomas are known to produce hyaluronic acid, in contrast to most pulmonary adenocarcinomas, which produce neutral mucin. CD44H (also known as CD44S) is the major cell surface receptor for hyaluronic acid. CD44H is expressed in both mesothelioma and mesothelial hyperplasia, and in a proportion of adenocarcinomas; some studies advocate the use of CD44H as a possible discriminator between mesothelioma and adenocarcinoma;[108] however, other authors have found the difference in staining between mesothelioma and adenocarcinoma only approached statistical significance.[109] Filie *et al.*[110] comment in a letter that the sensitivity and specificity are too low for this marker to have a practical use in the diagnosis of mesothelioma.

Wilms' tumour 1 gene (WT1)

The WT1 gene, a tumour suppressor gene located on chromosome 11p13, has been the subject of investigation with regard to its role in the development and pathogenesis of mesothelioma. Antibodies to the WT1 protein have been used both in frozen and in formalin-fixed, paraffin-embedded tissue,[111,112] but as yet there are insufficient published data to assess the future role of this antibody.

Parathyroid hormone related protein (PTHrP)

PTHrP is produced by many cancers and causes hypercalcaemia in malignancy. This protein has been demonstrated in malignant mesothelioma, but there are conflicting results regarding its expression in normal or reactive mesothelium. Relatively small numbers of pulmonary adenocarcinomas have shown positive staining; its potential role in distinguishing benign from malignant mesothelial proliferations, and in distinguishing mesothelioma from adenocarcinoma, is still being assessed.[113]

In summary, an approach using a panel of antibodies is necessary in the differential diagnosis of mesothelioma and adenocarcinoma. The International Mesothelioma Panel recommends inclusion of two positive markers for mesothelial cells and at least two exclusionary markers (positive in adenocarcinoma and negative in mesothelioma). Of the newer markers positive in mesothelioma, CK5/6 and calretinin appear to show the most promise, although it is still early in their assessment. Useful exclusionary markers include CEA, CD15, B72.3 and BG-8.

EM is the most useful ancillary test in cases where there are inconclusive or aberrant immunohistochemical findings.

Electron microscopy (EM)

Electron microscopy is of particular value in effusion samples, where there is usually abundant material available and clotted specimens can be set aside in glutaraldehyde, for ultrastructural assessment if needed. This ensures well preserved material and is not prone to the sampling problem which occurs in trying to divide small biopsy samples. If necessary, biopsy material can be examined by extraction from paraffin block material.

The role of EM in mesothelioma diagnosis has been controversial; it is considered by some to be the 'gold standard'[114] while others have claimed it to be of little or no value.[115,116] We have found EM to play an important role in the diagnosis of mesothelioma; however, with increasing emphasis on immunohistochemistry, the use of EM has generally declined due to perceived costs, availability of tissue, need for special preparation and technical expertise, and delay in obtaining results. It still plays an important role in cases in which immunohistochemical techniques fail to make a firm diagnosis. Cases included in clinical trials should ideally be confirmed by EM. In a recent editorial, Comin *et al.*[117] suggest the following as some of the guidelines for the use of EM in the differential diagnosis of mesothelioma:

- As a minimum, EM should be used for the differential diagnosis of epithelial mesothelioma when 1. the sample is small (e.g., those that are predominantly cytologic in character, including cell-block preparations); 2. the histologic appearances are atypical; or 3. there are discordant immunohistochemical findings.

Table 8.1. Comparison of features of mesothelioma and adenocarcinoma.

	Mesothelioma	**Adenocarcinoma**
Microvilli	Numerous, long, slender, sinuous, branching; luminal and abluminal	Less abundant, short and straight; luminal
Glycocalyx	Absent	Present
Microvillus core rootlets Terminal filamentous web	Absent	May be present
Secretory products	Hyaluronic acid (crystalloids, scroll-like structures in neolumen)	Mucous granules (60–75%) Lamellar bodies
Intermediate filaments	Abundant tonofibrillar bundles; perinuclear; insert into large desmosomes	May be present, usually less abundant than mesothelioma
Cellular junctions	Giant desmosomes may be present (>1 micron)	Giant desmosomes infrequent
Microvillus:stromal collagen interdigitation	Present	Absent

• EM has no role to play in the distinction between reactive mesothelial hyperplasia and mesothelioma.

Ultrastructural features useful in distinguishing adenocarcinoma from mesothelioma are presented in the Table 8.1.[33,118-120] These features are most easily recognised in well differentiated tumours.

Uncommon/unusual differential diagnostic issues: epithelioid mesothelioma

In the presence of adequate cytological or histological material, and reliable immuno-histochemistry and EM, there are relatively small numbers of cases where the distinction between mesothelioma and adenocarcinoma (or other tumours) remains difficult. Some of these differential diagnostic problems are discussed below.

Mesothelioma versus peritoneal and ovarian serous carcinomas

The histological distinction between epithelial peritoneal mesothelioma and papillary serous carcinoma diffusely involving the peritoneum may be difficult.[59,121] Metastasis of serous carcinoma to the pleural cavity may produce the same difficulties.[59] The distinction between mesothelioma and serous carcinoma is important in view of the important role of combination chemotherapy in the treatment of serous carcinomas, with potential long-term survival.[59] In distinguishing mesothelioma and serous carcinoma, the role of mucin stains is important, as some serous carcinomas will be positive.[122] However, mucin may not be detectable, and CEA is positive in only a minority of cases of serous carcinoma.[123,124] Panels of antibodies and EM may be useful in this setting. Khoury *et al.*[125] found that antibodies to CEA, CD15 and B72.3 were most useful in making the distinction, between serous carcinoma and mesothelioma, while Ordonez[126] recently examined panels of antibodies in the differential diagnosis of mesothelioma and serous carcinoma, and concluded that in this setting calretinin, thrombomodulin and keratin 5/6 are the best positive markers of mesothelioma, and MOC-31, B72.3, BerEp4, CA19-9 and LeuM1 are the best negative markers. In our experience B72.3 and Ber-EP4 are useful markers in distinguishing serous carcinomas (positive) from mesothelioma (negative).

EM distinction is based primarily on differences in microvilli, which are straight and generally short in serous carcinomas, versus long and wavy in mesothelioma; although long microvilli may be present in serous carcinomas, they are straighter and appear more rigid than the sinuous microvilli of mesotheliomas, and they usually possess an antennular glycocalyx.[59]

There are reports of malignant mesothelioma presenting as ovarian masses[127]; not surprisingly these cases were often initially misdiagnosed by the referring pathologist.

In view of the overlapping morphological appearances of serous carcinoma and mesothelioma, the diagnosis of mesothelioma in women always requires consideration of the possibility of genital tract malignancy in the differential diagnosis.

Large cell undifferentiated epithelioid malignancy involving the pleura

This term encompasses a problem group of primary and secondary malignant tumours involving the pleura in which the undifferentiated nature of the malignant cells means that distinction between mesothelioma and carcinoma may not be possible. These neoplasms will label with cytokeratins; however, neither glandular nor mesothelial markers are expressed. The ultrastructural features seen in well differentiated mesotheliomas and carcinomas are not present to enable distinction by EM. Definitive diagnosis in such cases is not possible.

Pseudomesotheliomatous (adeno)carcinoma of lung

This is a clinical and radiological mimic of mesothelioma that may also present pathological diagnostic problems. Some adenocarcinomas (and occasionally other primary carcinomas) of the lung may show diffuse infiltration of the pleura, in the form of plaques, nodules or a confluent rind, identical in macroscopic appearance to mesothelioma. These tumours usually have a small peripheral lung component which may be overlooked.[128-131] A subset of these tumours may also resemble mesothelioma in their histological appearance, with papillary, tubulopapillary or biphasic patterns of growth. The presence of neutral mucin has been emphasised in establishing a diagnosis of adenocarcinoma in this setting;[130] however, in view of the possibility of mucin-positive mesotheliomas[114] (see below), immunohistochemistry, and often EM, are essential in establishing the diagnosis in these cases. The prognosis for pseudomesotheliomatous adenocarcinoma is similar to that of mesothelioma, with a reported mean survival of 4.7 months.[130]

Localised mesothelioma

The diffuse growth pattern of mesothelioma can be useful in clinical and radiological diagnosis. However, in addition to the occasional mimicry of this diffuse growth pattern by adenocarcinoma (see above), there are instances where mesotheliomas grow as a localised mass. This pattern of growth has been described both in the pleura and the mediastinum, and has been observed in epithelial, biphasic and desmoplastic subtypes.[132-134] Knowledge of this unusual growth pattern should prompt consideration of mesothelioma when the histology fits the diagnosis of mesothelioma, but the radiological findings suggest other diagnoses. It also highlights the potential for confusion between mesothelioma and synovial sarcoma, as the localised growth pattern of the latter is an important feature in this differential diagnosis (see Biphasic mesothelioma section). Very rare cases of diffuse synovial sarcoma may also occur.

Mucin positive mesothelioma/glandular-marker positive mesothelioma

Some 60–70% of pulmonary adenocarcinomas produce epithelial mucin, a finding which is useful in the differential diagnosis with mesothelioma. In mesothelioma, stains for neutral mucin are generally negative, but acidic mucin as detected by Alcian blue staining may be present. However, there are small numbers of mesotheliomas which demonstrate staining for epithelial mucin;[114,135] in some of these tumours pre-treatment with hyaluronidase will abolish staining, but in other cases staining persists despite such pre-treatment.

A small proportion of mesotheliomas will stain positively (often weakly and focally) with one or more of the commonly used glandular markers (LeuM1, CEA, BerEP4), often in hyaluronate-rich cases.[57,136,137] Such findings highlight the importance of using panels of antibodies. The CEA staining that has been described in isolated cases of mesothelioma is a coarse granular cytoplasmic staining, which contrasts with the usual homogeneous staining of adenocarcinomas.[138] These glandular-marker positive cases can usually be correctly diagnosed by means of EM.[118]

It should be noted that glandular differentiation as identified by epithelial mucin or positive glandular markers is a relatively uncommon finding in mesothelioma and most pathologists will only encounter such variants on rare occasions.

Epithelioid vascular tumours of the serous membranes versus mesothelioma

Vascular tumours primarily involving the serous membranes are rare and often aggressive tumours and include the entities of epithelioid haemangioendothelioma and epithelioid angiosarcoma. The clinical and radiological picture (diffuse involvement of pleural, peritoneal or pericardial cavities) may closely mimic mesothelioma (and metastatic adenocarcinoma) and the similarity often extends to the histological appearances, where tubulo-papillary growth patterns may be prominent in some cases. Some tumours may demonstrate a biphasic pattern with both spindled and epithelioid areas, resembling biphasic mesothelioma. Abortive vessel formation and intra-cytoplasmic lumina containing red blood cells may be useful morphological clues to the vascular nature of the process.

Immunohistochemistry and/or EM are generally required to establish the diagnosis. CD31 staining in carcinomas and mesotheliomas is rare[139] and the use of this antibody, in combination with the generally weak or negative keratin staining seen in these vascular lesions, should enable the correct diagnosis.

Negative staining for glandular markers can heighten the similarity to mesothelioma, if a vascular lesion is not considered. Lin *et al.*[140] suggest that demonstration of immunoreactivity for two or more endothelial markers is essential in confirming the diagnosis.

We have seen a case of epithelioid haemangioendothelioma in a patient with a strong history of asbestos exposure, in which the tumour encased the lung in a rind-like fashion, highlighting how closely these tumours can mimic mesothelioma on clinical and radiological grounds. These vascular tumours are not associated with asbestos exposure. The prognosis of these tumours is generally poor with most patients surviving less than 12 months.

Biphasic mesothelioma

This form of mesothelioma, said to have behaviour intermediate between epithelial and sarcomatoid mesothelioma, is composed of both epithelioid and sarcomatoid elements, requiring at least 10% of either component for the diagnosis. Essentially this tumour can be considered together with the epithelial form of mesothelioma, and its main importance lies in the extensive differential diagnosis which must be considered when a biphasic tumour is seen within the pleura.

Mesothelioma is certainly the most common biphasic tumour in this site however, various tumours metastatic to the serosal surfaces may have a biphasic appearance. These include carcinosarcomas and sarcomatoid (spindle cell) carcinomas. Carcinosarcomas of the lung may involve the pleura either by metastasis or direct extension. Of particular note is sarcomatoid renal cell carcinoma; pleural metastasis of this tumour may be indistinguishable from mesothelioma by light microscopy and immunohistochemistry.

Metastatic melanoma may have epithelioid and spindle cell components, but clinical history, together with immunohistochemistry and/or EM, should enable the correct diagnosis.

Synovial sarcoma may be primary or secondary within the pleura. Important discriminators between this entity and mesothelioma include the usually younger age at presentation and lack of asbestos exposure in patients with synovial sarcoma. Circumscription and pseudoencapsulation are often seen in synovial sarcoma, with some cases even having a pedunculated appearance. In addition, the epithelial component of synovial sarcoma will often contain PAS positive, diastase-resistant material and stain with glandular markers such as Ber-EP4. Nicholson *et al.*[141] have recently commented on positive bcl-2 staining in the sarcomatous elements of pleural synovial sarcoma which may be of value in distinguishing this lesion from mesothelioma. In addition, many synovial sarcomas express CD99 but they are generally negative for CD34.[142] EM, together with the characteristic t(x;18)(p11.2;q11.2) chromosomal abnormality seen in synovial sarcoma, may also be useful in establishing the diagnosis.[143,144]

Other tumours which may rarely present in the pleura and have a biphasic appearance include neurogenic tumours such as malignant peripheral nerve sheath tumours,[145] desmoplastic small round cell tumour[146] and vascular tumours.

Sarcomatoid mesothelioma

Sarcomatoid mesothelioma is composed of keratin positive malignant spindle cells, sometimes associated with extensive collagen deposition. The term 'desmoplastic mesothelioma' is arbitrarily applied when >50% of the tumour is composed of hypocellular fibrous tissue.[57] Desmoplastic mesotheliomas comprise 5–10% of mesotheliomas and are usually pleura-based and sarcomatoid, but they may be biphasic or epithelioid.[147] The diagnosis of desmoplastic mesothelioma can be challenging, representing one of the most difficult areas in mesothelioma pathology. The diagnosis is highly dependent on sampling, often requiring thoracoscopic or open biopsy, which should preferably include adjacent tissues (skeletal muscle, fat) for assessment of invasion.

Although probably of little clinical relevance, distinction between poorly differentiated epithelioid mesothelioma and sarcomatoid mesothelioma can be difficult and there is often poor interobserver agreement in this area.

Cytokeratin-negative sarcomatoid mesotheliomas are said to exist and are diagnosed on the basis of their anatomical distribution, with a rind-like growth pattern. Cytokeratin-positive sarcomatoid mesotheliomas with various forms of heterologous differentiation (e.g., malignant fibrous histiocytoma, chondrosarcoma or osteosarcoma) are accepted as mesotheliomas, but tumours differentiating as pure liposarcoma, angiosarcoma or rhabdomyosarcoma are not recognised as mesothelioma. These are purely definitional distinctions.

Cytokeratin expression by a serosal-based sarcomatoid tumour is generally good evidence for the diagnosis of sarcomatoid mesothelioma, but the importance of clinical findings, e.g., the presence of an extrapleural primary tumour, cannot be overemphasised in this setting, because metastasis from tumours such as sarcomatoid renal cell carcinoma may be indistinguishable from sarcomatoid mesothelioma by light microscopy and immunohistochemistry.

Another spindle cell proliferation which may occur in the lung as a pleural based lesion, or in the serosal cavities (particularly the peritoneum), is inflammatory myofibroblastic tumour (also known as inflammatory pseudotumour, plasma cell granuloma, and numerous other names). These lesions are myofibroblastic proliferations associated with inflammatory infiltrates. Controversy exists as to whether they represent inflammatory/reactive processes or neoplasms, and the term probably encompasses a spectrum of lesions.[148] The clinical and radiological findings are usually different from those of mesothelioma, and the spindle cells in these myofibroblastic lesions are generally keratin negative.

Solitary fibrous tumours (previously known as pleural fibroma, localised (solitary) mesothelioma, submesothelial fibroma and localised fibrous mesothelioma) also demonstrate gross, histological and immunohistochemical features distinct from those of sarcomatoid mesothelioma, and they do not usually pose a significant problem in differential diagnosis. Solitary fibrous tumours were originally considered to be of mesothelial origin, derived from sub-mesothelial stromal cells. The term 'mesothelioma' has been discarded in the current terminology, as these tumours have been described in almost all sites in the body and are not of mesothelial origin.[149-151]

Malignant forms of this tumour, in pleural and other locations are described.[152,153]

Solitary fibrous tumour occurring in the pleura can usually be distinguished from sarcomatoid mesothelioma by its localisation (and often pedunculation), its varied but usually distinctive histological patterns, and its immunohistochemical profile (negative for cytokeratins and positive for CD34); bcl-2 is expressed in solitary fibrous tumours, but not in sarcomatoid mesothelioma and this finding has also been claimed to be of value in making the distinction between these tumours.[154] Solitary fibrous tumours also express CD99.[155]

Rare histological variants of mesothelioma

Mesothelioma is notorious for its diverse growth patterns, possibly related to its meso-dermal derivation. In addition to the more common subtypes, there are several rare variants, which are briefly discussed below.

Small cell mesothelioma

The small cell variant of mesothelioma is rare, but is important in view of the potential for misdiagnosis as small cell carcinoma. By analogy with desmoplastic mesothelioma, at least 50% of the tumour should display a small cell morphology to qualify for inclusion in this category. The 13 cases described by Mayall and Gibbs[156] contained areas of more typical mesothelioma when multiple blocks were examined; however, in 7 of their cases the small cell component comprised more than 90% of the tumour. The immunohis-tochemical profile was typical of mesothelioma. In addition, small cell mesothelioma does not display the haematoxyphilic nucleoprotein precipitates often seen in small cell carcinoma. Some cases of small cell mesothelioma described in post-mortem material may represent an artefact due to shrinkage and poor preservation of tumour cells.

Lymphohistiocytoid mesothelioma

This rare variant, comprising less than 1% of mesotheliomas, was first described in 1988,[157] with futher descriptions in 1989[120] and 1992.[158] Lymphohistiocytoid mesothe-liomas represent predominantly sarcomatoid or poorly differentiated epithelioid tumours, characterised by a background of histiocytoid neoplastic cells, obscured by intense lymphocytic infiltration. Mesothelial differentiation has been confirmed in the histiocytoid cells by immunohistochemistry (cytokeratin and vimentin co-expres-sion) and EM. By analogy with desmoplastic mesothelioma, at least 50% of the tu-mour should demonstrate a lymphohistiocytoid appearance for inclusion in this cat-egory. Recognition of areas of more conventional mesothelioma may be a useful pointer to the diagnosis. There is no prognostic significance associated with this diagnosis, its importance being related to the potential for misdiagnosis as a lymphoproliferative lesion (and, conversely, misdiagnosis of pleural lymphoma as mesothelioma). Aware-ness of the entity and appropriate use of immunohistochemical panels should prevent these potential pitfalls.

Deciduoid mesothelioma

Nascimento et al.[159] described two cases of epithelioid mesothelioma of the peritoneum in young women where the tumour cells were large with abundant glassy eosinophilic cytoplasm, reminiscent of decidual cells. The tumours followed an aggressive course. Orosz et al.[160] described an additional case in a 15-year-old girl who died 11 months after diagnosis. In our experience, mesotheliomas with a deciduoid appearance are restricted neither to females nor the peritoneum.

Desmoplastic small round cell tumour (DSRCT)

DSRCTs have characteristic clinico-pathological features, that differ from mesothelioma in many respects and DSRCT is not generally viewed as a mesothelioma variant. However, Gerald *et al.*,[161] in their initial description, suggested that these tumours may represent a primitive form of mesothelioma or 'mesothelioblastoma'. The recent description of such lesions occurring in a pleural location[144] further supports a relationship between desmoplastic small round cell tumour and mesothelial or submesothelial tissues. The presence of prominent epithelioid and papillary areas described in abdominal cases, together with the apparent 'biphasic' appearance (cellular islands within desmoplastic stroma), may occasionally render distinction from mesothelioma difficult. A superficial resemblance to small cell mesothelioma has also been noted. There is an important role for extensive immunohistochemical panels, EM and cytogenetics in such cases.

Benign/low grade mesothelial proliferations

This group of mesothelial proliferations almost invariably involve the peritoneal or pelvic cavities, occur more frequently in women, and are rare in the pleura.

Well differentiated papillary mesothelioma

This lesion usually occurs in the peritoneum of young women, but may rarely occur in the pleura.[57,162,163] The tumour is often found incidentally and presents as multiple peritoneal nodules. Histologically, all have a well developed papillary architecture lined by a single layer of uniform, cuboidal or flattened mesothelial cells, with bland nuclei. The prognosis is generally good, although occasionally the tumour may behave aggressively. The differential diagnosis includes serous tumours and malignant mesothelioma; in small lesions mesothelial hyperplasia may be considered.

These tumours do not usually occur in the pleura and diagnosis in this site requires classical benign morphology. We have seen a single case which involved peritoneal and pleural cavities simultaneously.[164]

Benign multicystic mesothelioma (peritoneal inclusion cysts)

This rare lesion arises within the pelvic peritoneum, usually in young women, and often following surgery; it may form a large multicystic mass, and its macroscopic appearance is a useful diagnostic clue. A similar lesion has been described in the pleura.[165] Controversy remains as to whether this represents a reactive or neoplastic process.[166-168] The differential diagnosis includes microcystic malignant mesothelioma and vascular tumours such as lymphangioma. Benign multicystic mesothelioma may recur and can result in death.

Adenomatoid tumour

This is a distinctive benign tumour of mesothelial origin, usually found in relation to the genital tract in both males and females. Originally thought to be of endothelial derivation, its mesothelial nature has now been proven.[57] Adenomatoid tumours have been described in the pleural cavities, discovered as incidental lesions in patients undergoing lung resection for other reasons.[169]

Summary

The diagnosis of mesothelioma continues to present many challenges to pathologists. This is due in part to the range of morphological appearances that may be seen in mesothelioma and hence the potential for confusion with other malignancies involving the pleura. In addition there are benign and reactive mesothelial processes that may be mistaken for mesothelioma; conversely there are mesotheliomas that are cytologically bland or paucicellular that may be confused with a benign process.

In this chapter we have sought to highlight some of the common diagnostic difficulties seen in routine practice. We have emphasised the importance of close attention to morphological features in both cytological and histological specimens, as well as the critical role of ancillary studies in establishing the diagnosis.

While it is often possible to diagnose mesothelioma in cytological specimens and small (core) biopsies, these sample types are not always appropriate and there is sometimes a need for directed thoracoscopic and even open biopsy in a small proportion of cases.

A multidisciplinary approach involving clinicians, radiologists and pathologists is essential to optimise sampling and facilitate diagnosis.

References

1. Whitaker, D. Laboratory diagnosis of malignant mesothelioma on serous effusion. AIMLS Broadsheet No. 13. *Aust J Med Lab Sci* 1989; **10**: 81–86.
2. Whitaker, D., Papadimitriou, J.M. Mesothelial healing: morphological and kinetic investigations. *J Pathol* 1985; **145**: 159–175.
3. Connell, N.D., Rheinwald, J.G. Regulation of the cytoskeleton in mesothelial cells: reversible loss of keratin and increase in vimentin during rapid growth in culture. *Cell* 1983; **34**: 245–253.
4. Bolen, J.W., Hammar, S.P., Mcnutt, M.A. Reactive and neoplastic serosal tissue. A light-microscopic, ultrastructural and immunohistochemical study. *Am J Surg Pathol* 1986; **10**: 34–47.
5. Yokoi, T., Mark, E.J. Atypical mesothelial hyperplasia associated with bronchogenic carcinoma. *Hum Pathol* 1991; **22**: 695–699.
6. Nosanchuk, J.S., Naylor, B. A unique cytologic picture in pleural fluid from patients with rheumatoid arthritis. *Am J Clin Pathol* 1968; **50**: 330–335.
7. Kelley, S., McGarry, P., Hutson, Y. Atypical cells in pleural fluid characteristic of systemic lupus erythematosis. *Acta Cytol* 1971; **15**: 357–362.
8. Henderson, D.W., Shilkin, K.B., Whitaker, D. Reactive mesothelial hyperplasia vs mesothelioma, including mesothelioma in situ. *Am J Clin Pathol* 1998; **110**: 397–404.

9. Ruffie, P., Feld, R., Cormier, Y. *et al.* Diffuse malignant mesothelioma of the pleura in Ontario and Quebec: a retrospective study of 332 patients. *J Clin Oncol* 1989; **7**: 1157–1168.

10. Boutin, C., Rey, F. Thoracoscopy in pleural malignant mesothelioma: a prospective study of 188 consecutive patients. *Cancer* 1993; **72**: 389–393.

11. Whitaker, D., Sterrett, G., Shilkin, K. Early diagnosis of malignant mesothelioma: the contribution of effusion and fine needle aspiration cytology and ancillary techniques. In: Peters, G.A., Peters, B.J., eds. *Asbestos medical research. Sourcebook on asbestos diseases: medical legal and engineering aspects.* New York: Garland, 1989; **4**: 71–115.

12. Whitaker, D., Sterrett, G.F., Shilkin, K.B. Cytological appearances of malignant mesothelioma. In: Henderson DW, Shilkin KB, Langlois S Le P, Whitaker D., eds. *Malignant mesothelioma.* New York: Hemisphere, 1992: 167–182.

13. Whitaker, D., Shilkin, K. Diagnosis of pleural malignant mesothelioma in life – a practical approach. *J Pathol* 1984; **143**: 147–175.

14. Leong, A.S-Y., Stevens, M.W., Mukherjee, T.M. Malignant mesothelioma: cytologic diagnosis with histologic, immunohistochemical and ultrastructural correlation. *Semin Diagn Pathol* 1992; **9**: 141–150.

15. Whitaker, D., Sterrett, G., Shilkin, K.B. Mesotheliomas. In: Gray W, ed. *Diagnostic cytopathology.* New York: Churchill Livingstone, 1995: 195–224.

16. Whitaker, D. Cell aggregates in malignant mesothelioma. *Acta Cytol* 1977; **21**: 236–239.

17. Becker, S.N., Pepin, D.W., Rosenthal, D.L. Mesothelial papilloma: a case of mistaken identity in pericardial effusion. *Acta Cytol* 1976; **20**: 266–268.

18. Spriggs, A.L., Jerome, D.W. Benign mesothelial proliferation with collagen formation in pericardial fluid. *Acta Cytol* 1979; **23**: 428–430.

19. Luthringer, D.J., Virmani, R., Weiss, S.W., Rosai, J. A distinctive cardiovascular lesion resembling histiocytoid (epithelioid) hemangioma. *Am J Surg Pathol* 1990; **14**: 993–1000.

20. Veinot, J.P., Tazelaar, H.D., Edwards, W.D., Colby, T.V. Mesothelial/monocytic incidental cardiac excrescences: cardiac MICE. *Mod Pathol* 1994; **7**: 9–16.

21. Kho-Duffin, J., Tao, L-C., Cramer, H. *et al.* Cytologic diagnosis of malignant mesothelioma, with particular emphasis on the epithelial noncohesive cell type. *Diagn Cytopathol* 1999; **20**: 57–62.

22. Stevens, M.W., Leong, A.S-Y., Fazzalari, N.L. *et al.* Cytopathology of malignant mesothelioma. A step-wise logistic regression analysis. *Diagn Cytopathol* 1992; **8**: 333–341.

23. Henderson, D.W., Whitaker, D., Shilkin, K.B. The differential diagnosis of mesothelioma: a practical approach to diagnosis during life. In: Henderson, D.W., Shilkin, K.B., Langlois, S., Le. P., Whitaker. D., eds. *Malignant mesothelioma.* New York: Hemisphere, 1992: 183–197.

24. Hsu, C. Cytologic detection of malignancy in pleural effusion: a review of 5255 samples from 3811 patients. *Diagn Cytopathol* 1987; **3**: 8.

25. Nance, K.V., Shermer, R.W., Askin, F.B. Diagnostic efficiency of pleural biopsy as compared with that of pleural fluid examination. *Mod Pathol* 1991; **4**: 320–324.

26. Colby, T.V. Benign mesothelial cells in lymph node. *Adv Anat Pathol* 1999; **6**: 41–48.

27. Argani, P., Rosai, J. Hyperplastic mesothelial cells in lymph nodes. *Hum Pathol* 1998; **29**: 339–346.

28. Marshall, R.J., Herbert, A., Braye, S.G., Jones, D.B. Use of antibodies to carcinoembryonic antigen and human milk fat globule to distinguish carcinoma, mesothelioma, and reactive mesothelium. *J Clin Pathol* 1984; **37**: 1215–1221.

29. To, A., Coleman, D.V., Dearnaley, D.P. *et al.* Use of antisera to epithelial membrane antigen for the cytodiagnosis of malignancy in serous effusions. *J Clin Pathol* 1981; **34**: 1326–1332.

30. To, A., Dearnaley, D.P., Ormerod, M.G. *et al.* Epithelial membrane antigen. Its use in the cytodiagnosis of malignancy in serous effusions. *Am J Clin Pathol* 1982; **78**: 214–219.
31. Van der Kwast, Th.H., Versnel, M.A., Delahaye, M. *et al.* Expression of epithelial membrane antigen on malignant mesothelioma cells. *Acta Cytol* 1988; **32**: 169–174.
32. Heyderman, E., Ridley, P.D. Malignant mesothelioma. *J R Soc Med* 1989; **82**: 571–572.
33. Henderson, D.W., Shilkin, K., Whitaker, D. The pathology of mesothelioma, including immunohistology and ultrastructure. In: Henderson DW, Shilkin KB, Langlois SL, Whitaker D, eds. *Malignant mesothelioma*. New York: Hemisphere, 1992: 69–139.
34. Leong, A.S-Y., Parkinson, R., Milios, J. 'Thick' cell membranes revealed by immunocytochemical staining: a clue to the diagnosis of mesothelioma. *Diagn Cytopathol* 1990; **6**: 9–13.
35. Esposito, V., Baldi, A., De Luca, A., *et al.* p53 immunostaining in differential diagnosis of pleural mesothelial proliferations. *Anticancer Res* 1997; **17**: 733–736.
36. Cote, R.J., Jhanwar, S.C., Novick, S., Pellicer, A. Genetic alterations of the p53 gene are a feature of malignant mesotheliomas. *Cancer Res* 1991; **51**: 5410–5416.
37. Mayall, J., Goddard, H., Gibbs, A.R. p53 immunostaining in the distinction between benign and malignant mesothelial proliferations using formalin-fixed paraffin sections. *J Pathol* 1992; **168**: 377–381.
38. Ramael, M., Lemmens, G., Eerdedekens, C. *et al.* Immunoreactivity for p53 protein in malignant mesothelioma. *J Pathol* 1992; **168**: 371–375.
39. Kafiri, G., Thomas, D.M., Shepherd, N.A. *et al.* p53 expression is common in malignant mesothelioma. *Histopathology* 1992; **21**: 331–334.
40. Walts, A.E., Said, J.W., Koeffler, H.P. Is immunoreactivity for p53 useful in distinguishing benign from malignant effusions? Localization of p53 gene product in benign mesothelial and adenocarcinoma cells. *Mod Pathol* 1994; **7**: 462–468.
41. Stoetzer, O.J., Munker, R., Darsow, M., Wilmanns, W. p53 immunoreactive cells in benign and malignant effusions: diagnostic value using a panel of monoclonal antibodies and comparison with CEA-staining. *Oncol Res* 1999; **6**: 455–458.
42. Mayall, F.G., Goddard, H., Gibbs, A.R. The frequency of p53 immunostaining in asbestos-associated mesotheliomas and non-asbestos-associated mesotheliomas. *Histopathology* 1993; **22**: 383–386.
43. Eposito, V., Baldi, A., De Luca, A. *et al.* Role of PCNA in differentiating between malignant mesothelioma and mesothelial hyperplasia: prognostic considerations. *Anticancer Res* 1997; **17**: 601–604.
44. Ramael, M., Jacobs, W., Weyler, J. *et al.* Proliferation in malignant mesothelioma as determined by mitosis counts and immunoreactivity for proliferating cell nuclear antigen (PCNA). *J Pathol* 1994; **172**: 247–253.
45. Ayres, J.G., Crocker, J.G., Skilbeck, N.Q. Differentiation of malignant from normal and reactive mesothelial cells by the argyrophil technique for nucleolar organiser region associated proteins. *Thorax* 1988; **43**: 366–370.
46. Soosay, G.N., Griffiths, M., Papadaki, L. *et al.* The differential diagnosis of epithelial-type mesothelioma from adenocarcinoma and reactive mesothelial proliferations. *J Pathol* 1991; **163**: 299–305.
47. Wolanski, K.D., Whitaker, D., Shilkin, K.B., Henderson, D.W. The use of epithelial membrane antigen and silver-stained nucleolar organizer regions testing in the differential diagnosis of mesothelioma from benign reactive mesothelioses. *Cancer* 1998; **82**: 583–590.
48. Burmer, G.C., Rabinovitch, P.S., Kuander, B.G. *et al.* Flow cytometric analysis of malignant pleural mesotheliomas. *Hum Pathol* 1989; **20**: 777–783.

49. Pyrhnen, S., Laasonen, A., Tammilehto, L. *et al.* Diploid predominance and prognostic significance of S-phase cells in malignant mesothelioma. *Eur J Cancer* 1991; **27**: 197–200.
50. El-Naggar, A.K., Ordonez, N.G., Garnsey, L., Batsakis, J.G. Epithelioid pleural mesotheliomas and pulmonary adenocarcinomas: a comparative DNA flow cytometric study. Hum Pathol 1991; **22**: 972–978.
51. Frierson, H.F., Mills, S.E., Legier, J.F. Flow cytometric analysis of ploidy in immunohistochemically confirmed samples of malignant epithelial mesothelioma. *Am J Clin Pathol* 1988; **90**: 240–243.
52. Lee, W.C., Testa, J.R. Somatic genetic alterations in human malignant mesothelioma. *Int J Oncol* 1999; **14**: 181–188.
53. Popescu, N.C., Chahinian, A.P., DiPaulo J.A. Nonrandom chromosome alterations in human malignant mesothelioma. *Cancer Res* 1988; **48**: 142–147.
54. Balsara, B.R., Bell, D.W., Sonoda, G. Comparative genomic hybridization and loss of heterozygosity analyses identify a common region of deletion at 15q11.1–15 in human malignant mesothelioma. *Cancer Res* 1999; **59**: 450–454.
55. Mangano, W.E., Cagle, P.T., Churg, A. *et al.* The diagnosis of desmoplastic malignant mesothelioma and its distinction from fibrous pleurisy. A histologic and immunohistochemical analysis of 31 cases including p53 immunostaining. *Am J Clin Pathol* 1998; **110**: 191–199.
56. Stout, A. Biological effects of asbestos. *Ann N Y Acad Sci* 1965; **132**: 680–682.
57. Battifora, H., McCaughey, W.T.E. *Tumors of the serosal membranes.* Atlas of tumor pathology. 3rd series, fascicle 15. Washington, DC: Armed Forces Institute of Pathology, 1995.
58. Roggli, V.L., Sanfilippo, F., Shelburne, J.D. Mesothelioma. In: Roggli VL, Greenberg SD, Pratt PC, eds. *Pathology of asbestos-associated diseases.* Boston: Little, Brown, 1992: 109–164.
59. Henderson, D.W., Comin, C.E., Hammar, S.P. *et al.* Malignant mesothelioma of the pleura: current surgical pathology. In: Corrin B, ed. *Pathology of lung tumors.* New York, NY: Churchill Livingstone, 1997: 241–280.
60. Lilis, R. Mesothelioma. In: Merchant, J.A., Boehlecke, B.A., Taylor, G., Pickett-Harner, M., eds. *Occupational respiratory diseases.* National Institute for Occupational Safety and Health (NIOSH) publication no. 86–102. Washington, DC: US Department of Health and Human Services, 1986: 682.
61. Whitaker, D., Henderson, D.W., Shilkin, K.B. The concept of mesothelioma in situ: implications for diagnosis and histogenesis. *Semin Diagn Pathol* 1992; **9**: 151–161.
62. Willis, R.A. *Pathology of tumours.* 4th ed., London: Butterworths, 1967: 181–183.
63. Andrion, A., Magnani, C., Betta, P-G. *et al.* Malignant mesothelioma of the pleura: interobserver variability. *J Clin Pathol* 1995; **48**: 856–860.
64. Leigh, J., Rogers, A.J., Ferguson, D.A. *et al.* Lung asbestos fiber content and mesothelioma cell type, site and survival. *Cancer* 1991; **68**: 135–141.
65. De Pangher Manzini, V., Brollo, A., Franceschi S *et al.* Prognostic factors of malignant mesothelioma of the pleura. *Cancer* 1993; **72**: 410–417.
66. Beer, T.W., Buchanan, R., Matthews, A.W. Prognosis in malignant mesothelioma related to MIB 1 proliferation index and histological subtype. *Hum Pathol* 1998; **29**: 246–251.
67. Ordonez, N.G. The immunohistochemical diagnosis of epithelial mesothelioma. *Hum Pathol* 1999;**30**:313–323.
68. Roboz, J., Greaves, J., Silides, D. *et al.* Hyaluronic acid content of effusions as a diagnostic aid for malignant mesothelioma. *Cancer Res* 1985; **445**: 1850–1854.
69. Pettersson, T., Froseth, B., Riska, H., Klockars, M. Concentration of hyaluronic acid in pleural fluid as a diagnostic aid for malignant mesothelioma. *Chest* 1988; **94**: 1037–1039.

70. Azumi, N., Underhill, C.B., Kagan, E., Sheibani, K. A novel biotinylated probe specific for hyaluronate. *Am J Surg Pathol* 1992; **16**: 116–121.
71. Weiss, S.W., Enzinger, F. Mesothelioma. In: *Soft tissue tumors.* 3rd ed. Mosby ,1995: 787–819.
72. Wang, N-S., Huang, S-N., Gold, P. Absence of carcinoembryonic antigen-like material in mesothelioma. An immunohistochemical differentiation from other lung cancers. *Cancer* 1979; **44**: 937–943.
73. Wick, M.R. Immunophenotyping of malignant mesothelioma. *Am J Surg Pathol* 1997; **21**: 1395–1398.
74. Brown, R.W., Clark, G.M., Tandon, A.K., Allred, D.C. Multiple marker immunohistochemical phenotypes distinguishing malignant pleural mesothelioma from pulmonary adenocarcinoma. *Hum Pathol* 1993; **24**: 347–354.
75. Kawai, T., Suzuki, M., Torikata, C., Suzuki, Y. Expression of carbohydrate antigens in human pulmonary adenocarcinoma. *Cancer* 1993; **72**: 1581–1587.
76. Bedrossian, C.W.M., Bonsib, S., Moran, C. Differential diagnosis between mesothelioma and adenocarcinoma: a multimodal approach based on ultrastructure and immunocytochemistry. *Semin Diagn Pathol* 1992; **9**: 124–140.
77. Garcia-Prats, M.D., Ballestin. C., Sotelo, T. *et al.* A comparative evaluation of immunohistochemical markers for the differential diagnosis of malignant pleural tumours. *Histopathology* 1998; **32**: 462–472.
78. Dejmek, A., Hjerpe, A. Immunohistochemical reactivity in mesothelioma and adenocarcinoma: a stepwise logistic regression analysis. *APMIS* 1994; **102**: 255–264.
79. Weiss, L.M., Battifora, H. The search for the optimal immunohistochemical panel for the diagnosis of malignant mesothelioma. *Hum Pathol* 1993; **24**: 345–346.
80. Wick, M.R., Loy, T., Mills, S.E. *et al.* Malignant epithelioid pleural mesothelioma versus peripheral pulmonary adenocarcinoma: a histochemical, ultrastructural and immunohistologic study of 103 cases. *Hum Pathol* 1990; **21**: 759–766.
81. Ordonez, N.G. Value of the MOC-31 monoclonal antibody in differentiating epithelial pleural mesothelioma from lung adenocarcinoma. *Hum Pathol* 1998; **29**: 166–169.
82. Sosolik, R.C., McGaughty, V.R., De Young, B.R. Anti-MOC-31: a potential addition to the pulmonary adenocarcinoma versus mesothelioma immunohistochemistry panel. *Mod Pathol* 1997; **10**: 716–719.
83. Kuenen-Boumeester, V., van Loenen, P., de Bruijn, E.M.C.A. *et al.* Quality control of immunocytochemical staining of effusions using a standardized method of cell processing. *Acta Cytol* 1996; **40**: 475–479.
84. DiLoreto, C., Puglisi, F., Di Lauro, V *et al.* TTF-1 protein expression in pleural malignant mesotheliomas and adenocarcinomas of the lung. *Cancer Lett* 1998; **124**: 73–78.
85. Leers, M.P.G., Aarts, M.M.J., Theunissen, P.H.M.H. E-cadherin and calretinin: a useful combination of immunochemical markers for differentiation between mesothelioma and metastatic adenocarcinoma. *Histopathology* 1998; **32**: 209–216.
86. Peralta-Soler, A., Knudsen, K.A., Jaurand, M.C. *et al.* The differential expression of N-cadherin and E-cadherin distinguished pleural mesotheliomas from lung adenocarcinomas. *Hum Pathol* 1995; **26**: 1363–1369.
87. Han, A.C., Peralta-Soler, A., Knudsen, K.A. *et al.* Differential expression of N-cadherin in pleural mesotheliomas and E-cadherin in lung adenocarcinomas in formalin-fixed paraffin-embedded tissues. *Hum Pathol* 1997; **28**: 641–645.
88. Singh, G., Whiteside, T.L., Dekker, A. Immunodiagnosis of mesothelioma. Use of antimesothelial cell serum in an indirect immunofluorescence assay. *Cancer* 1979; **43**: 2288–2296.

89. Donna, A., Betta, P-G., Jones, J.S.P. Verification of the histologic diagnosis of malignant mesothelioma in relation to the binding of an antimesothelial cell antibody. *Cancer* 1989; **63**: 1331–1336.

90. Hsu, S-M., Hsu, P-L., Zhao, X. *et al.* Establishment of human mesothelioma cell lines (MS-1,-2) and production of a monoclonal antibody(Anti-MS) with diagnostic and therapeutic potential. *Cancer Res* 1988; **48**: 5228–5236.

91. O'Hara, C.J., Corson, J.M., Pinkus, G.S. *et al.* ME1. A monoclonal antibody that distinguishes epithelial-type malignant mesothelioma from pulmonary adenocarcinoma and extrapulmonary malignancies. *Am J Pathol* 1990; **136**: 421–428.

92. Moll, R., Dhouailly, D., Sun, T-T. Expression of keratin 5 as a distinctive feature of epithelial and biphasic mesotheliomas. An immunohistochemical study using monoclonal antibody AE14. *Virchows Archiv B Cell Pathol* 1989; **58**: 129–145.

93. Clover, J., Oates, J., Edwards, C. Anti-cytokeratin 5/6: a positive marker for epithelioid mesothelioma. *Histopathology* 1997; **31**: 140–143.

94. Ordonez, N.G. Value of cytokeratin 5/6 immunostaining in distinguishing epithelial mesothelioma of the pleura from lung adenocarcinoma. *Am J Surg Pathol* 1998; **22**: 1215–1221.

95. Nagel, H., Hemmerlein, B., Ruschenburg, I. *et al.* The value of anti-calretinin antibody in the differential diagnosis of normal and reactive mesothelia versus metastatic tumours in effusion cytology. *Pathol Res Pract* 1998; **194**: 759–764.

96. Doglioni, C., Dei Tos, A.P., Laurino, L. *et al.* Calretinin: a novel immunocytochemical marker for mesothelioma. *Am J Surg Pathol* 1996; **20**: 1037–1046.

97. Gotzos, V., Vogt, P., Celio, M.R. The calcium binding protein calretinin is a selective marker for malignant pleural mesotheliomas of the epithelial type. *Pathol Res Pract* 1996; **192**: 137–147.

98. Riera, J.R., Astengo-Osuna, C., Longmate, J.A., Battifora, H. The immunohistochemical diagnostic panel for epithelial mesothelioma. A reevaluation after heat-induced epitope retrieval. *Am J Surg Pathol* 1997; **21**: 1409–1419.

99. Dei Tos, A.P., Doglioni, C. Calretinin: a tool for diagnostic immunohistochemistry. *Adv Anat Pathol* 1998; **5**: 61–66.

100. Sheibani, K., Esteban, J.M., Bailey, A. *et al.* Immunopathologic and molecular studies as an aid to the diagnosis of malignant mesothelioma. *Hum Pathol* 1992; **23**: 107–116.

101. Ordonez, N.G. Value of antibodies 44-3A6, SM3, HBME-1 and thrombomodulin in differentiating epithelial pleural mesothelioma from lung adenocarcinoma: a comparative study with other commonly used antibodies. *Am J Surg Pathol* 1997; **21**: 1399–1408.

102. Attanoos, R.L., Goddard, H., Gibbs, A.R. Mesothelioma-binding antibodies: thrombomodulin, OV632 and HBME-1 and their use in the diagnosis of malignant mesothelioma. *Histopathology* 1996; **29**: 209–215.

103. Kennedy, A.D., King, G., Kerr, K.M. HBME-1 and antithrombomodulin in the differential diagnosis of malignant mesothelioma of pleura. *J Clin Pathol* 1997; **50**: 859–862.

104. Miettinen, M., Kovatich, A.J. HBME-1 – a monoclonal antibody useful in the differential diagnosis of mesothelioma, adenocarcinoma, and soft tissue and bone tumours. *Appl Immunohistochem* 1995; **3**: 115–122.

105. Ordonez, N.G. Value of thrombomodulin immunostaining in the diagnosis of mesothelioma. *Histopathology* 1997; **31**: 25–30.

106. Geiger, B., Ayalon, O. Cadherins. *Annu Rev Cell Biol* 1992; **8**: 307–332.

107. Peralta-Soler, A., Knudsen, K.A., Tecson-Miguel, A. *et al.* Expression of E-cadherin and N-cadherin in surface epithelial-stromal tumors of the ovary distinguishes mucinous from serous and endometrioid tumors. *Hum Pathol* 1997; **28**: 734–739.

108. Attanoos, R.L., Webb, R., Gibbs, A.R. CD44H expression in reactive mesothelium, pleural mesothelioma and pulmonary adenocarcinoma. *Histopathology* 1997; **30**: 260–263.

109. Afify, A.M., Stern, R., Jobes, G. *et al.* Differential expression of CD44S and hyaluronic acid in malignant mesotheliomas, adenocarcinomas, and reactive mesothelial hyperplasias. *Applied Immunohistochem* 1998; **6**: 11–15.

110. Filie, A.C., Abati, A., Fetsch, P. *et al.* Hyaluronate binding probe and CD44 in the differential diagnosis of malignant effusions: disappointing results in cytology material (letter). *Diagn Cytopathol* 1998; **18**: 473–474.

111. Amin, K.M., Litzky, L.A., Smythe, W.R. *et al.* Wilms' tumor 1 susceptibility gene products are selectively expressed in malignant mesothelioma. *Am J Pathol* 1995; **146**: 344–356.

112. Kumar-Singh, S., Segers, K., Rodeck, U. *et al. WT1* mutation in malignant mesothelioma and WT1 immunoreactivity in relation to p53 and growth factor receptor expression, cell-type transition, and prognosis. *J Pathol* 1997; **181**: 67–74.

113. Clark, S.P., Chou, S.T., Martin, T.J., Danks, J.A. Parathyroid hormone-related protein antigen localization distinguishes between mesothelioma and adenocarcinoma of the lung. *J Pathol* 1995; **176**: 161–165.

114. Hammar, S.P., Bockus, D.E., Remington, F.L., Rohrbach, K.A. Mucin-positive epithelial mesotheliomas: a histochemical, immunohistochemical and ultrastructural comparison with mucin-producing adenocarcinomas. *Ultrastruct Pathol* 1996; **20**: 293–325.

115. Naylor, B. Pleural, peritoneal and pericardial fluids. In: Bibbo M, ed. *Comprehensive cytopathology*. Philadelphia: Saunders, 1991: 541–614.

116. Churg, A. Diseases of the pleura. In: Thurlbeck WM, Churg AM. 2nd ed. *Pathology of the lung*, 2ed. New York: Thieme Medical, 1995: 1080–1109.

117. Comin, C.E., de Klerk, N.H., Henderson, D.W. Malignant mesothelioma: current conundrums over risk estimates and whither electron microscopy for diagnosis? *Ultrastruct Pathol* 1997; **21**: 315–320.

118. Oury, T.D., Hammar, S.P., Roggli, V.L. Ultrastructural features of diffuse malignant mesotheliomas. *Hum Pathol* 1998; **29**: 1382–1392.

119. Henderson, D.W., Papadimitriou, J.M., Coleman, M. Mesothelial tumours. In: *Ultrastructural appearances of tumours*. Edinburgh: Churchill Livingstone, 1986: 133–138.

120. Coleman, M., Henderson, D.W., Mukherjee, T.M. The ultrastructural pathology of malignant pleural mesothelioma. *Pathol Annu* 1989; **24**(pt 1): 303–353.

121. Fox, H. Primary neoplasia of the female peritoneum. *Histopathology* 1993; **23**: 103–110.

122. Foyle, A., Al-Jabi, M., McCaughey, W.T.E. Papillary peritoneal tumours in women. *Am J Surg Pathol* 1981; **5**: 241–249.

123. Bollinger, D.J., Wick, M.R., Dehner, L.P. *et al.* Peritoneal malignant mesothelioma versus serous papillary adenocarcinoma. A histochemical and immunohistochemical comparison. *Am J Surg Pathol* 1989; **13**: 659–670.

124. Raju, U., Fine, G., Greenawald, K.A., Ohorodnik, J.M. Primary papillary serous neoplasia of the peritoneum: a clinicopathological and ultrastructural study of eight cases. *Hum Pathol* 1989; **20**: 426–436.

125. Khoury, N., Raju, U., Crissman, J.D. *et al.* A comparative immunohistochemical study of peritoneal and ovarian serous tumours and mesotheliomas. *Hum Pathol* 1990; **21**: 811–819.

126. Ordonez, N.G. Role of immunohistochemistry in distinguishing epithelial peritoneal mesotheliomas from peritoneal and ovarian serous carcinomas. *Am J Surg Pathol* 1998; **22**: 1203–1214.

127. Clement, P.B., Young, R.H., Scully, R.E. Malignant mesotheliomas presenting as ovarian masses. A report of nine cases, including two primary ovarian mesotheliomas. *Am J Surg Pathol* 1996; **20**: 1067–1080.

128. Harwood, T.R., Gracey, D.R., Yokoo, H. Pseudomesotheliomatous carcinoma of the lung: a variant of peripheral lung cancer. *Am J Clin Pathol* 1976; **65**: 159–167.

129. Dessy, E., Pietra, G.G. Pseudomesotheliomatous carcinoma of the lung. An immunohistochemical and ultrastructural study of three cases. *Cancer* 1991; **68**: 1747–1753.
130. Koss, M., Travis, W., Moran, C., Hochholzer, L. Pseudomesotheliomatous adenocarcinoma: a reappraisal. *Semin Diagn Pathol* 1992; **9**: 117–123.
131. Koss, M.N., Fleming, M., Przygodzki, R.M. *et al.* Adenocarcinoma simulating mesothelioma: a clinicopathologic and immunohistochemical study of 29 cases. *Ann Diagn Pathol* 1998; **2**: 93–102.
132. Myers, J., Tazelaar, H., Katzenstein, A-L. *et al.* Localized malignant epithelioid and biphasic mesothelioma of the pleura. Clinicopathologic, immunohistochemical, and flow cytometric analysis of 3 cases. *Lab Invest* 1992; **66**: 115A.
133. Crotty, T.B., Myers, J.L., Katzenstein, A-L. Localized malignant mesothelioma: a clinicopathologic and flow cytometric study. *Am J Surg Pathol* 1994; **18**: 357–363.
134. Crotty, T.B., Colby, T.V., Gay, P.C., Pisani, R.J. Desmoplastic mesothelioma masquerading as sclerosing mediastinitis: a diagnostic dilemma. *Hum Pathol* 1992; **23**: 79–82.
135. MacDougall, D.B., Wang, S.E., Zibar, B.L. Mucin-positive epithelial mesothelioma. *Arch Pathol Lab Med* 1992; **116**: 874–880.
136. Robb, J.A. Mesothelioma versus adenocarcinoma: false positive CEA and LeuM1 staining due to hyaluronic acid. (Letter). *Hum Pathol* 1989; **20**: 400.
137. Gaffey, M.J., Mills, S.E., Swanson, P.E. *et al.* Immunoreactivity for BerEP4 in adenocarcinomas, adenomatoid tumours, and malignant mesotheliomas. *Am J Surg Pathol* 1992;**16**:593–599.
138. Stirling, J.W., Henderson, D.W., Spagnolo, D.V., Whitaker, D. Unusual granular reactivity for carcinoembryonic antigen in malignant mesothelioma. (Letter). *Hum Pathol* 1990; **21**: 678–679.
139. De Young, B.R., Frierson, H.F., Ly, M.N. *et al.* CD31 immunoreactivity in carcinomas and mesotheliomas. *Am J Clin Pathol* 1998; **110**: 374–377.
140. Lin, B.T.Y., Colby, T., Gown, A.M. *et al.* Malignant vascular tumours of the serous membranes mimicking mesothelioma: a report of 14 cases. *Am J Surg Pathol* 1996; **20**: 1431–1439.
141. Nicholson, A.G., Goldstraw, P., Fisher, C. Synovial sarcoma of the pleura and its differentiation from other primary pleural tumours: a clinicopathological and immunohistochemical review of three cases. *Histopathology* 1998; **33**: 508–513.
142. Fisher, C. Synovial sarcoma. *Ann Diagn Pathol* 1998; **2**: 401–421.
143. Gaertner, E., Zeran, E.H., Fleming, M.V. *et al.* Biphasic synovial sarcomas arising in the pleural cavity. *Am J Surg Pathol* 1996; **20**: 36–45.
144. Jawahar, D.A., Vuletin, J.C., Gorecki, P. *et al.* Primary biphasic synovial sarcoma of the pleura. *Respir Med* 1997; **91**: 568–570.
145. Ordonez, N.G., Tornos, C. Malignant peripheral nerve sheath tumor of the pleura with epithelial and rhabdomyoblastic differentiation: report of a case clinically simulating mesothelioma. *Am J Surg Pathol* 1997; **21**: 1515–1521.
146. Parkash, V., Gerald, W.L., Parma, A. *et al.* Desmoplastic small round cell tumor of the pleura. *Am J Surg Pathol* 1995; **19**: 659–665.
147. Cantin, R., Al-Jabi, M., McCaughey, W.T. Desmoplastic diffuse mesothelioma. *Am J Surg Pathol* 1982; **6**: 215–222.
148. Coffin, C.M., Humphrey, P.A., Dehner, L.P. Extrapulmonary inflammatory myofibroblastic tumor: a clinical and pathologic survey. *Semin Diagn Pathol* 1998; **15**: 85–101.
149. Chan, J.K.C. Solitary fibrous tumour-everywhere, and a diagnosis in vogue. *Histopathology* 1997; **31**: 568–576.

150. Suster, S., Nascimento, A.G., Miettinen, M. *et al.* Solitary fibrous tumour of soft tissue. *Am J Surg Pathol* 1995; **19**: 1257–1266.
151. Chang, Y.L., Lee, Y.C., Wu, C.T. Thoracic solitary fibrous tumour: clinical and pathological diversity. *Lung Cancer* 1999; **23**: 53–60.
152. Moran, C.A., Suster, S., Koss, M.N. The spectrum of histologic growth patterns in benign and malignant fibrous tumours of the pleura. *Semin Diagn Pathol* 1992; **9**: 169–180.
153. Vallat-Deccouvelaere, A.-V., Dry, S.M., Fletcher, C.D.M. Atypical and malignant solitary fibrous tumors in extrathoracic locations. Evidence of their comparability to intra-thoracic tumors. *Am J Surg Pathol* 1998; **22**: 1501–1511.
154. Chilosi, M., Facchetti, F., Dei Tos, A.P. bcl-2 expression in pleural and extra-pleural solitary fibrous tumours. *J Pathol* 1997; **181**: 362–367.
155. Mentzel, T., Bainbridge, T.C., Katencamp, D. Solitary fibrous tumour: clinicopathological, immunohistochemical, and ultrastructural analysis of 12 cases arising in soft tissues, nasal cavity and nasopharynx, urinary bladder and prostate. *Virchows Arch* 1997; **430**: 445–453.
156. Mayall, F.G., Gibbs, A.R. The histology and immunohistochemistry of small cell mesothelioma. *Histopathology* 1992; **20**: 47–51.
157. Henderson, D.W., Attwood, H.D., Constance, T.J. *et al.* Lymphohistiocytoid mesothelioma: a rare lymphomatoid variant of predominantly sarcomatoid mesothelioma. *Ultrastruct Pathol* 1988; **12**: 367–384.
158. Henderson, D.W., Shilkin, K.B., Whitaker, D. *et al.* Unusual histological types and anatomic sites of mesothelioma. In: Henderson, D.W., Shilkin, K.B., Langlois, S.L., Whitaker, D., eds. *Malignant mesothelioma.* New York: Hemisphere, 1992: 140–166.
159. Nascimento, A.G., Keeney, G.L., Fletcher, C.D.M. Deciduoid peritoneal mesothelioma: an unusual phenotype affecting young females. *Am J Surg Pathol* 1994; **18**: 439–445.
160. Orosz, Z., Nagy, P., Szentirmay, Z. *et al.* Epithelial mesothelioma with deciduoid features. *Virchows Arch* 1999; **434**: 263–266.
161. Gerald, W.L., Miller, H.K., Battifora, H. *et al.* Intra-abdominal desmoplastic small round cell tumor. Report of 19 cases of a distinctive type of high grade polyphenotypic malignancy affecting young individuals. *Am J Surg Pathol* 1991; **15**: 499–513.
162. Daya, D., McCaughey, W.T.E. Well differentiated papillary mesothelioma of the peritoneum. A clinicopathologic study of 22 cases. *Cancer* 1990; **65**: 292–296.
163. Raju, U., Fine, G., Greenawald, K.A. Primary papillary serous neoplasia of the peritoneum: a clinicopathologic and ultrastructural study of eight cases. *Hum Pathol* 1989; **20**: 426–436.
164. Shilkin, K.B. Well differentiated papillary mesothelioma of the pleura and peritoneum. Short course on tumours and tumour-like disorders of serosal membranes. XXI International Congress, International Academy of Pathology, Budapest, 1996.
165. Ball, N.J., Urbanski, S.J., Green, F.H.Y., Kieser, T. Pleural multicystic mesothelial proliferation. The so-called multicystic mesothelioma. *Am J Surg Pathol* 1990; **14**: 375–378.
166. Weiss, S.W., Tavassoli, F.A. Multicystic mesothelioma. An analysis of pathologic findings and biologic behaviour in 37 cases. *Am J Surg Pathol* 1988; **12**: 737–746.
167. Ross, M.J., Welch, W.R., Scully, R.E. Multilocular peritoneal inclusion cysts (so-called cystic mesothelioma). *Cancer* 1989; **64**: 1336–1346.
168. Clement, P.B. Reactive tumor-like lesions of the peritoneum (Editorial). *Am J Clin Pathol* 1995; **103**: 673–676.
169. Kaplan, M.A., Tazelaar, H.D., Hayashi, T. *et al.* Adenomatoid tumors of the pleura. *Am J Surg Pathol* 1996; **20**: 1219–1223.

= 9 =

Surgery and Staging of Malignant Mesothelioma

Joseph B. Shrager, Daniel Sterman, and Larry Kaiser

Surgery for malignant mesothelioma falls into one of three categories: diagnostic, palliative or potentially curative. Until very recently, there was little interest in surgery for this disease beyond the diagnostic and palliative procedures, as therapeutic nihilism has been the typical attitude of physicians towards this difficult disease. In the past several years, however, there has been renewed interest in combining radical cytoreductive surgery in selected mesothelioma patients with adjuvant therapies. The results of these aggressive approaches have been impressive in patients with localised, epithelioid mesothelioma and have begun to moderate the pessimism with which this disease has been viewed.

This chapter will review the staging of mesothelioma and discuss the available and currently most widely accepted surgical approaches for the various stages. It should be understood that the field is currently in flux, with new staging systems and new combined-modality therapeutic approaches having been recently advanced. Some of these may be on the verge of widespread application. We will attempt to differentiate between concepts which are reasonably well accepted and those which remain controversial or experimental.

Staging

In the past 25 years, at least 5 staging systems have been proposed for malignant mesothelioma.[1-5] The lack of a uniform, single staging system has made it difficult to predict survival, guide management, and evaluate outcome of new therapies in this disease. Without a standard staging system, it has not been possible to perform valid intergroup or interstudy comparisons. Efforts at developing useful staging systems have been hindered by mesothelioma's long latent period, which has made information about the natural history of the disease difficult to obtain, and its plate-like growth pattern, which has rendered it difficult to determine tumour volumes and degree of local invasion.

To unify the various previously proposed staging systems, the International Mesothelioma Interest Group (IMIG) developed a system in 1994 based on an analysis of

Table 9.1. The International Mesothelioma Interest Group Staging System.

T1	T1a	Tumour limited to the ipsilateral parietal pleura, including mediastinal and diaphragmatic pleura
		No involvement of the visceral pleura
	T1b	Tumour involving the ipsilateral parietal pleura, including mediastinal and diaphragmatic pleura
		Scattered foci of tumour also involving the visceral pleura

T2 Tumour involving each of the ipsilateral pleural surfaces (parietal, mediastinal, diaphragmatic, and visceral pleura) with at least one of the following features:
 involvement of diaphragmatic muscle
 confluent visceral pleural tumour (including the fissures) or extension of tumour from visceral pleura into the underlying pulmonary parenchyma

T3 Describes locally advanced but potentially resectable tumour
Tumour involving all of the ipsilateral pleural surfaces (parietal, mediastinal, diaphragmatic, and visceral pleura) with at least one of the following features:
 involvement of the endothoracic fascia
 extension into the mediastinal fat
 solitary, completely resectable focus of tumour extending into the soft tissues of the chest wall
 nontransmural involvement of the pericardium

T4 Describes locally advanced technically unresectable tumour
Tumour involving all of the ipsilateral pleural surfaces (parietal, mediastinal, diaphragmatic, and visceral) with at least one of the following features:
 diffuse extension or multifocal masses of tumour in the chest wall, with or without associated rib destruction
 direct transdiaphragmatic extension of tumour to the peritoneum
 direct extension of tumour to the contralateral pleura
 direct extension of tumour to one or more mediastinal organs
 direct extension of tumour into the spine
 tumour extending through to the internal surface of the pericardium, with or without a pericardial effusion; or
 tumour involving the myocardium

N-Lymph nodes
 NX Regional lymph nodes cannot be assessed
 N0 No regional lymph node metastases
 N1 Metastases in the ipsilateral bronchopulmonary or hilar lymph nodes
 N2 Metastases in the subcarinal or the ipsilateral mediastinal lymph nodes, including the ipsilateral internal mammary nodes
 N3 Metastases in the contralateral mediastinal, contralateral internal mammary, ipsilateral, or contralateral supraclavicular lymph nodes

M-Metastases
 MX Presence of distant metastasis cannot be assessed
 M0 No distant metastasis
 M1 Distant metastasis present

Stage	Description	Stage	Description	Stage	Descr
Stage I		Stage III	Any T3M0	Stage IV	Any T4
I a	T1aN0M0		Any N1M0		Any N3
I b	T1bN0M0		Any N2M0		Any M1
Stage II	T2N0M0				

the then emerging information about the impact of tumour and nodal status on survival (Table 9.1). This system is notable for its recognition of several aspects of mesothelioma. First, it reflects improved survival of patients with T1N0 disease, classifying these patients as stage I. Second, it separates these stage I patients into Ia, with tumours that involve only the parietal pleura, and Ib, with tumours that also involve the visceral pleura. This distinction is surgically important, as Ia disease is amenable to resection by parietal pleurectomy alone, while Ib and stage II disease (which reflect increasing visceral pleural burdens) require both parietal and visceral pleurectomy or extrapleural pneumonectomy (removal of the entire lung and pleura) if there is to be any hope of resecting all gross disease. T3 in this system describes locally advanced tumours covering all ipsilateral pleural surfaces with extension through the pleura in at least one location. These tumours are on the borderline of what might be considered resectable by extrapleural pneumonectomy. T4 tumours are clearly unresectable, with either diffuse chest wall involvement, transdiaphragmatic extension, transpericardial extension, spinal extension, mediastinal organ extension, or contralateral pleural involvement. Nodal disease is classified as in the current system for staging of non-small cell lung cancer.

The IMIG staging system does stratify patients appropriately according to prognosis (Figure 9.1).[6] Even with this new system, however, it often remains difficult to assign the correct stage to individual patients. Computed tomography (CT) of the chest cannot distinguish parietal from visceral pleural involvement or accurately distinguish between abutment and invasion of adjacent structures. Magnetic resonance

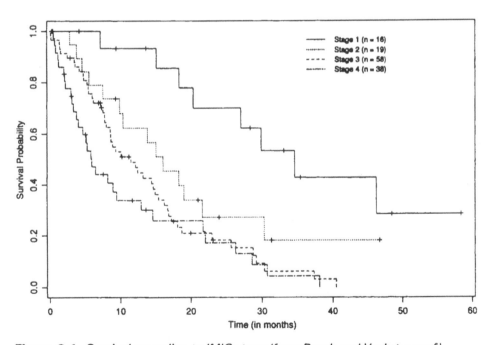

Figure 9.1. *Survival according to IMIG stage (from Rusch and Venkatraman[6]).*

imaging (MRI) adds more accuracy, but it remains imperfect in these regards. Both CT and MRI can determine whether there is mediastinal lymph node enlargement, but enlarged nodes may not be involved by tumour, and large portions of the mediastinum are often obscured by bulky tumour. Complete pre-resectional assessment, therefore, may require thoracoscopy for evaluation of T status and mediastinoscopy for evaluation of enlarged mediastinal lymph nodes.

Sugarbaker *et al.* have proposed another staging system for malignant mesothelioma (Table 9.2).[7] This system has allowed stratification of survival by stage among patients undergoing a protocol of extrapleural pneumonectomy followed by chemotherapy and radiation therapy (to be discussed further below). This system can only be applied to patients undergoing extrapleural pneumonectomy, as it depends upon careful pathological evaluation of the resected specimen. It differs in many respects from the International Staging System and may become the standard system for those undergoing resective surgery.

None of the current staging systems recognise the numerous pathological and biological variables that affect survival. These include histology, age, gender, performance status, type of symptoms, histologic subtype, and platelet count. Nevertheless, adherence to a common system will, it is hoped, allow stratification of patients to aid in resolving controversy over choices of therapy for this disease.

Diagnostic surgery

Surgical procedures may be indicated to establish a diagnosis of malignant mesothelioma or to evaluate extent of disease in a patient with an established diagnosis. These procedures may include video thoracoscopy (VATS), open pleural biopsy via a small incision, mediastinoscopy, and/or laparoscopy (Table 9.3).

If less invasive diagnostic procedures such as cytologic analysis of pleural fluid obtained by thoracentesis or closed pleural biopsy have failed to achieve a histological diagnosis in a patient suspected of having mesothelioma, the most appropriate next step is usually a

Table 9.2. Sugarbaker's staging system for mesothelioma.

Stage	Description
I	Disease completely resected within the capsule of the parietal pleura without adenopathy: ipsilateral pleural, lung, pericardium, diaphragm, or chest wall disease limited to previous biopsy sites
II	All of stage I with positive resection margins and/or intrapleural adenopathy
III	Local extension of disease into the chest wall or mediastinum; heart, or through diaphragm, peritoneum; or with extrapleural lymph node involvement
IV	Distant metastatic disease

Note: Patients with Butchart stage II and III disease are combined into stage III. Stage I represents patients with resectable disease and negative nodes. Stage II indicates resectable disease but positive nodes.

Table 9.3. Surgical options in the management of malignant mesothelioma (see text for descriptions).

1.	**Diagnostic**
a)	Thoracoscopy
b)	Open (small incision) pleural biopsy
c)	Mediastinoscopy
d)	Laparoscopy
2.	**Palliative**
a)	Chest tube and pleurodesis
b)	Thoracoscopy and pleurodesis
c)	Pleuroperitoneal shunt
d)	Pleurectomy
3.	**Potentially curative**
a)	Pleurectomy/decortication
b)	Extrapleural pneumonectomy

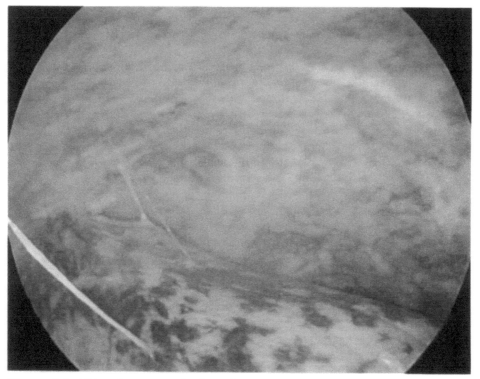

Figure 9.2. Video thoracoscopic view of mesothelioma involving parietal but largely sparing visceral pleura.

VATS exploration and pleural biopsy. Often using only one or two 3-cm-long intercostal incisions, the pleural space can be visualised by video camera (Figure 9.2), and generous biopsies of the diseased pleura can be obtained, from which pathologists generally have no trouble determining a specific diagnosis. At the same time, information about local extent of disease (T status), including whether the tumour covers both visceral and parietal pleurae, whether it invades deeply into fissures, and whether it is likely to be growing into lung, can be obtained. This information is important in determining the suitability of an individual for surgical debulking and which procedure is likely to be required.

Often, a patient will clearly not be a candidate for aggressive surgical resection due to overall medical status or imaging studies showing frank invasion of chest wall or mediastinal organs. In these cases, additional VATS staging information is not critical, and thus a surgical biopsy may be obtained with a single, 3-cm-long incision through which one can cut down on the parietal pleura at the site of greatest pleural thickening on CT. This may be considered less invasive than VATS, since the pleural space need not be entered and the patient does not require placement of a double-lumen endotracheal tube.

It has become clear in recent years that improved survival can be expected in patients with the epithelial versus sarcomatous or mixed histological types.[8] The differentiation between these types is difficult by cytological analysis or from small, closed pleural biopsy specimens. This renders it more important to obtain generous, surgical biopsies in order to plan management, and surgeons are therefore being increasingly called upon to perform these procedures.

Mediastinoscopy may also add important staging information. As with carcinoma of the lung, it is not clear whether routine mediastinoscopy is appropriate in patients with mesothelioma or whether only those with enlarged nodes by imaging studies should undergo the procedure. Nevertheless, virtually all surgeons would consider patients with histologically documented N3 disease (stage IV) to be excluded from consideration for attempted curative resections. Aggressive management of those with N2 (stage III) disease is controversial and should probably be reserved for the youngest patients with the best performance status.

Finally, laparoscopy may also be useful in the staging work-up of a patient with known mesothelioma. In particular, when MRI suggests transdiaphragmatic invasion, laparoscopy should be performed to confirm or refute this finding in a patient who is being considered for pleurectomy or extrapleural pneumonectomy. If the tumour is found to have transdiaphragmatic extension, the lesion is T4 (stage IV), and the patient is not a candidate for radical surgical excision. We generally perform the laparoscopy under the same anaesthetic as the planned pleurectomy or extrapleural pneumonectomy. If transdiaphragmatic extension is documented, the planned procedure is aborted.

Palliative surgery

Although often determination of resectability can be made only at the time of exploratory thoracotomy, in some cases the overall medical status of the patient combined with the staging information described above indicates that radical extirpative procedures should not be performed. For example, consider a 75-year-old patient with stage III disease (N2 by mediastinoscopy and confluent T3 pleural disease by VATS) in the right hemithorax. Such a patient would require a right extrapleural pneumonectomy for a chance of complete resection, but he would not be considered for this procedure and the associated adjuvant treatment because of the morbidity of the treatment in this age group. In cases like this one, however, one form or another of surgery may provide the most effective form of palliation by controlling the malignant pleural effusion and resulting dyspnoea (Table 9.3).

The simplest form of palliative treatment that a surgeon may offer a patient with mesothelioma is chest tube placement and pleurodesis. Once an effusion has developed, it is persistent and returns rapidly following thoracentesis such that several litres may be removed in a matter of weeks. Complete drainage and full re-expansion of the lung are necessary for chemical sclerosing agents to induce adhesions which obliterate the pleural space and reduce the possibility of recurrent effusion. This is difficult to achieve late in the course of mesothelioma because of the constricting tumour rind which usually creates a trapped lung at this point in the disease. Thus, if drainage and chemical pleurodesis is to be effective, it must be applied when there is a free-flowing effusion and minimal visceral pleural tumour burden.

If chest tube placement achieves complete drainage of the pleural fluid and full re-expansion of the lung, 5 g of talc in a slurry are placed through the tube into the pleural space. The tube is replaced to suction overnight and removed when drainage is less than approximately 200 cc in 24 hours. If drainage persists at a high volume, repeat talc administration is performed. Talc appears to be the most effective of the several materials which have been used for this purpose,[9] and reported success rates with talc slurry pleurodesis are in the range of 60–95%.

Some have favoured VATS evacuation of fluid and insufflation of talc in its powdered form over chest tube placement and talc slurry, even in patients with free-flowing effusions. Advocates of this approach claim that the talc can be more reliably distributed throughout the pleural space in this manner, resulting in a more effective pleurodesis. A prospective, randomised study of chest tube slurry versus VATS talc for all forms of malignant pleural effusion, however, did not bear this out.[10] A larger, multi-institutional study of the same issue is ongoing. Certainly, in patients in whom a diagnosis has been unobtainable by fluid cytology and who for this reason are undergoing diagnostic VATS, talc should be insufflated at the time of the procedure if the patient is not a candidate for debulking surgery.

If the pleural fluid has become loculated following repeated thoracenteses, as is often the case, and a single chest tube does not effect complete drainage, then VATS deloculation and pleurodesis is indicated. Through 3 port sites under general anaesthesia, the loculations are broken down under direct vision and all of the fluid and organising debris are removed. Talc is then insufflated to cover all pleural surfaces and the lung is re-expanded. Again, this procedure will only be effective if there is no tumour encasing the lung and restricting its expansion. If such restricting visceral pleural disease is present, the patient must be considered for either formal decortication via thoracotomy or placement of a pleuroperitoneal shunt.

We have found pleuroperitoneal shunting to be suboptimal on a number of fronts and therefore feel that it has a limited role in palliation of mesothelioma patients. This procedure involves placement of a catheter which is tunnelled subcutaneously from the pleural space into the peritoneal cavity. A one-way valve is left beneath the skin, which the patient must pump on a regular basis in order to convey fluid from the pleural space to the abdomen. The procedure can usually be performed under local anaesthesia and the pump is well tolerated although inconvenient to patients and somewhat annoying. The major shortcomings of the shunts, however, include frequent occlusion of the catheter,[11] and the theoretical concern, borne out by anecdotal reports, of rapid spread of tumour to the abdomen.[12]

Pleurectomy, which will be discussed below as a potentially curative procedure, can also be employed in a strictly palliative manner. That is, patients who have stage III or IV disease which is not felt to be completely resectable for potential cure may nevertheless undergo pleurectomy with the understanding that gross disease will remain after the procedure. This is in some cases a reasonable approach because pleurectomy is the most effective means of reducing the recurrence of pleural effusion, and it is the only effective means (other than a pleuroperitoneal shunt) when the lung is restricted in its expansion by visceral pleural disease. Furthermore, the procedure is generally well tolerated, with significantly less morbidity than an extrapleural pneumonectomy (EPP), and therefore a patient who is not felt to be a candidate for the latter may be a candidate for pleurectomy.

Pleurectomy is performed through a generous posterolateral thoracotomy. An extrapleural plane of dissection is entered and the pleura along most of the mediastinum and chest wall can be removed. The diaphragmatic pleura generally cannot be completely resected. An attempt is made to decorticate as much diseased visceral pleura as possible off the lung without injuring the underlying lung parenchyma. As the intention in palliative cases is not to remove all tumour, aggressive visceral pleural decortication into the fissures or in areas where the tumour is densely adherent to the lung is not performed. Blood replacement is frequently necessary. Two large chest tubes are left in place at the conclusion of the procedure.

The mortality following pleurectomy is 1–2%. Major complications are unusual but may include prolonged air leaks, haemorrhage, pneumonia, subcutaneous emphysema, empyema, and vocal cord paralysis.[13,14] It remains an open question whether a patient who has no chance for cure should undergo a thoracotomy for palliative pleurectomy. In situations where the less invasive options for controlling pleural effusion are felt to have a good chance of being effective, these should probably be attempted first.

Potentially curative surgery

Procedures which are performed with the intention of cure include pleurectomy and the significantly more aggressive procedure, extrapleural pneumonectomy. When these are performed with curative intent, the goal is removal of all gross disease, understanding that it is highly likely that there will be residual microscopic disease remaining in the hemithorax. These procedures are, therefore, typically followed by adjuvant treatments aimed at eliminating the residual microscopic disease.

Much judgement is required in determining, first, which patients have potentially resectable tumours, and second, which operation (pleurectomy or EPP) is required to achieve as close to a complete resection as possible. Multiple different adjuvant treatments have been tried, including chemotherapy, radiation therapy, combined chemotherapy and radiation therapy, photodynamic therapy, and intrapleural chemotherapy. The small numbers of patients in the various trials and the persistent problem of accurate and uniform staging continue to make interpretation of the outcomes of these therapies difficult. Nevertheless, it appears that some strides have been made against mesothelioma by these aggressive, combined approaches in selected patients.

Before a patient is considered for operation, assessment should be directed at whether the patient can tolerate pleurectomy or EPP. Cardiac and general medical status should be routinely evaluated as for any other thoracic procedure, with a low threshold for stress testing in a patient being considered for extrapleural pneumonectomy. Echocardiography should be performed to evaluate ventricular function, particularly if cardiotoxic adjuvant chemotherapies may be employed, and to rule out pericardial effusion.

Mesothelioma patients often have underlying abnormalities of pulmonary function secondary to coexisting asbestosis, pleural fibrosis, and chronic obstructive pulmonary disease.[14] For patients being considered for EPP, if pulmonary function testing demonstrates a forced expiratory volume in 1 second (FEV1) of less than 2 L, a quantitative ventilation-perfusion scan should be performed in order to determine the postoperative predicted FEV1. A predicted postoperative FEV1 of less than 1 L is a contraindication to the procedure. Resting hypoxia or hypercarbia are relative contraindications.

Imaging studies such as CT and MRI are useful in making an initial determination of a patient's candidacy for surgical resection, but the ultimate determination can only be made at the time of surgery. A tumour of any size, if confined to one hemithorax, demonstrating minimal invasion of diaphragm, pericardium and chest wall, and without evidence of mediastinal lymph node involvement, may be resectable. Video thoracoscopy, mediastinoscopy, and laparoscopy may be applied in selected cases, as described above, to help make these determinations prior to thoracotomy.

The CT and MRI criteria for resectability include preserved extrapleural fat planes, normal CT attenuation values and MRI signal intensities adjacent to the tumour, absence of extrapleural soft tissue masses, and smooth diaphragmatic surfaces. Separation of ribs by tumour or obvious bone destruction suggests it cannot be resected. Any tumour that extends through the diaphragm or diffusely invades the chest wall (other than at a previous biopsy site) or mediastinal organs is considered likely to be unresectable.[15] Positron emission tomography (PET) scanning with 18-fluoro-2-deoxyglucose is an emerging modality for the evaluation of mesothelioma, but its utility awaits direct comparison with the more common modalities and with surgical specimens.[16]

Patients with distant metastases are not candidates for resection. Although 50% of patients with mesothelioma have distant metastases at autopsy, these metastases are rarely the cause of death, and local intrathoracic extension is the predominate cause of symptoms during life. The most common sites of distant metastasis are liver (25%), bone (16%), adrenal (14%), and kidney (13%). Brain metastasis is distinctly unusual.[17] The preoperative work-up should therefore include a CT scan of the upper abdomen performed at the same time as the chest CT, and a bone scan.

Pleurectomy (sometimes called pleurectomy/decortication) may be attempted with curative intent in patients with IMIG stage I disease and selected patients with stage II disease. The procedure is performed as described above for palliative pleurectomy cases, except that every attempt is made to remove all gross disease. This may include tedious decortication of tumour from within the fissures, along the mediastinum, and deep into the costodiaphragmatic recesses. Results with this approach combined with various adjuvant protocols are listed in Table 9.4. If, during pleurectomy, it is found that gross tumour cannot be removed without a concomitant pneumonectomy, and if the patient's pulmonary function and comorbidities allow the more extensive procedure to be performed, then the pneumonectomy should be performed. This possibility should be discussed with all patients before the procedure.

EPP is a significantly more radical procedure. It removes, en bloc, the entire parietal pleura, visceral pleura, lung, pericardium, and hemidiaphragm.[18] The diaphragm is replaced with a prosthetic patch, as is the ipsilateral pericardium. This procedure should allow resection of all gross disease in stages I, II, and selected stage III patients. Most would not consider the procedure in patients with stage III lesions with N2 disease that can be identified preoperatively.

Since EPP is associated with significant rates of morbidity and mortality, it should be carried out in institutions with significant experience with the procedure,[19] and selection of patients who are good surgical candidates is critical. Supraventricular arrhythmia is the most common complication, occurring in 25–40% of patients, but this can generally be controlled with medication. Other complications include those listed for pleurectomy. The additional, life-threatening complications beyond those of pleurectomy which can occur following EPP stem from the pulmonary resection itself and include bronchial stump dehiscence and postpneumonectomy respiratory distress syndrome (ARDS). As following pneumonectomy, bronchial stump leak is more common following

Table 9.4. Results of selected trials of pleurectomy/decortication.

Year	Author	N	Median survival (mo)	2-year survival %
1997	Pass	39	14.5	—
1996	Rusch	51	18.3	40
1994	Allen	56	9	8.9
1989	Achatzy	46	10	11
1984	Law	28	20	32
1982	Chahinian	30	13	27
1976	Wanebo	33	16.1	—
	Totals	525	13.4	

Table 9.5. *Results of selected trials of extrapleural pneumonectomy.*

Year	Author	N	Median survival (mo)	2-year survival %
1999	Sugarbaker	183	19	38
1997	Pass	39	9.4	—
1996	Rusch	50	9.9	—
1994	Allen/Faber	40	13.3	22.5
1982	Chahinian	6	18	33
1976	Butchart	29	4.5	10.3
	Totals	376	12.9	

right than left EPP. It may be managed by reoperation and reclosure of the stump if it occurs early in the postoperative period, but requires open window thoracostomy as initial treatment if it occurs late postoperatively. In either case, significant morbidity and an approximately 20% mortality result. This complication may be more likely when local adjuvant therapies such as radiation, photodynamic therapy, or intrapleural chemotherapy are employed. Postpneumonectomy ARDS occurs in unpredictable fashion following EPP as it does following pneumonectomy. It is managed with supportive care typically involving intubation, antibiotics, and diuresis and has been reported to have a mortality of up to 50%. There is no proven way to avoid this complication.

Table 9.5 lists the results of selected trials of EPP with or without adjuvant therapies. EPP alone has never been shown to significantly prolong survival. Thus, more recent studies have combined EPP with adjuvant therapies of various types – 'combined modality' therapy.

In an early report, Butchart *et al.*[3] documented a median survival of only 4.5 months following EPP without adjuvant treatment. Importantly, however, it was noted that there were 2 long-term survivors and that epithelial histology was associated with a better prognosis. Allen and Faber compared EPP with pleurectomy in 96 patients, many of whom received adjuvant chemotherapy or radiation therapy. Operative mortality was slightly higher in the EPP group (7.5% versus 5.4%), but there was a non-statistically significant trend toward increased survival in the EPP patients.[20-22] The Lung Cancer Study Group (LCSG)[23] reported 20 patients who underwent EPP with a 15% mortality rate. Recurrence-free survival was significantly longer in those undergoing EPP than those undergoing more limited operation, but there was no difference in overall survival. Rusch *et al.* reported 101 resections evenly split between EPP and pleurectomy.[6] Local recurrence occurred mainly after the latter, while distar t metastasis was more likely to occur following EPP. Median survival was greater following pleurectomy (9.9 versus 18.7 months), suggesting that the inherent biology of the individual tumours plays a greater role than the type of resection in determining survival.

Given the failure of the single modality surgery to effect cure or even prolong life for more than a few months, surgery has frequently been combined with adjuvant therapies. Traditionally, the adjuvant treatments have consisted of various combinations of preoperative or postoperative chemotherapy and/or radiotherapy. The newest adjuvants tried have been intrapleural chemotherapy and photodynamic therapy. On the horizon as adjuvants to surgery are gene therapy and immunotherapy.

The combination of pleurectomy with postoperative intrapleural brachytherapy and/or external beam radiation without chemotherapy has been reported to increase survival in several studies.[13,24,25] In the Memorial Sloan-Kettering study the external beam dose was 4500 cGy, and median survival for the entire group was 12.6 months with a 2-year survival of 35%. Those with pure epithelial histology without gross residual tumour had a median survival of 22.5 months and a 2-year survival of 41%. Most complications were radiation-related, including pneumonitis, pulmonary fibrosis, oesophagitis, and pericardial effusion. The pulmonary toxicity of radiation is a major reason why many groups have moved towards EPP over pleurectomy, thereby allowing greater doses of radiation to be administered to the hemithorax after surgery.

Several investigators have combined EPP with sequential postoperative chemotherapy and up to 5500 cGy of radiotherapy to the operated hemithorax. Using a regimen of doxorubicin, cyclophosphamide, and cisplatin initially, and paclitaxel and carboplatin in later patients, the Brigham and Women's Hospital/Dana Farber Cancer Institute group has reported the most dramatic results.[26] Patients with resectable disease in Butchart stage I with epithelial histology and no mediastinal lymph node involvement had a 39% 5-year survival rate. Patients with sarcomatous or mixed histology or tumours invading the full-thickness of the diaphragm had a much poorer prognosis. Only 4% of patients developed extrathoracic metastases, and the most common sites of tumour recurrence were the ipsilateral chest, the peritoneal cavity, and the contralateral chest. The latest data from this group show that in patients with epithelial cell type, negative resection margins, and absence of mediastinal lymph node metastasis, the 5-year survival is 46%![7] Operative mortality in the entire group of patients undergoing EPP was only 3.8%. More recently, this group has followed surgery with intrapleural chemotherapy.

Those who have already reported trials of cytoreductive surgery followed by intrapleural chemotherapy with variable results include the LCSG,[27] UCLA[28] and Fox Chase Cancer Center.[29] In LCSG trial 882, pleurectomy/decortication was followed by intrapleural cisplatin and mitomycin with a median survival of 17 months. Locoregional disease was the most common site of relapse. At UCLA, a similar protocol substituting cytosine arabinoside for mitomycin was associated with low morbidity, but there was no significant prolongation of survival. The Fox Chase study added systemic chemotherapy and demonstrated significant toxicity and again no survival advantage.

Photodynamic therapy (PDT) is a novel adjuvant treatment whereby light-sensitive photosensitisers which localise in neoplastic cells are administered systemically and produce toxic oxygen free-radicals within these cells in response to light of a particular wavelength. The light is typically applied within the involved hemithorax intraoperatively, immediately following resection. Since most mesothelioma recurrences are local, this sort of local adjuvant treatment which directly attacks the residual microscopic tumour has been felt to be most promising as a surgical adjuvant. Some success has been achieved using PDT with the photosensitiser Porfimer sodium as adjuvant therapy in patients with low tumour burden.[30,31] A phase III trial, however, demonstrated no survival or local control advantage for patients undergoing PDT with this first-generation photosensitiser.[32] Others have reported a high morbidity rate following adjuvant PDT, with increased rates of bronchopleural fistulae, oesophageal perforation, and empyema[33,34] New, hopefully safer and more effective, photosensitisers are currently under investigation.

Other therapies on the horizon but which have not yet been tried in any systematic way as adjuvants to surgical debulking include gene therapy, immunotherapy, immunoconjugate therapy, and chemohyperthermia.

Summary

We have reviewed the most commonly used staging systems for malignant mesothelioma and described currently accepted surgical treatments for the various stages. Whereas until recently surgery had been primarily applied in diagnostic or palliative fashion, recent encouraging reports of cytoreductive pleurectomy or EPP combined with adjuvant therapies have somewhat alleviated the nihilistic approach to this disease which has been dominant for many years. Until emerging therapies such as gene therapy demonstrate effectiveness against the disease, the best hope for patients who can tolerate an aggressive approach is currently surgical cytoreduction followed by adjuvant chemotherapy and radiation therapy. For reasonably healthy patients with epithelial cell type mesotheliomas and limited disease confirmed by the currently available surgical staging procedures described herein, EPP followed by aggressive adjuvant therapy would appear to be the treatment of choice. For others, surgical palliation in the form of pleurectomy, VATS pleurodesis, or chest tube drainage and pleurodesis may be applied selectively.

References

1. Chahinian, A.P. Therapeutic modalities in malignant pleural mesothelioma. In: Chretien, J., Hirsch, A., eds. *Diseases of the pleura*. New York: Masson, 1983; 224–236.
2. Sugarbaker, D.J., Strauss, G.M., Lynch, T.J., *et al.* Node status has prognostic significance in the multimodality therapy of diffuse, malignant mesothelioma. *J Clin Oncol* 1993; **11**: 1172–1178.
3. Butchart, E.G., Ashcroft, T., Barnsley, W.C. *et al.* Pleuropneumonectomy in the management of diffuse malignant mesothelioma of the pleura. Experience with 29 patients. *Thorax* 1976; **31**: 15–24.
4. Mattson, K. Natural history and clinical staging of malignant mesothelioma. *Eur J Respir Dis* 1982; **63**(Suppl 124): 87.
5. Rusch, V.W., Ginsberg, R.J. New concepts in the staging of mesotheliomas. In: Deslauriers J, Lacquet LK, eds. *Thoracic surgery: surgical management of pleural diseases*. St. Louis: Mosby, 1990; 336–343.
6. Rusch, V.W., Venkatraman, E. The importance of surgical staging in the treatment of malignant pleural mesothelioma. *J Thorac Cardiovasc Surg* 1996; **111**: 815–826.

7. Sugarbaker, D.J., Flores, R.M., Jaklitsch, M.T., Richards, W.G., Strauss, G.M. *et al.* Resection margins, extrapleural nodal status, and cell type determine postoperative long-term survival in trimodality therapy of malignant pleural mesothelioma: results in 183 patients. *J Thorac Cardiovasc Surg* 1999; **117**: 54–65.

8. Rice, T.W., Adelstein, D.J., Kirby, T.J., Saltarell, M.G., Murthy, S.R, Van Kird, M.A., Wiedemann, H.P., Weick, J.K. Aggressive multimodality therapy for malignant pleural mesothelioma. *Ann Thorac Surg* 1994; **58**: 24–29.

9. Zimmer, P.W, Hill, M., Casey, K. *et al.* Prospective randomized trials of talc slurry vs. bleomycin in pleurodesis for symptomatic malignant pleural effusions. *Chest* 1997; **112**(2): 430–434.

10. Yim, A.P., Chan, A.T., Lee, T.X. *et al.* Thoracoscopic talc insufflation versus talc slurry for symptomatic malignant pleural effusion. *Ann Thorac Surg* 1996; **62**(6):1655–1658.

11. Tsang, V., Fernando, H.C., Goldstraw, P. Pleuroperitoneal shunt for recurrent malignant pleural effusion. *Thorax* 1990; **45**: 369–374.

12. Prior, A.J., Ball, A.B. Intestinal obstruction complicating malignant mesothelioma of the pleura. *Respir Med* 1993; **87**: 147–148.

13. Aisner, J. Current approach to malignant mesothelioma of the pleura. *Chest* 1995; **107**: 332S–344S.

14. Pass, H.I., Pogrebniak, H.W. Malignant pleural mesothelioma. *Curr Prob Surg* 1993; **30**: 921–1012.

15. Patz, E.F., Jr., Shaffer, K., Piwnica-Worms, D.R. *et al.* Malignant pleural mesothelioma: value of CT and MR imaging in predicting resectability. *Am J Roentgenol* 1992; **159**: 961–966.

16. Bénard, F., Sterman, D.H., Smith, R.J. *et al.* Metabolic imaging of malignant pleural mesothelioma with fluorine-18-deoxyglucose positron emission tomography. *Chest* 1998; **114**: 712–722.

17. King, J.A., Tucker, J.A., Wong, S.W. Mesothelioma: a study of 22 cases. *South Med J* 1997; **90**(2): 199–205.

18. Sugarbaker, D.J., Mentzer, S.J., Straus, G. Extrapleural pneumonectomy in the treatment of malignant pleural mesothelioma. *Ann Thorac Surg* 1992; **54**: 941–946.

19. Sugarbaker, D.J., Jaklitsch, M.T., Soutter, A.D., *et al.* Multimodality therapy of malignant mesothelioma. In: Roth, J.A., Ruckdeschel, J.C., Weisenburger, T.H. eds, *Thoracic oncology* 2nd edn Philadelphia: W.B. Saunders, 1995; 538–555.

20. Allan, K.B., Faber, L.P., Warren, W.H. Malignant pleural mesothelioma. Extrapleural pneumonectomy and pleurectomy. *Chest Surg Clin North Am* 1994; **4**: 113–126.

21. Faber, L.P. Extrapleural pneumonectomy for diffuse, malignant mesothelioma. *Ann Thorac Surg* 1994; **58**: 1782–1783.

22. Faber, L.P. Surgical treatment of asbestos-related disease of the chest. *Surg Clin North Am* 1988; **68**: 525–543.

23. Rusch, V.W., Piantadosi, S., Holmes, E.C. The role of extrapleural pneumonectomy in malignant pleural mesothelioma. A Lung Cancer Study Group trial. *J Thorac Cardiovasc Surg* 1991; **102**: 1–9.

24. Hilaris, B.S., Nori, D., Kwong, E. *et al.* Pleurectomy and intraoperative brachytherapy and postoperative radiation in the treatment of malignant pleural mesothelioma. *Int J Radiat Oncol Biol Phys* 1984; **10**: 325–331.

25. Martini, N., McCormack, P.M, Bains, M.S. *et al.* Pleural mesothelioma. *Ann Thorac Surg* 1987; **43**: 113–120.

26. Sugarbaker, D.J., Norberto, J.J. Multimodality management of malignant pleural mesothelioma. *Chest* 1998; **113**: 61S–65S.

27. Rusch, V. N. Trials in malignant mesothelioma. LCSG 851 and 882. *Chest* 1994; **106**: 359S–362S.

28. Lee, J.D, Perez, S., Wang, H.J. *et al.* Intrapleural chemotherapy for patients with incompletely resection malignant mesothelioma: the UCLA experience. *J Surg Oncol* 1995; **60**: 262–267.

29. Sauter, E.R., Langer, C., Coia, L.R. *et al.* Optimal management of malignant mesothelioma after subtotal pleurectomy: revisiting the role of intrapleural chemotherapy and postoperative radiation. *J Surg Oncol* 1995; **60**: 100–105.

30. Pass, H.I., Donington, J.S. Use of photodynamic therapy for the management of pleural malignancies. *Semin Surg Oncol* 1995; **11**: 360–367.

31. Ris, H.B., Altermatt, H.J., Nachbur, B. *et al.* Intraoperative photodynamic therapy with *m*-tetrahydroxphenylchlorin for chest malignancies. *Las Surg Med* 1996; **18**: 39–45.

32. Pass, H.I., Temeck, B.K, Kranda, K. *et al.* Phase III randomized trial of surgery with or without intraoperative photodynamic therapy and postoperative immunochemotherapy for malignant pleural mesothelioma. *Ann Surg Oncol* 1997; **4**: 628–633.

33. Takita, H., Mang, T.S., Loewen, G.M. *et al.* Operation and intracavitary photodynamic therapy for malignant pleural mesothelioma: a phase II study. *Ann Thorac Surg* 1994; **58**: 995–998.

34. Luketich, J.D., Westkaemper, J., Sommers, K.E. *et al.* Bronchoesophagopleural fistula after photodynamic therapy for malignant mesothelioma. *Ann Thorac Surg* 1996; **62**: 283–284.

=10=

Imaging in Mesothelioma

Jack G. Rabinowitz

Imaging occupies a vital role in the diagnosis and treatment of malignant pleural mesothelioma (MPM). In this respect the conventional chest x-ray, although limited in its scope, still remains an important modality. It can suggest or render a diagnosis of existing disease or at least recognise abnormalities affecting the lungs and/or the pleura.

More recently, additional imaging modalities such as computed tomography (CT), high resolution tomography and magnetic resonance imaging (MRI) have proven to be not only important adjuncts but more efficient in outlining the features of both asbestosis and mesothelioma. These techniques more readily distinguish pleural disease from normal pleura, accurately stage and determine tumour extent, and easily identify the optimal site for biopsy as well as aid in the biopsy procedure itself. High resolution tomography has been shown to be well in advance in demonstrating fine interstitial disease and plays an important role in distinguishing emphysematous destruction from the interstitial changes of asbestosis.[1,2] However, it does not appear to be of any greater use in the evaluation of mesothelioma.[1] Because of the partial volume effect on curved surfaces, the plate-like growth of mesothelioma is poorly demonstrated on CT.[3] MRI has been shown to be a more sensitive detector and may prove vital in predicting surgical resectability.

Since exposure to asbestos is highly responsible for the development of MPM, the detection of asbestos-related disease on the chest x-ray is helpful in establishing a diagnosis. Pleural plaques indicate significant past exposure to asbestos and are detected approximately 20 years after the initial exposure.[4] The asbestos fibres settle beneath the surface of the parietal pleura where they incite a fibrogenic reaction resulting in sclerosis and calcification. There is no evidence to date to suggest that the plaques themselves are premalignant.[5]

The plaques are located predominantly in the basilar portions of the chest wall, diaphragm, and mediastinum and appear as smooth lesions that rarely exceed 1 cm in thickness (Fig. 10.1). Until the fibrous component becomes sufficiently thickened, non-calcified plaques may be difficult to see on conventional chest x-ray.[4] They generally

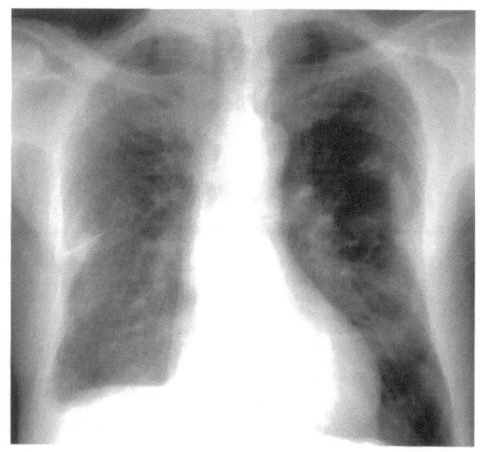

Figure 10.1. *Asbestosis. Chest shows multiple calcific plaques involving the chest wall bilaterally. The lungs are emphysematous and minimally fibrotic.*

follow the rib contours and diaphragmatic surface. Along the chest wall they can be mistaken for muscle shadows and in this respect oblique views are required for better demonstration. The shape of the plaque varies from flange-like when small to oval and protuberant when large.[6]

The CT appearance is quite similar with a slight variation. Asbestos plaques have been described as thickened skip areas of uniform density although the medial margin may be of higher density. However, in extensive asbestosis, the pleural masses may be irregularly thick and lobular. This feature can be confused with the development of mesothelioma.[6] Apparently a pleural plaque may grow and alter its configuration. Although the exact mechanism is unknown, it is thought that the continual migration and fragmentation of asbestos fibres produces active inflammatory changes that stimulate growth.

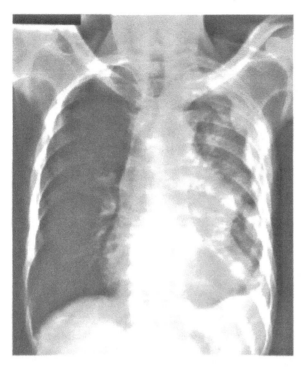

Figure 10.2. A. Mesothelioma. Chest shows multiple nodular masses of irregular size that encase the entire pleural surface that includes mediastinal and cardiac structures. In addition there is extension of the tumour into the axilla between the 2nd and 3rd ribs. There is also a decrease of volume on this side. **B.** CT demonstrates the total encasement by irregular nodular masses. Tumor extension between the ribs is also noticed.

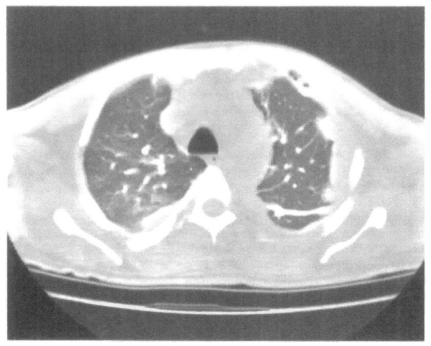

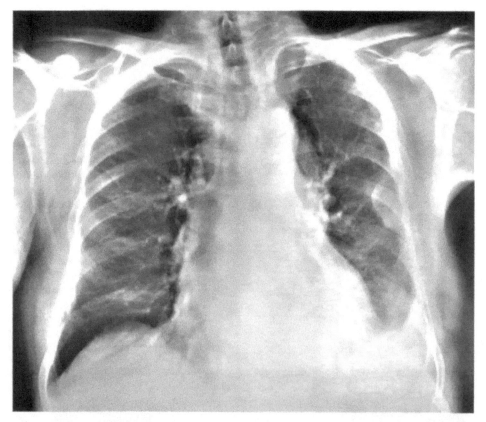

Figure 10.3. *Mesothelioma. Chest shows the left hemithorax is somewhat decreased in volume and is associated with some pleural effusion. A pleural-based mass of moderate size occupies the mid-portion of the lateral chest wall, resembling loculated fluid.*

Calcification occurs within the plaques in a large percentage of cases and is probably the most striking feature. These are seen as linear or slightly oval calcified densities in areas of pleural thickening along the rib cage surface of the diaphragm or mediastinum adjacent to the cardiac structure.

The radiographic features of mesothelioma are, in general, quite distinctive although not specific. Malignant mesothelioma is a diffuse lesion involving both pleural surfaces in contrast to a so-called benign variety which presents as a solitary mass. The latter arises spontaneously, is not related to asbestos exposure, and is probably pathogenetically different.[7] The major feature of MPM noted on plain film and on CT, is the presence of extensive, lobular thickened pleural based masses. The latter vary in size and thickness but can be uniform and encase the lung as a thickened pleural rind (Fig. 10.2).

Although malignant mesothelioma frequently encases the entire lung, its greatest growth occurs along the surface of the lower lobes where the pleural plaques of asbestosis predominate. In most cases, encasement of the pleural compartments by the tumour results in decreased volume of the involved hemithorax (Fig. 10.2). This finding is recognised easily on the conventional chest film and more so on CT studies. On conventional x-rays, the intercostal spaces are narrowed, causing a decrease in the slope of the rib cage and on CT the overall volume is small when compared to the opposite side. The mediastinum is generally fixed or frozen in the majority of cases in both CT and plain radiographs. This is thought to be characteristic for mesothelioma. Occasionally, a shift to the ipsilateral or even the contralateral side may occur, the latter as a result of a large pleural effusion or the presence of bulky masses.[8]

Pleural effusion is an important diagnostic feature found in 30–95% of patients with mesothelioma. Although benign pleural effusion can be seen in asbestosis, its occurrence is less common; it occurs well before other manifestations of asbestos-related disease, often within the first 10 years after exposure.[5] However, of greater importance is the occurrence of unilateral pleural effusion in patients with known asbestosis (Fig. 10.3). This presentation is highly suspect for mesothelioma and is probably the most frequent manifestation of the tumour. The amount of fluid varies and can be loculated or quite massive, obscuring the underlying tumour masses (Fig. 10.4). This can be problematic if one is unaware of any previous history of asbestos exposure. Occasionally the pleural fluid has been known to regress as the tumour enlarges. Pleural effusions are easily identified on conventional chest x-rays. The supine position can be confusing on CT and it is recommended that the decubitus position be used when mesothelioma is suspected in patients with asbestosis.

The above features are quite characteristic but not pathognomonic for mesothelioma since a similar pattern may be found in patients with advanced metastatic carcinoma.[6] In fact only electron microscopy and/or histochemical studies may allow for differentiation. Moreover, advanced asbestos disease with extensive and somewhat large plaques can simulate mesothelioma, rendering differentiation somewhat difficult. CT studies on these patients similarly demonstrate irregular lobular masses that resemble mesothelioma. Involvement of the interlobar fissures, however, is an important differentiating finding since it occurs in 40–86% of patients with mesothelioma.[3] The inflammatory reaction associated with asbestosis occurs principally in submesothial tissues and therefore spares the visceral pleura. Consequently, any growth or alteration of the fissures should be considered suspect for developing mesothelioma.

MRI plays an important role in determining the extent of malignant mesothelioma before therapy.[9,10] Malignant mesothelioma and particularly advanced tumour is known to invade the chest wall, pericardium, diaphragm and the abdomen. The tumour most frequently extends through the intercostal spaces into the surrounding soft tissue, often sparing the ribs (Fig. 10.2B). However, rib invasion can occur as a complication of advanced disease. In one series, contrast enhanced T_1 MRI demonstrated oedema of the intercostal ribs and therefore invasion of the bony structures by tumour in 30% of the cases.[3] In general, contrast enhanced T_1 weighted images are more reliable than CT in

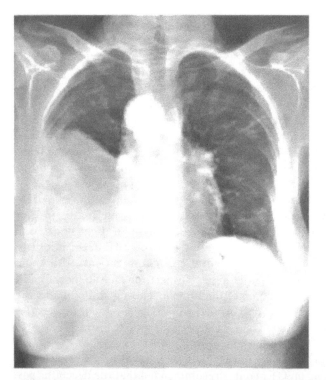

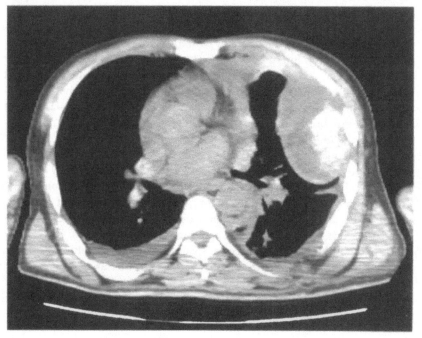

Figure 10.4. A. Mesothelioma resembling loculated pleural effusion. Chest PA shows multiple large bulky masses involving the lower left thoracic cage consisting of loculated pleural fluid and tumour mass. **B.** CT confirms the presence of the bulky tumours surrounding the entire hemithorax and associated with loculated pleural effusion.

predicting resectability by better showing pleural and chest wall changes.[3] MRI provides images in multiple planes and readily delineates tumorous lesions from normal structures. The most reliable finding indicative of resectability is a clear fat plane between the inferior diaphragmatic surface and the adjacent abdominal organs as well as a smooth inferior diaphragmatic surface.[9] This feature was less frequently manifested on CT and therefore is less reliable. Preservation of normal mediastinal fat without tumour infiltration of soft tissues and involvement of less than 50% of a mediastinal structure are additional findings suggesting resectability.

Rounded atelectasis is another mass that is associated with asbestosis and can be confused with mesothelioma. Unfortunately, it can rarely coexist with mesothelioma.[11] Rounded atelectasis has nevertheless certain unique characteristics, which, if noted, easily distinguish this lesion from most pleural masses. It is, however, often preceded by a pleural effusion most often caused by asbestosis, although other causes may be responsible. The lesion forms as the effusions develop into localised fibrosis fixing a portion of lung to the pleura. The fixed part of lung rotates into a rounded mass as the lung surrounding it re-expands. It presents as a rounded peripheral mass with a comet tail that arises usually inferiorly from the rounded mass and extends toward the hilum. The latter consists of the bronchi and vessels exiting from the lung mass. Rounded atelectasis is not associated with a large pleural effusion or chest wall invasion.

Positron emission tomography (PET) imaging, although used sporadically, may prove to be an important modality in the diagnosis and evaluation of malignant mesothelioma. In one recent study, 2-fluoro-2-dioxy-D-glucose (FDR) provided excellent delineation of the active tumour sites.[12] In fact hypermetabolic lymph node involvement was noted in 12 patients, 9 of which appeared normal on CT scans.

References

1. Gamsu, G., Aberli, D.R., Lynch, D. Computed tomography in the diagnosis of asbestos related thoracic disease. *J Thoracic Imaging* 1989; **4**(1): 61–67.
2. Aberli, D.R., Balmes, J.R. Computed tomography of asbetos-related pulmonary parenchymal and pleural diseases. *Clin Chest Med* 1991; **3**(1): 115–131.
3. Knuuttila, A., Halme, M., Kivisaari, L., Kivisaari, A., Salo, J., Mattson, K. The clinical importance of magnetic resonance imaging versus computed tomography in malignant pleural mesothelioma. *Lung Cancer* 1998; **2**: 215–225.
4. Hillerdal, G. Pleural plaques and risk for bronchial carcinoma and mesothelioma. *Chest* 1994; **105**:144–150.
5. McCloud, T.C. Conventional radiography in the diagnosis of asbestos related disease. *Radiol Clin North Am* 1992; **30**: 1178–1189.
6. Rabinowitz, J.G., Efremidis, S.C., Cohen, B., Dan, S., Efremides, A., Chahinian, A.P., Teirstein, A.S. A comparative study of mesothelioma and asbestosis using computed tomography and conventional radiography. *Radiology* 1982; **144**: 453–460.
7. Khan, J.H., Rahman, S.B., Clary-Macy, C. *et al.* Giant solitary fibrous tumor of the pleura. *Ann Thorac Surg* 1998; **65**: 1461–1464.

8. Dynes, M.C., White, E.M., Fry, W.A., Ghahremani, G.G. Imaging manifestations of pleural tumors. *Radiographics* 1992; **12**: 1191–1201.
9. Patz, E.F., Shaffer, K., Piwnica-Worms, D.R., Jochelson, M., Sarin, M., Sugarbaker, D.J., Pugatch, R.D. Malignant pleural mesothelioma: Value of CT & MR imaging in predicting resectability. *AJR* 1992; **159**: 961–966.
10. McCloud, T.C. CT & MR in pleural disease. *Clin Chest Med* 1998; **19**(2): 261–276.
11. Munden RF, Libshitz HI. Rounded alectatasis and mesothelioma. *AJR* 1998; **170**: 1519–1522.
12. Benard, F., Sterman, D., Smith, R.J., Kaiser, L.R., Albelda, S.M., Alavi, A. Metabolic imaging of malignant pleural mesothelioma with fluorodeoxy glucose positron emission tomography. *Chest* 1998; **114**(3): 713–722.

=11=

Treatment of Malignant Mesothelioma: Radiotherapy and Chemotherapy

A. Philippe Chahinian

The treatment of malignant mesothelioma (MM) is a particular challenge for the physician. The diffuse nature of the disease makes it difficult for the surgeon to perform a radical resection. Even if technically possible, such extensive resections are usually not curative. The role of two other treatment modalities, radiotherapy and chemotherapy, will be discussed in this chapter.

Radiotherapy

In the past, only anecdotal reports provided some insight on the efficacy of radiotherapy for pleural MM.[1] Elmes stated that radiotherapy was avoided because it seemed 'to cause the tumor to grow more rapidly through the chest wall and to involve the skin'.[2] The first systematic trial of radiotherapy was published in France by Eschwege and Schlienger in 1973.[3] These authors gave a total dose of 3500–7500 cGy delivered by a 23 MeV betatron in individual doses of 330 cGy three times per week in 14 patients with pleural MM. Anterior and posterior portals were used to include the entire hemithorax, the diaphragm, axillary and supraclavicular areas, and two-thirds of the adjacent mediastinum. Most patients received a total of 4500 cGy. Portals were reduced after that dose in patients who continued radiotherapy. Despite this large volume and the risk of radiation pneumonitis, as well as cardiac and spinal cord injury, tolerance was reported to be acceptable and a favourable effect on pain was noted. Median survival after onset of radiotherapy was 15 months, with a range of 1 to 37 months.

Shortly thereafter, Voss *et al.* in Germany reported their results using similar doses (4000–6000 cGy to the hemithorax and adjacent mediastinum with telecobalt or a 42 MeV betatron) in 14 patients with pleural MM.[4] The favourable effect on pain, which disappeared in 10 patients, was confirmed, but the survival was shorter, with a mean of 10 months.

Gordon *et al.* in Boston evaluated results of radiotherapy using a 4 MeV or 8 MeV linear accelerator (at daily doses of usually 200 cGy) according to two distinct groups.[5]

The 'radical' radiotherapy group included 6 patients with pleural MM treated with curative intent at doses ranging from 2200 to 5600 cGy to the hemithorax following partial pleurectomy. Three patients also received doxorubicin-based chemotherapy. Median survival for that group was 11.5 months, with a range of 6 to 13 months in 5 patients. One patient remained alive without evidence of disease at 5 years. The 'palliative' radiotherapy group included 17 patients treated with total doses of 800 to 5700 cGy for relief of symptoms. Some also received chemotherapy. The median survival of this group was similar (12 months), with a range of 3 to 60 months. Even though these groups are heterogeneous and somewhat artificially separated, the authors concluded that 'whole lung external beam irradiation for control of gross MM is not effective, and that conventional doses of radiation therapy delivered in a safe fashion did not control 1-2 mm nodules distributed over the visceral pleura'. Adequate palliation was achieved with doses at or above 4000 cGy in 4 weeks. The use of interstitial or radiocolloid treatment, given to a few patients by Gordon et al., was limited by the large surfaces to be treated and the problems posed by effective diffusion and widespread distribution of the agent.[5]

A major obstacle to radiotherapy has been the usual anatomical extent of the disease, involving the entire pleural surface as well as interlobar fissures. Complex and sophisticated techniques using combined photon-electron beam treatments, customised blocks and CT scan for treatment planning have been described with little evidence of any clear-cut benefit in terms of survival.[6,7] Holsti et al. in Finland have evaluated six different fractionation schedules of hemithoracic irradiation in 57 patients with mesothelioma.[8] They included conventional fractionation (2000 cGy in 10 fractions over 12 days), split-course radiotherapy (5500 cGy in 25 fractions of 220 cGy over 7 weeks with a two-week rest halfway, followed by a boost dose of 1500 cGy over 8 days to the major tumour volume), hyperfractionation (7000 cGy over 7 weeks, 125 cGy twice daily with a 6-hour interval and a 10-day rest halfway) and hypofractionation (3850 cGy over 15 days), as well as complex schedules of combined hyperfractionation and hypofractionation, or combined conventional radiotherapy and hypofractionation. They concluded that the pattern of progression was similar in each treatment group.

One possible benefit of radiotherapy has been its prophylactic use in a small field to prevent seeding along the track of invasive procedures such as needle pleural biopsy, chest tube sites, or thoracoscopy incisions. In France, Boutin et al. randomised 40 patients with pleural mesothelioma after such procedures to no radiotherapy (20 patients) or radiotherapy to these sites (three daily sessions of 700 cGy 10 to 15 days after the procedure).[9] None of the radiotherapy-treated patients developed entry tract tumour seeding, which occurred in 8 (40%) of patients not so treated.

Interstitial radiotherapy has also been evaluated in some patients with pleural mesothelioma. Radioactive colloidal gold has been administered intrapleurally and resulted in some good long-term results in a cumulative review of 18 cases.[10] Two patients survived 3.5 years and one 11 years.

Another way to attempt to improve these results has been the use of combined modalities. Several Phase II trials have combined radiotherapy with concomitant chemotherapy.[11] Interestingly, an earlier report from Falkson et al. in South Africa had suggested that procarbazine added to radiation resulted in subjective and objective improvement in 14 out of 26 patients with pleural mesothelioma.[12] Median survival was 23.5 months for responders and 10 months for non-responders. Alberts *et al.,*[7] also from South Africa, have observed only a slight prolongation of survival by adding procarbazine (median survival 10.9 months in 14 patients, with only two partial responses) or cyclophosphamide (median survival 10.8 months in 33 patients) as opposed to radiotherapy alone (median survival 7.8 months in 13 patients). The use of doxorubicin, however, yielded a median survival of 22.6 months in 10 patients, but with no objective responses. Two other trials combining doxorubicin and radiotherapy have not confirmed these results. One by Chahinian *et al.*[13] resulted in a median survival of 10 months in 14 patients, and the other by Sinoff *et al.*[14] yielded a very similar figure of 11 months median survival in 10 patients. Such apparently divergent results could be attributed to the small number of patients in these Phase II trials. Linden *et al.* in Sweden have treated 31 patients with pleural mesothelioma with hemithoracic radiotherapy alone (total dose 4000 cGy in daily fractions of 200 cGy) and observed only one partial response.[15] Median survival was 6 months. In another subgroup of 16 patients with good performance status and below 70 years of age, concomitant chemotherapy with doxorubicin and cyclophosphamide was administered. There were only 2 partial responses, but the median survival was 13 months, probably because of more favourable prognostic factors in this group. They concluded that hemithoracic irradiation was not useful.

Whereas the discussion of surgery is beyond the scope of this chapter, it should be mentioned that various techniques of external and interstitial radiotherapy have also been combined with surgery.[16] Hilaris *et al.* have reported the results of palliative pleurectomy combined with intraoperative brachytherapy (using either 125 I, 192 Ir, or 32 P),[17] followed by postoperative external radiotherapy combining electron and photon beams (at doses of 4500 cGy in 4.5 weeks). The median survival was 21 months in 41 patients. At the time of the report, 17 patients were still alive, a fact which could have favorably influenced these actuarial survival data. The median disease-free survival was 11 months. Sugarbaker *et al.* have combined extrapleural pneumonectomy with radiation to the hemithorax and chemotherapy with cyclophosphamide, doxorubicin and cisplatin in 120 selected patients.[18] Overall survival was 45% at 2 years and 22% at 5 years.

Interestingly, a complete response to fast neutron therapy has been reported in London in a patient with a bulky pleural mesothelioma localised to the lower half of the pleural cavity.[19] Seven months later, a relapse at the lower border of the field regressed after cobalt radiation, and this patient remained free of recurrent disease up to 78 months after treatment.

Much less data are available on results of radiotherapy in peritoneal mesothelioma, but it is intriguing that some long-term survivals have nevertheless been described. Among four patients treated by intraperitoneal instillation of 32 P followed by external radiotherapy to the entire abdomen (1000 to 3000 cGy in 3 to 4 weeks), and a boost to the pelvis (1000 to 2500 cGy in 2 to 3 weeks), two patients survived more than 10 years.[20] Three of these patients also received chemotherapy with cyclophosphamide with or without vincristine. In a cumulative review of the literature including a total of 10 patients, some good long-term results have been reported with the use of intraperitoneal radioactive colloidal gold, with 3 complete responses lasting more than 2.5, 3.5 and 5 years, respectively.[10]

Chemotherapy

Our knowledge of the effects of various chemotherapeutic agents has gradually increased over the past 20 years, although it is still very limited because of the small number of patients, which precludes the systematic evaluation of new agents as well as the conduct of large Phase III type clinical trials. Mesothelioma is a disease which has been poorly responsive to chemotherapy, and there is as yet no standard chemotherapy regimen. In view of the rarity of the disease, the use of laboratory models such as the nude mouse human xenograft system[21-23] is particularly helpful in selecting the most active agents for clinical trials. These models have generally confirmed the well-known clinical fact that this tumour is resistant to most drugs. There are, however, regimens which have produced occasional good responses, and which do not justify the attitude of total nihilism so common to many oncologists dealing with mesothelioma patients.

Few studies have addressed the issue of chemotherapy resistance in mesothelioma cells. It has been shown, however, that the mRNA for the multidrug resistance-associated protein (MRP) and for gamma-glutamylcysteine synthetase, but not for the P-glycoprotein of multidrug resistance (MDR1), are overexpressed in chemotherapy-naive human mesothelioma cell lines.[24] Expression of MRP was correlated with doxorubicin resistance.

Single agents

The activity of many single agents has now been evaluated in mesothelioma. The cumulative response rates to these drugs is shown in Tables 11.1 and 11.2 depending on the num-

Table 11.1. Single agents in mesothelioma, more than 40 patients.

Agent	Number of			
	Patients	Complete response	All responses	Response rate
Doxorubicin	112	6	17	15%
Dihydro-azacytidine	104	1	8	9%
Carboplatin	97	2	12	12%
Etoposide	96	0	5	5%
Cisplatin	74	2	10	14%
Epirubicin	69	0	8	12%
Mitoxantrone	64	1	3	5%
Methotrexate high	60	1	22	37%
Trimetrexate	51	0	6	12%
Ifosfamide	43	0	6	14%
Pirarubicin	43	1	6	14%
Acivicin	43	0	0	0%
Gemcitabine	43	1	8	19%

ber of evaluable patients per drug (more or less than 40 evaluable patients, respectively). These data are summarised from Chahinian and Rusch,[11] with updates given in this text.

Response rates to single agents are usually very low, varying from 0% to 15% in most trials. Results in Table 11.1 indicate that the response rates to anthracyclines (doxorubicin, epirubicin) and platinum compounds (cisplatin, carboplatin) have now been evaluated in a relatively large number of patients and are roughly similar, varying between 12% and 15%. It is remarkable that a few complete responses have been observed, most notably with doxorubicin. It is posssible, however, that this is due to response assessment by plain chest x-rays rather than CT scans, since trials with that drug are somewhat older. Most single agent studies have yielded median survivals of 5 to 9 months only.[11]

Dihydro-azacytidine was selected for its unusual toxicity for serosal surfaces (pericarditis, pleuritis), leading to the expectation that this agent might be particularly active for mesothelioma. Results have been rather disappointing, with an overall response rate of 9% in a total of 104 patients. Although the Cancer and Leukemia Group B trial of dihydro-azacytidine yielded a response rate of 17% and a median survival of 6.3 months in 41 patients,[25] an identical trial by the Southwest Oncology Group in 51 patients resulted in a 4% response rate only, with a median survival of 4.0 months.[26]

Similar comments can be made about the new agent gemcitabine, a pyrimidine analogue, which has been evaluated recently. Preliminary resuts in the United States showed only one minor regression in the first 13 patients.[27] On the other hand, a response rate of 31% was seen in Germany in 16 patients (1 complete and 4 partial responses),[28] and of 21% in 14 patients in Belgium.[29] Further evaluation is desirable for this new agent, and the activity of gemcitabine combined with cisplatin is described below.

High-dose methotrexate was evaluated largely in one study from Finland (3 g total dose with citrovorum factor rescue).[30] The relatively high response rate (37%)

Table 11.2. *Single agents in mesothelioma, less than 40 patients.*

Agent	Number of			Response rate
	Patients	Complete response	All responses	
Vindesine	38	0	1	3%
Cyclophosphamide	34	0	3	9%
Pcnu	34	0	0	0%
Vinorelbine	29	0	7	24%
Cisplatin high	26	0	8	31%
Paclitaxel (Taxol)	26	0	2	8%
Fluorouracil	25	4	5	20%
Vincristine	23	0	0	0%
Bleomycin	22	0	2	9%
Topotecan	22	0	0	0%
Detorubicin	21	2	9	43%
Edatrexate	20	1	5	25%
Diaziquone	20	0	0	0%
Vinblastine	20	0	0	0%
Mitomycin	19	0	4	21%

and a median survival of 11 months both deserve confirmation. Etoposide has been evaluated by the European Organisation for Research and Treatment of Cancer by both the intravenous and the oral route and has been largely ineffective,[31] despite an initial case report which described a good response to that agent.[32]

Results shown in Table 11.2 pertain to small numbers of patients (less than 40 per drug) and are not definitive. Some trends are emerging, however. The new agent paclitaxel (Taxol) has a low response rate of 8% so far in 26 patients.[33,34] Similarly, other microtubule inhibitors such as the vinca alkaloids (vindesine, vincristine, vinblastine) have been inactive, with the exception of vinorelbine, which has produced a 21% response rate.[34a] The new topoisomerase 1 inhibitor topotecan was evaluated by the North Central Cancer Treatment Group and produced no objective response in 22 patients.[35]

More noticeable results have been seen with high-dose cisplatin (either 40 mg/m^2 daily for 5 days, or 80 mg/m^2 weekly for 6 weeks), fluorouracil, edatrexate and mitomycin. Further evaluation of these agents appears highly desirable. The response rate to detorubicin is unusual. It emanated from a single group in France and is at great variance with the results observed with its parent drug, doxorubicin.

Suramin has been reported to be effective *in vitro* against human mesothelioma cell lines[36] and is of interest because of its ability to inhibit DNA synthesis as well as the action of various growth factors including PDGF, which plays an important role in the growth of mesothelioma. Results in human mesothelioma xenografts in nude mice did not confirm such activity.[37] It is of interest, however, that suramin was successful when given intraperitoneally in a patient with peritoneal mesothelioma.[38]

Onconase is a ribonuclease isolated from the eggs of the leopard frog and has been reported to produce 4 partial responses in 25 patients with mesothelioma.[39] There is currently a randomised trial under way prospectively comparing that agent with doxorubicin. It is also intriguing that lovastatin, a lipid lowering agent and inhibitor of coenzyme A reductase, has the ability to induce apoptosis of human mesothelioma cells *in vitro*.[40]

Combination chemotherapy

Although many regimens of combination chemotherapy have been evaluated,[11] there is no clear-cut clinical evidence that they are superior to single agents. Whereas older trials included mainly doxorubicin in combination with cyclophosphamide with or without other agents, most current regimens have included cisplatin combined with another drug. The relative rarity of the disease precludes the conduct of large randomised Phase III trials to definitely address that issue.

Laboratory models such as the nude mouse system have clearly shown that some combinations of drugs are superior to the same drugs given as single agents.[23] This was the case for the combination of mitomycin and cisplatin, which was more effective than mitomycin or cisplatin alone,[21] and the combination of paclitaxel and cisplatin, similarly superior to paclitaxel or cisplatin alone.[37] Based on these results, a randomised Phase II trial was conducted by the Cancer and Leukemia Group B (CALGB) using cisplatin (75 mg/m^2) combined with either mitomycin (10 mg/m^2) (CM), or with doxorubicin (60 mg/m^2) (CD), repeated every 4 weeks.[41] There were 35 evaluable patients in each arm. The response rate was

26% for CM, including 2 complete responses, and 14% for CD, with no complete response. As expected with these levels of response, no significant difference in median survival was observed (7.7 months for CM and 8.8 months for CD). It is, however, encouraging that a response rate greater than 20% was seen in a cooperative group study for CM, thereby justifying the use of a predictive model (in this case the nude mouse system) to select regimens for clinical trials in this rare disease. A preliminary report of high-dose cisplatin (105–120 mg/m^2) and doxorubicin (90 mg/m^2) produced two complete remissions and one partial remission in 4 patients.[42] Of note is that three other trials using more conventional doses of doxorubicin and cisplatin produced response rates which are inversely correlated with the number of evaluable patients: 67% in 6 patients, 42% in 19 patients, and 25% in 24 patients.[11] In the CALGB trial indicated above on 35 patients, the response rate was even lower, 14%. Hence results in small series should await confirmation by larger trials.

Other doublets including cisplatin have been evaluated. The combination of VP16 and cisplatin resulted in only 3 partial responses among 26 patients (12% response rate).[43] The combination of dihydro-5-azacytidine with cisplatin in 29 patients produced only a 17% response rate, with a median survival of 6.4 months.[44] The combination of cisplatin and vinblastine resulted in a 25% response rate (with one complete response) in 20 patients.[45] Promising results were observed with the combination of gemcitabine and cisplatin in Australia, with a response rate of 47.6% (all partial) among 21 patients, and a median survival of 41 weeks.[46] Most responses were seen in patients with the epithelial subtype. Symptomatic improvement was correlated with response. The combination of a new topoisomerase 1 inhibitor irinotecan (CPT-11) with cisplatin was evaluated in Japan and produced a 40% partial response rate in 15 patients.[47] Both CPT-11 and its active metabolite SN-38 were detected in the pleural fluid 1 hour after intravenous injection of CPT-11, at respective concentrations of 36.5% and 75.8% of plasma levels. Another apparently active new combination which requires further evaluation includes cisplatin and a novel experimental multi-targeted antifolate (called MTA or LY231514), which produced 4 responses among 7 patients.[48]

The combination of paclitaxel and carboplatin has been evaluated in only two small series, with interesting preliminary results. One trial on 7 patients yielded 4 partial responses,[49] and another one, also of 7 patients, resulted in 1 complete and 1 partial response.[50] These results tend to confirm the activity of such a combination seen in nude mice[37] and provide a rationale for further evaluation of this regimen, which is now widely used in patients with non-small cell lung cancer.

Triple drug combinations have been evaluated without any proof so far that they are superior to two-drug combinations. Cisplatin, doxorubicin and vindesine combined did not result in any objective response in 11 patients.[51] Methotrexate (at a regular dose of 30 mg/m^2) and vinblastine were effective when combined with cisplatin, producing responses in 8 out of 11 patients and an overall median survival of 14 months.[52] Again, confirmation is necessary in view of the small number of patients. The CAP combination, including cyclophosphamide, doxorubicin (Adriamycin) and cisplatin, resulted in 30% partial responses in 23 patients, with an overall median survival of 60 weeks.[53]

Several trials have added a third agent to the mitomycin-cisplatin (MP) as described above, being initially discovered to be effective in nude mice and which resulted in a 26% response rate in CALGB, representing the highest response rate among all the chemotherapy trials conducted in that cooperative group. Doxorubicin was added to MP in Italy and resulted in 22% partial responses in 23 patients, with an overall median survival of 45.5 weeks.[54] Vinblastine was added to MP in Britain with an objective response rate of 20% in 39 patients, a 62% symptomatic improvement and 79% pain response.[55] Interferon was also added to MP in Turkey, following the discovery in the nude mouse model that this biological agent, basically inactive by itself, was able to increase the antitumor activity of chemotherapy in human mesothelioma xenografts.[56] Twenty patients were treated with mitomycin, cisplatin and intramuscular alpha-interferon and two showed a partial response.[57] Whereas the response rate was not apparently better than with mitomycin and cisplatin, the median survival of 15 months was somewhat better than expected.

Even more complex multi-drug regimens have been evaluated. The combination of cisplatin, doxorubicin, bleomycin and mitomycin, together with systemic and intrapleural hyaluronidase, has been given to 27 patients in France, with a response rate of 44%, including 2 complete ones, and an overall median survival of 15 months.[58] The combination of cisplatin, mitomycin, 5-fluorouracil with leucovorin, and etoposide (PMFE) was given to 50 patients with a 34% partial response rate and an overall median survival of 16 months.[59]

Intracavitary chemotherapy

Because malignant effusions, whether pleural or peritoneal, are common presenting manifestations of mesothelioma, the use of intracavitary chemotherapy represents a logical approach. Various regimens have been used, most of them also based on cisplatin.[11]

That agent given alone at doses of 90–100 mg/m^2, together with intravenous thiosulphate to lessen its systemic toxicity, produced 1 response in 8 patients with pleural mesothelioma, and 1 complete, 2 partial responses and reduction of ascites in 6 cases among 13 patients with peritoneal mesothelioma.[60,61] A combined modality approach with debulking surgery, intraperitoneal doxorubicin plus cisplatin and external whole abdominal radiotherapy up to 30 Gy was used in 5 patients with early peritoneal mesothelioma and resulted in median survival of more than 18 months.[62]

The combination of mitomycin and cisplatin, which has been evaluated somewhat extensively by the intravenous route following the identification of its effectiveness in nude mice,[21] has also been given by the intracavitary route both in pleural and peritoneal mesothelioma at the Memorial Sloan-Kettering Cancer Center in New York. That combination was effective in controlling ascites in 6 of 11 patients with peritoneal mesothelioma, and two of these patients remained without evidence of recurrent disease in the peritoneal cavity for periods of over 32 and 41 months.[63,64] A median survival of 17 months was obtained in 27 patients with pleural mesothelioma treated initially with surgery (pleurectomy or decortication) followed by intrapleural and systemic mitomycin and cisplatin, first intrapleurally and then systemically.[65] In a similar approach at the Cleveland Clinic, where 19 patients underwent either pleurectomy or pleuropneumonectomy followed by intracavitary and systemic chemotherapy with cisplatin alone or in combination with mitomycin, a median survival of 13 months was observed.[66]

The exact role of intracavitary chemotherapy as well as its use in combined modality therapies remains to be further defined by prospective trials.

Other therapies

Although immunotherapy is discussed in Chapter 18, it should be mentioned that the nude mouse model first showed that the antitumour effect of chemotherapy (cisplatin or mitomycin) against human mesothelioma xenografts was augmented by the addition of human recombinant alpha-interferon (IFN), whereas that agent by itself had very little activity in that model.[56] Similar findings were observed *in vitro* in human mesothelioma cell lines.[67] This is another demonstration that the addition of an agent with little or no activity by itself could increase the effectiveness of active drugs.

Clinical trials have since been conducted using mainly combinations of cisplatin and alpha-IFN. The combination of cisplatin (60 mg/m^2 intravenously weekly) and alpha-IFN (3 mU subcutaneously on days 1–4) for either 5 weeks on/3 weeks off or 4 weeks on/4 weeks off produced a 40% response rate in 25 patients in France, with an overall median survival of 12 months.[68] Patients with epithelial cell type had the highest response rate (50%), and weight loss and thrombocytosis were poor prognostic factors. A similar combination, with a different dose and schedule of cisplatin (25 mg/m^2 4 times weekly) and of alpha-IFN (5 mU/m^2 subcutaneously 3 times weekly) with the addition of tamoxifen (20 mg orally twice a day, in an attempt to decrease drug resistance), resulted in a 19% response rate in 36 patients, with a median survival of 8.7 months at the National Cancer Institute in Bethesda.[69] Again, thrombocytosis and non-epithelial histology resulted in poor prognosis. More recently a very similar trial in France using weekly cisplatin (60 mg/m^2) and weekly alpha-IFN (at a higher dose of 6 mU daily for 4 days) given 4 weeks on/4 weeks off produced one complete response and 4 partial responses in 12 evaluable patients, with a median overall survival of 16.5 months.[70]

In view of the paucity of active regimens for mesothelioma, such results provide a basis for further trials of combined chemotherapy-IFN in that disease.

In conclusion, the experience with chemotherapy in MM is now steadily increasing and it is clear that some regimens have produced both acceptable objective response rates for such a refractory disease, as well as noticeable symptomatic improvement. These data no longer justify the therapeutic nihilism which has been such a common attitude in many physicians toward this disease.

References

1. Chahinian, A.P., Holland, J.F. (1978): Treatment of diffuse malignant mesothelioma: A review. *Mt. Sinai J. Med.*, **45**: 54–67.
2. Elmes, P.C. (1973): The natural history of diffuse mesothelioma. In: *Biological Effects of Asbestos*, P. Bogovoski, J.C. Gilson, V. Timbrell, and J.C. Wagner, eds, Lyon, France, International Agency for Research on Cancer, p. 267.

3. Eschwege, S., Schlienger, M. (1973): La radiothérapie des mésotheliomes pleuraux malins. A propos de 14 cas irradiés a doses élevées. *J. Radiol. Electrol. (Paris)*, **54**: 255–259.
4. Voss, A.C., Wollgens, P., Untucht, H.J. (1974). Das Pleuramesotheliom aus strahlentherapeutischer Sicht. *Strahlentherapie*, **148**: 329–332.
5. Gordon, W., Antman, K.H., Greenberger, J.S., Weichselbaum, R.R., Chaffey, J.T. (1981): Radiation therapy in the management of patients with mesothelioma. *Int. J. Radiat. Oncol. Biol. Phys.*, **8**: 19–25.
6. Kutcher, G.J., Kestler, R.T., Greenblatt, D., Brenner, H., Hilaris, B.S., Nori, D. (1987): Technique for external beam treatment for mesothelioma. *Int J. Radiat. Oncol. Biol. Phys.*, **13**: 1747–1752.
7. Alberts, A.S., Falkson, G., Goedhals, L., Vorobiof, D.A, Van Der Merwe, C.A. (1988): Malignant pleural mesothelioma: A disease unaffected by current therapeutic maneuvers. *J. Clin. Oncol.*, **6**: 527–535.
8. Holsti, L.R., Pyrhonen, S., Kajanti, M., Mantyla, M., Mattson, K., Maasilta, P., Kivisaari, L. (1997): Altered fractionation of hemithorax irradiation for pleural mesothelioma and failure patterns after treatment. *Acta Oncol*, **36**: 397–405.
9. Boutin, C., Rey, F., Viallat, J.R. (1995): Prevention of malignant seeding after invasive diagnostic procedures in patients with pleural mesothelioma. A randomized trial of radiotherapy. *Chest*, **108**: 754–758.
10. Legha, S.S., Muggia, F.M. (1977): Therapeutic approaches in malignant mesothelioma. *Cancer Treat. Rev.*, **4**: 13–23.
11. Chahinian, A.P., Rusch, V.W. (1997): Malignant mesothelioma. In Holland, J.F., Frei, E., III., Bast, R.C., Kufe, D.W., Morton, D., Weichselbaum, R.R., eds, "Cancer Medicine", 4th Ed., Williams & Wilkins, Baltimore, pp1805–1826.
12. Falkson, G., Falkson, H.C., Fichart, T. (1970): Radiosensitization by procarbazine in the treatment of malignant mesothelioma. In: "Radiation Protection and Sensitization", Moroson H, Quintiliani M, eds, Taylor & Francis, London, pp 499–502.
13. Chahinian, A.P., Pajak, T.F., Holland, J.F., Norton, L., Ambinder, R.M., Mandel, E.M. (1982): Diffuse malignant mesothelioma. Prospective evaluation of 69 patients. *Ann. Intern. Med.*, **96**: 746–755.
14. Sinoff, C., Falkson, G., Sandison, A.G., De Muelenaere, G. (1982). Combined doxorubicin and radiation therapy in malignant pleural mesothelioma. *Cancer Treat. Rev.*, **66**: 1605–1607.
15. Linden, C.J., Mercke, C., Albrechtsson, U., Johansson, L., Ewers, S.B. (1996): Effect of hemithorax irradiation alone or combined with doxorubicin and cyclophosphamide in 47 pleural mesotheliomas. A nonrandomized phase II study. *Eur. Respir. J.*, **9**: 2565–2572.
16. McCormack, P.M., Nagasaki, F., Hilaris, B.S., Martini, N. (1982): Surgical treatment of pleural mesothelioma. *J. Thorac. Cardiovasc. Surg.*, **84**: 834–842.
17. Hilaris, B.S., Nori, D., Kwong, E., Kutcher, G.J, Martini, N. (1984): Pleurectomy and intraoperative brachytherapy and postoperative radiation in the treatment of malignant pleural mesothelioma. *Int. J. Radiat. Oncol. Biol. Phys.*, **10**: 325–331.
18. Sugarbaker, D.J., Garcia, J.P., Richards, W.G., Harpole, D.H. Jr, Healy-Baldini, E., DeCamp, M.M. Jr, Mentzer, S.J., Liptay, M.J., Strauss, G.M., Swanson, S.J. (1996): Extrapleural pneumonectomy in the multimodality therapy of malignant pleural mesothelioma. Results in 120 consecutive patients. *Ann. Surg.*, **224**: 288–294.
19. Blake, P.R., Catteral, M., Emerson, P.A. (1985): Pleural mesothelioma treated by fast neutron therapy. *Thorax*, **40**: 72–73.
20. Rogoff, E.E., Hilaris, B.S., Huvos, A.G. (1973): Long term survival in patients with malignant peritoneal mesothelioma treated with irradiation. *Cancer*, **32**: 656–664.

21. Chahinian, A., Norton, L., Holland, J.F., Szrajer, L., Hart, R.D. (1984): Experimental and clinical activity of mitomycin C and cis-diamminedichloroplatinum in malignant mesothelioma. *Cancer Res.*, **44**: 1688–1692.

22. Chahinian, A.P., Kirschner, P.A., Gordon, R.E., Szrajer, L., Holland, J.F. (1991): Usefulness of the nude mouse in mesothelioma based on a direct patient xenograft comparison. *Cancer*, **68**: 558–560.

23. Chahinian, A.P. (1993): The nude mouse model in mesothelioma research and therapy. *Eur. Respir. Rev.*, **3**: 204–207.

24. Ogretmen, B., Bahadori, H., McCauley, M., Boylan, A., Green, M., Safa, A.R. (1998): Co-ordinated over-expression of the MRP and gamma-glutamylcysteine synthetase genes, but not MDR1, correlates with doxorubicin resistance in human malignant mesothelioma cell lines. *Int. J. Cancer*, **75**: 757–761.

25. Vogelzang, N.J., Herndon, J.E. II, Cirrincione, C., Harmon, D.C., Antman, K.H., Corson, J.M., Suzuki, Y., Citron, M.L., Green, M.R. (1997): Dihydro-5-azacytidine in malignant mesothelioma. A Phase II trial demonstrating activity accompanied by cardiac toxicity. *Cancer*, **79**: 2237–2242.

26. Bavisetto, L.M., Rankin, C., Behrens, B.C., Gandara, D.R., Rivkin, S.E., Balcerzak, S.P., Antman, K. (1998) : A Phase II Southwest Oncology Group study of dihydroxyazacytidine for mesothelioma. *Cancer Ther.*, **1**: 18–20.

27. Millard, F.E., Herndon, J., Vogelzang, N.J, Green, M.R. (1997): Gemcitabine for malignant mesothelioma. A phase II study of the Cancer and Leukemia Group B (CALGB 9530). *Proc. Am. Soc. Clin. Oncol.*, **16**: 475a.

28. Bischoff, H.G., Manegold, C., Knopp M., Blatter, J., Drings, P. (1998): Gemcitabine (Gemzar) may reduce tumor load and tumor associated symptoms in malignant pleural mesothelioma. *Proc. Am. Soc. Clin. Oncol.*, **17**: 464a.

29. Van Meerbeeck, J., Debruyne, C., Postmus, P.E., Groen, H.J.M., Manegold, C., Baas, P., Van Zandwijk, N., Pennucci, A.M.C., Gridelli, C., Galdermans, D., Lentz, M., Giaccone, G. (1996): Sequential phase 2 studies with paclitaxel and gemcitabine in malignant pleural mesothelioma. *Eur. Respir. J.*, **9**: 400s.

30. Solheim, O.P., Saeter, G., Finnanger, A.M., Stenwig, A.E. (1992): High-dose methotrexate in the treatment of malignant mesothelioma of the pleura. A phase II study. *Br. J. Cancer*, **65**: 956–960.

31. Sahmoud, T., Postmus, P.E., Van Pottelsberghe, C., Mattson, K., Tammilehto, L. Splinter, T.A., Planting, A.S., Sutedja, T., Van, Pawel, J., Van Zandwijk, N., Baas, P., Roozendaal, K.J., Schrijver, M., Kirkpatrick, A., Van Glabbeke, M., Ardizzoni, A., Giaccone, G. (1997): Etoposide in malignant pleural mesothelioma. Two phase II trials of the EORTC Lung Cancer Cooperative Group. *Eur. J. Cancer*, **33**: 2211–2215.

32. Smit, E.F., Berendson, H.H., Postmus, P.E. (1990): Etoposide and mesothelioma. *J. Clin. Oncol.*, **8**: 1281.

33. Vogelzang, N.J., Herndon, J., Clamon, G.H., Mauer, A.M., Cooper, M.R., Green, M.R. (1994): Paclitaxel (Taxol) for malignant mesothelioma. A Phase II study of the Cancer and Leukemia Group B. *Proc. Am. Soc. Clin. Oncol.*, **13**: 405.

34. Van Meerbeeck, J.P., Postmus, P.E., Oliva, C., Van Zandwijk, N., Giaccone, G. (1994): A Phase II trial of Taxol in malignant pleural mesothelioma. *Lung Cancer*, **11** (Suppl 1):191.

34a. Steele, J.P., Shamash, J., Evans, M.T., Gower, N.H., Tischkowitz, M.D., Rudd, R.M. (2000): Phase II study of vinorelbine in patients with malignant pleural mesothelioma. *J. Clin. Oncol.*, **18**: 3912–3917.

35. Maksymiuk, A.W., Marschke, R.F. Jr, Tazelaar, H.D., Grill, J., Nair, S., Marks, R.S., Brooks, B.J., Mailliard, J.A., Burton, G.M., Jett, J.R. (1998): Phase II trial of topotecan for the treatment of mesothelioma. *Am. J. Clin. Oncol.*, **21**: 610–613.

36. Morocz, I.A., Lauber, B., Schmitter, D., Stahel, R.A. (1993): Effect of suramin treatment on mesothelioma and other lung cancer derived cell lines. *Eur. Respir. Rev.*, 3: 213–215.

37. Chahinian, A.P., Mandeli, J.P., Gluck, H., Naim, H., Teirstein, A.S., Holland, J.F. (1998): Effectiveness of cisplatin, paclitaxel, and suramin against human malignant mesothelioma xenografts in athymic nude mice. *J. Surg. Oncol.*, 67: 104–111.

38. Westermann, A.M., Dubbelman, R., Moolenaar, W.H., Beijnen, J., Rodenhuis, S. (1997): Successful intraperitoneal suramin treatment of peritoneal mesothelioma. *Ann. Oncol.*, 8: 801–802.

39. Costanzi, J., Darzynkiewicz, Z., Chun, H., Mittelman, A., Panella, T., McCachren, S., Puccio, C., Taub, R., Shogen, K., Mikulski, S. (1997): The use of Onconase for patients with advanced malignant mesothelioma. Fourth International Mesothelioma Conference, International Mesothelioma Interest Group, Philadelphia, May 13–15.

40. Rubins, J.B., Greatens, T., Kratzke, R.A., Tan, A.T., Polunovsky, V.A., Bitterman, P. (1998): Lovastatin induces apoptosis in malignant mesothelioma cells. *Am. J. Respir. Crit. Care, Med* 157: 1616–1622.

41. Chahinian, A.P., Antman, K., Goutsou, M., Corson, J.M., Suzuki, Y., Modeas, C., Herndon, J.E., Aisner, J., Ellison, R.R., Leone, L., Vogelzang, N.J., Green, M.R. (1993): Randomized Phase II trial of cisplatin with mitomycin or doxorubicin for malignant mesothelioma by the Cancer and Leukemia Group B. *J. Clin. Oncol.*, 11: 1559–1565.

42. Stewart, D.J., Gertler, S.Z., Tomiak, A., Shamji, F., Goel, R., Evans, W.K. (1994): High dose doxorubicin plus cisplatin in the treatment of unresectable mesotheliomas. Report of four cases. *Lung Cancer*, 11: 251–258.

43. Eisenhauer, E.A., Evans, W.K., Murray, N., Kocha, W., Wierzbicki, R., Wilson, K. (1988): A phase II study of VP16 and cisplatin in patients with unresectable malignant mesothelioma. An NCI of Canada Clinical Trials Group study. *Invest New Drugs*, 6: 327–329.

44. Samuels, B.L., Herndon, J.E., Harmon, D.C., Carey, R., Aisner, J., Corson, J.M., Suzuki, Y., Green, M.R., Vogelzang, N.J. (1998): Dihydro-5-azacytidine and cisplatin in the treatment of malignant mesothelioma. A phase II study by the Cancer and Leukemia Group B. *Cancer*, 82: 1578–1584.

45. Tsavaris, N., Mylonakis, N., Karvounis, N., Bacoyiannis, C., Briasoulis, E., Skarlos, D., Pavlidis, N., Stamatelos, G., Kosmidis, P. (1994): Combination chemotherapy with cisplatin-vinblastine in malignant mesothelioma. *Lung Cancer*, 11: 299–303.

46. Byrne, M.J., Davidson, J.A., Musk, A.W., Dewar, J., Van Hazel, G., Buck, M., De Klerk, N.H, Robinson, B.W.S. (1999): Cisplatin and gemcitabine treatment for malignant mesothelioma. A phase II study. *J. Clin. Oncol.*, 17: 25–30.

47. Nakano, T., Chahinian, A.P., Shinjo, M., Togawa, N., Tonomura, A., Miyake, M., Ninomiya, K., Yamamoto, T., Higashino, K. (1999): Cisplatin in combination with irinotecan in the treatment of patients with malignant pleural mesothelioma: a pilot phase II clinical trial and pharmacokinetic profile. *Cancer*, 85: 2375–84.

48. Thodtmann, R., Kemmerich, M., Depenbrock, H., Blatter, J., Ohnmacht, U., Hanauske, A.R. (1998): Phase I study of MTA (Multi-Targeted Antifolate, LY231514) plus cisplatin in patients with advanced solid tumours. *Proc. Am. Soc. Clin. Oncol.*, 17: 254a.

49. Hoffman, K.R. (1996): Paclitaxel and carboplatin combination chemotherapy is an effective palliative treatment for malignant mesothelioma. *Proc. Am. Soc. Clin. Oncol.*, 15: 1425.

50. Bednar, M.E, Chahinian, A.P. (1999): Paclitaxel and carboplatin for malignant mesothelioma. *Proc. Am. Soc. Clin. Oncol.*, 18: 496a.

51. Nakano, T., Miyake, M., Takenaka, N., Iwahashi, N., Hada, T., Higashino, K. (1993): A pilot Phase II study of cisplatin, doxorubicin, and vindesine for the treatment of malignant pleural mesothelioma. *Eur. Respir. Rev.*, 3(Rev 11): 211–212.

52. Hunt, K.J., Longton, G., Williams, M.A., Livingston, R.B. (1996): Treatment of malignant mesothelioma with methotrexate and vinblastine, with or without platinum chemotherapy. *Chest*, **109**: 1239–1242.
53. Shin, D.M., Fossella, F.V., Umsawasdi, T., Murphy, W.K., Chasen, M.H., Walsh, G., Komaki, R., McMurtrey, M.J., Hong, W.K. (1995): Prospective study of combination chemotherapy with cyclophosphamide, doxorubicin, and cisplatin for unresectable or metastatic malignant pleural mesothelioma. *Cancer*, **76**: 2230–2236.
54. Pennucci, M.C., Ardizzoni, A., Pronzato, P., Fioretti, M., Lanfranco, C., Verna, A., Giorgi, G., Vigani, A., Frola, C., Rosso, R. (1997): Combined cisplatin, doxorubicin, and mitomycin for the treatment of advanced pleural mesothelioma. A phase II FONICAP trial. *Cancer*, **79**: 1897–1902.
55. Middleton, G.W., Smith, I.E., O'Brien, M.E., Norton, A., Hickish, T., Priest, K., Spencer, L., Ashley, S. (1998): Good symptom relief with palliative MVP (mitomycin-C, vinblastine and cisplatin) chemotherapy in malignant mesothelioma. *Ann. Oncol.*, **9**: 269–273.
56. Sklarin, N.T., Chahinian, A.P., Feuer, E.J., Lahman, L.A., Szrajer, L., Holland, J.F. (1988): Augmentation of activity of cis-diamminedichloroplatinum (II) and mitomycin C by interferon in human malignant mesothelioma xenografts in nude mice. *Cancer Res.*, **48**: 64–67.
57. Tansan, S., Emri, S., Selcuk, T., Koc, Y., Hesketh, P., Heeren, T., McCaffrey, R.P., Baris, Y.I. (1994): Treatment of malignant pleural mesothelioma with cisplatin, mitomycin C and alpha interferon. *Oncology*, **51**: 348–351.
58. Breau, J.L., Boaziz, C., Morere, J.F., Sadoun, D., Israel, L. (1993): Chemotherapy with cisplatin, adriamycin, bleomycin and mitomycin C, combined with systemic and intrapleural hyaluronidase in stage II and III pleural mesothelioma. *Eur. Respir. Rev.*, **3 (Rev 11)**: 223–225.
59. Kasseyet, S., Boutin, C., Astoul, P., Frenay, C. (1997): Malignant pleural mesothelioma. Results of a phase II trial of chemotherapy. Fourth International Mesothelioma Conference, International Mesothelioma Interest Group, Philadelphia, May 13–15.
60. Pfeifle, C.E., Howell, S.B., Markman, M. (1985): Intracavitary cisplatin chemotherapy for mesothelioma. *Cancer Treat. Rev.*, **69**: 205–207.
61. Markman, M., Cleary, S., Pfeifle, C., Howell, S.B. (1986): Cisplatin administered by the intracavitary route as treatment for malignant mesothelioma. *Cancer*, **58**: 18–21.
62. Antman, K., Klegar, K.L., Pomfret, E.A., Osteen, R.T., Amato, D.A., Larson, D.A., Corson, J.M. (1985): Early peritoneal mesothelioma: A treatable malignancy. *Lancet*, **2** 977–981.
63. Markman, M., Kelsen, D. (1989): Intraperitoneal cisplatin and mitomycin as treatment for malignant peritoneal mesothelioma. *Reg. Cancer Treat.*, **2**: 49–53.
64. Markman, M., Kelsen, D. (1992): Efficacy of cisplatin-based intraperitoneal chemotherapy as treatment of malignant peritoneal mesothelioma. *J. Cancer Res. Clin. Oncol.*, **118**: 547–550.
65. Rusch, V.W., Saltz, L., Venkatraman, E., Ginsberg, R. McCormack, P., Burt, M., Markman, M., Kelsen, D. (1994): A phase II trial of pleurectomy/decortication followed by intrapleural and systemic chemotherapy for malignant pleural mesothelioma. *J. Clin.Oncol.*, **12**: 1156–1163.
66. Rice, T.W., Adelstein, D.J., Kirby, T.J., Saltarelli, M.G., Murthy, S.R., Van Kirk, M.A., Wiedemann, H.P., Weick, J.K. (1994): Aggressive multimodality therapy for malignant pleural mesothelioma. *Ann. Thorac. Surg.*, **58**: 24–29.
67. Hand, A.M.S., Husgalvel-Pursiainen, K., Pelin, K., Vallas, M., Suitiala, T., Ekman, A., Mattson, M., Mattson, K., Linnainmaa, K. (1992): Interferon-α and -γ in combination with chemotherapeutic drugs. In vitro sensitivity studies in four human mesothelioma cell lines. *Anti-Cancer Drugs*, **3**: 687–694.

68. Soulié, P., Ruffié, P., Trandafir, L., Monnet, I., Tardivan, A., Terrier, P., Cvitkovic, E., Le Chevalier, T., Armand, J.P. (1996): Combined systemic chemoimmunotherapy in advanced diffuse malignant mesothelioma. Report of a Phase I–II study of weekly cisplatin/interferon alfa-2a. *J. Clin. Oncol.*, **14**: 878–885.

69. Pass, H.W., Temeck, B.K., Kranda, K., Steinberg, S.M., Pass, H.I. (1995): A phase II trial investigating primary immunochemotherapy for malignant pleural mesothelioma and the feasibility of adjuvant immunochemotherapy after maximal cytoreduction. *Ann. Surg. Oncol.*, **2**: 214–220.

70. Purohit, A., Moreau, L., Dietemann, A., Seibert, R., Pauli, G., Wihlm, J.M., Quoix, E. (1998): Weekly systemic combination of cisplatin and interferon alpha-2a in diffuse malignant pleural mesothelioma. *Lung Cancer,* **22**: 119–125.

=12=

Gene Therapy for Malignant Mesothelioma – 'Suicide Gene' and Immunological Approaches

Daniel H. Sterman, Steven M. Albelda, Sutapa Mukherjee and
Bruce W. S. Robinson

In the absence of other reliably effective therapies for malignant mesothelioma, several groups are investigating the evolving technology of gene therapy. There are several characteristics that make mesothelioma an attractive target for gene therapy. First is the absence of any effective standard therapy. Second is its unique accessibility in the pleural space for vector delivery, biopsy, and subsequent analysis of treatment effects. A surgical 'debulking' procedure to remove gross disease, followed by gene therapy to remove residual disease would thus be technically feasible. Third, local extension of disease, rather than distant metastases, is responsible for much of the morbidity and mortality associated with this neoplasm. Thus, unlike other more widespread neoplasms, small increments of improvement in local control could engender significant improvements in palliation or survival. Accordingly, a number of gene therapy trials aimed at treating mesothelioma using a wide variety of approaches have begun or are in the planning stages (Table 12.1). Mesothelioma appears to be, at least to some extent, susceptible to immunotherapy, so gene therapy approaches aimed at efficiently stimulating host anti-mesothelioma immune responses may be effective.

The HSV*tk* studies were supported by Grant No. P01 CA66726 from the National Cancer Institute and Grant MO1-RR00040 to the General Clinical Research Center of the University of Pennsylvania Medical Center from the National Gene Vector Laboratories, the Nicolette Asbestos Trust, and the Samuel H. Lunenfeld Charitable Foundation. Institutional support was provided by the University of Pennsylvania Cancer Center.

The Immunological gene therapy studies were supported by Grants from the National Health and Medical Research Council of Australia, James Hardie Industries Molecular Biology Fellowship, the Insurance Commission of Western Australia, the Cancer Foundation of Western Australia and an Australian Lung Foundation/Dust Diseases Board of NSW Grant.

Table 12.1. *Gene therapy approaches for mesothelioma.*

Strategy	Therapeutic gene	Molecular mechanism	Location
'Suicide gene'	Herpes simplex thymidine kinase	Delivery of enzyme capable of generating toxic metabolite after exposure to ganciclovir	University of Pennsylvania Medical Center, Philadelphia
Genetic immuno-potentiation	Cytokines (IL-2, GM-CSF, IL-12, etc.) Anti-sense TGF-β (planned)	Augmentation of immune response to tumor	Queen Elizabeth II Medical Center, Perth, Australia
Combination suicide gene/ tumor vaccine	Herpes simplex virus thymidine kinase (delivered by modified, irradiated ovarian carcinoma cell line)	Delivery of enzyme capable of generating toxic metabolite, killing tumour cells and stimulating anti-tumour immune response	Louisiana State University Medical Center, New Orleans
Mutation compensation	Anti-sense SV40 TAg wild-type p16/p21	Inhibition of dominant oncogenes Augmentation of tumor suppressers.	No protocols approved
Replicating virus	Replication-competent Adenoviral vector (with HSV*tk* gene) Herpes simplex virus-1 mutants such as HSV-1716	Replication-restricted virus capable of lysing tumour cells with or without ganciclovir	No protocols yet approved

I. Gene therapy using the herpes simplex virus thymidine kinase gene

One promising approach in current experimental cancer gene therapy is the introduction of a toxic or 'suicide' gene into mesothelioma cells, facilitating their destruction (molecular chemotherapy). One such 'suicide' gene approach involves the transduction of a neoplasm with a cDNA encoding for the enzyme herpes simplex virus thymidine kinase (HSV*tk*) that would render its cells sensitive to a 'benign' drug, ganciclovir (GCV).[1] HSV*tk* catalyses GCV to GCV monophosphate, which is then rapidly converted by mammalian kinases to the triphosphate form. GCV triphosphate is a toxic analogue which is a potent inhibitor of DNA polymerase and competes with nucleosides for DNA replication.[2] A 'bystander' effect, in which neighbouring, non-transduced tumour cells are also killed, appears to be an important component of this system and results from: 1) passage of toxic GCV metabolites from transduced to non-transduced cells via gap junctions or apoptotic vesicles;[3] and 2) induction of an antitumour immune response capable of killing cells at a distance from those transduced with HSV*tk*.[4]

Experiments have shown that replication-deficient adenovirus encoding HSV*tk* efficiently transduced mesothelioma cells both in tissue culture and in animal models,[5-7] and that infection with this vector rendered human mesothelioma cells sensitive to doses of GCV that were 2–4 logs lower that the doses required to kill cells infected with control virus.[5] Subsequently, the Ad.HSV*tk* vector was used to treat established human mesothelioma tumours and human lung cancers growing within the peritoneal cavities of SCID mice.[8,9]

Based on these efficacy data in animals and on successful preclinical toxicity testing, an initial Phase I clinical trial for patients with mesothelioma began in November 1995 at the University of Pennsylvania Medical Center in conjunction with Penn's Institute for Human Gene Therapy. In this protocol, patients with mesothelioma who had patent pleural cavities underwent intrapleural administration of one dose of increasing concentrations of Ad.HSV*tk* vector followed by 2 weeks of intravenous GCV therapy.[10] The protocol was designed as a dose-escalation study, starting with a vector dose of 1×10^9 plaque forming units (pfu) and increasing in half-log intervals to the current dose level of 1×10^{12} pfu. At the completion of the 14-day GCV course, patients were discharged from hospital for outpatient follow-up that included biochemical and haematological testing and a computed tomography scan of the chest performed on study day 30. Throughout the study, the patients were carefully evaluated for evidence of toxicity, viral shedding, immune responses to the virus and radiographic evidence of tumour response.

Between November 1995 and November 1997, 26 (21 male, 5 female) patients were enrolled in the study.[11] Clinical toxicities of the Ad.HSV*tk*/GCV gene therapy were minimal and a maximally tolerated dose (MTD) was not achieved. Detectable gene transfer was documented in 17 of 25 evaluable patients in a dose-related fashion by either DNA-polymerase chain reaction (PCR), reverse transcription-PCR, *in situ* hybridisation, and/or immunohistochemistry (IHC) using a murine monoclonal antibody directed against HSV*tk*. All patients treated at dose levels of 3.2×10^{11} pfu or greater demonstrated evidence of *tk* protein on post-treatment biopsies via immunoblot or IHC, with positive staining on the latter of tumour 40–50 cell layers below the mesothelial surface (Table 12.2).[11]

Strong anti-adenoviral humoral and cellular immune responses were noted, including acute neutrophil-predominant intratumoral inflammation in the post-treatment biopsy sections; generation of high titres of anti-adenoviral neutralising antibodies in serum and pleural fluid; significant increases in inflammatory cytokine production (TNF-α, IL-6) in pleural fluid; generation of serum antibodies against adenoviral structural proteins; and increased lymphocyte proliferative responses to adenoviral proteins.[12]

The anti-tumour effects of Ad.HSV*tk*/GCV gene therapy were difficult to gauge because of the diffuse nature of mesothelioma and the design of the Phase I trial, which was focused on safety and toxicity. This was made more difficult because of the heterogeneity of the patient population in terms of age, stage, histology and vector dose. Given these caveats, there was at least one partial tumour response in the initial trial seen on follow-up CT scan of a patient with Stage 1 sarcomatoid mesothelioma. This patient

Table 12.2. Results of UPENN Phase I clinical trials of Ad.HSVtk/GCV gene therapy for mesothelioma.

Patient age/sex	Stage/ cell type	Vector dose (pfu)	Survival after ℞ (months)	Gene transfer	Tumour response
1 62/M	IA/E*	1×10^9	66	-	SD x 2 yrs
2 56/M	III/E	1×10^9	8‡	-	—
3 69/M	III/B	1×10^9	20‡	+	—
4 66/M	II/E	3.2×10^9	10.5‡	-	—
5 71/M	IA/E	3.2×10^9	58‡	-	SD x 3 yrs
6 71/M	II/B	1×10^{10}	4‡	+	—
7 70/M	II/E	1×10^{10}	6‡	-	—
8 60/M	II/E	1×10^{10}	27‡	+	—
9 74/M	II/B	3.2×10^{10}	2‡	NP	—
10 60/M	III/E	3.2×10^{10}	9‡	-	—
11 37/F	IV/E	1×10^{11}	16‡	-	—
12 37/M	III	1×10^{11}	2‡	-	—
13 65/F	III/E	1×10^{11}	10‡	+	—
14 66/F	IA/E	3.2×10^{11}	50‡	+	SD x 2 yrs
15 60/M	IV/B	3.2×10^{11}	5‡	+	—
16 69/M	IB/E	3.2×10^{11}	8‡	+	—
17 70/F	IB/E	3.2×10^{11}	15‡	+	—
18 69/F	IB/E	3.2×10^{11}	3.5‡	+	—
19 75/M	II/E	3.2×10^{11}	7.5‡	+	—
20 68/M	IV/B	3.2×10^{11}	0.5‡	+	—
21 71/M	IB/E	3.2×10^{11}	41‡	+	—
22 76/M	IB/E	3.2×10^{11}	33‡	+	—
23 81/M	II/E	3.2×10^{11}	25‡	+	—
24 71/M	II/E	1×10^{12}	21‡	+	—
25 65/M	II/E	1×10^{12}	5‡	+	—
26 67/M	IA/S	1×10^{12}	22‡	+	PR (CT)
27 67/M*	III/B	1×10^{11}	7‡	+	—
28 53/M*	III/E	1×10^{11}	13‡	+	—
29 30/F*	I/E	5×10^{11}	32.5	+	SD
30 56/F*	IA/E	5×10^{11}	32	+	SD
31 66M*	II/E	5×10^{11}	9‡	+	—
32 74M*	I/E	5×10^{11}	19‡	+	PR (PET)
33 64M*†	I/E	5×10^{11}	10‡	+	—
34 69/M*†	II/E	5×10^{11}	21	NP	—

E=epithelioid; B=biphasic; NP=test not performed; SD=stable disease (CT +/- PET); PR=partial response.
* Received third-generation E1/E4-deleted adenoviral vector.
† Received 15 mg/kg/day GCV for 14 days.
‡ Deceased.
§ Received adjuvant corticosteroids.

later died from intra-abdominal disease progression. In addition, patients in the initial Phase I study remained clinically stable for at least 2 years, with no evidence of tumour growth on serial chest radiographs and chest CT scans, before demonstrating evidence of progression.[11] Overall, 25 of the initial 26 patients have died, with a median survival after treatment of 11 months, and no fatal complications attributable to the gene therapy protocol. One early-stage patient remained without evidence of disease for 31 months after completing the protocol, before developing a local recurrence which was treated with pleurectomy and intrapleural photodynamic therapy. He is now without evidence of active disease 66 months after enrolment in the gene therapy protocol. Included within the initial Phase I gene therapy trial was a substudy in five patients involving concomitant administration of systemic corticosteroids. This demonstrated mitigation of acute, vector-induced inflammatory responses with no decrement in anti-adenoviral humoral or cellular responses and no improvement in degree of intratumoral gene transfer.[13]

This initial Phase I trial indicated that intrapleural Ad.HSV*tk* gene therapy was safe, could effectively deliver transgene to superficial areas of mesothelioma tumour nodules, and might be leading to some degree of tumour reduction.[11] Nevertheless, improved intratumoral gene transfer will likely be necessary for significant clinical responses. This can be achieved by: 1) using higher intrapleural doses of Ad.HSV*tk*; 2) intrapleural injection of Ad.HSV*tk* after surgical debulking; 3) repeated intrapleural dosing of vector; and 4) direct intratumoral vector injections. Additional phase I trials involving all of these approaches are planned. We have initiated two new Phase I clinical rials in the past 3 years, including a clinical trial continuing the dose-escalation protocol with a less immunogenic and hepatotoxic adenoviral vector deleted in the E1 and E4 early gene regions. To date, 5 patients have been treated with this new vector. Preliminary analysis shows detectable gene transfer with less systemic toxicity and lower increases in hepatic enzyme levels. Two patients at the higher dose level have shown radiographically stable disease for over 30 months after completion of the gene therapy protocol with the E1/E4 deleted vector, with one demonstrating a dramatic decrease in tumour metabolic activity on serial 18-fluorodeoxyglucose (FDG) PET scans.

We have also started a Phase I clinical trial using stable doses of the same E1/E4-vector, but with dose escalation of the GCV substrate. After enrolment of the first cohort of three patients, we have confirmed that GCV dosing up to 7.5 mg/kg twice daily for 14 days is well tolerated, with no increase in hepatic or haematological toxicities. One patient had evidence of a significant, but transitory, decrease in tumour metabolic activity on 18-FDG PET scan after treatment, but later died from disease progression and pulmonary embolism 19 months after completion of the protocol.

II. Gene therapy using immunomodulatory approaches

Using gene therapy to augment the immune response to tumours is another active area for cancer gene therapy research, since systemic and/or intrapleural administration of cytokines may partially overcome mesothelioma's resistance to immune destruction, but clinical applications are limited by significant associated toxicity.[14,15] Investigators at Queen Elizabeth II Hospital in Perth, Australia, evaluated intratumoral delivery of cytokine genes in their murine model of mesothelioma as a means of stimulating anti-tumour immune responses without systemic toxicity. Based upon successful tumour reduction in animals, they conducted a Phase I clinical trial in pleural mesothelioma using a recombinant vaccinia virus (VV) expressing the human IL-2 gene.[16,17] VV was chosen as the vector because of its large genome, proven safety in human vaccines, and the availability of anti-VV antibodies for diagnostic use.

The VV-IL-2 vector was injected intratumorly into palpable chest wall masses of 6 patients with advanced stage malignant mesothelioma on a repeated basis. VV-IL-2 mRNA was detected in serial tumour biopsies for 3–6 days after injection, but uniformly declined to low levels by day 8. Significant serum anti-VV IgG antibody titres were induced in all patients by intratumoral injection of recombinant VV, but, interestingly, did not have any bearing on the pattern or duration of VV-IL-2 mRNA expression. The presence of anti-VV neutralising antibodies did correlate, however, with an inability to be able to culture live VV from tumour biopsy samples. Toxicities were minimal aside from fever, and there was no clinical or serological evidence of spread of VV to patient contacts. No significant tumour regressions were seen in any of the patients, and only minimal intratumoral cellular immune responses were detected.[16,17] In future gene therapy approaches to mesothelioma, VV-IL-2 may prove more efficacious in a more replication competent form, or as part of a 'cocktail' of cytokine genes delivered via VV (i.e., IL-2, IL-12, and GM-CSF).[16]

Another immunomodulatory approach to gene therapy of mesothelioma under investigation is intratumoral delivery of a gene encoding for the bacterial heat shock protein, HSP-65, one of the most immunogenic molecules known. This 'molecular chaperone' is involved in protein folding and transport, and mediates increased presentation of tumour antigens. Animal experiments in murine mesothelioma models conducted at the National Heart and Lung Institute in London, involving intraperitoneal delivery of HSP-65 using polycationic liposomes, demonstrated a dose-dependent decrease in tumour size and significant prolongation of survival compared to controls, with some mice living as long as 1 year after treatment.[18]

Preclinical data

Mesothelioma represents one of the few animal models of cancer in which the mouse tumour is similar to the human tumour. This has been confirmed in a number of studies of the clinical behaviour, histopathology, antigen expression, immunobiological behaviour, tumour suppressor gene lesions, oncogene mutations, etc., studied.[19] Murine mesothelioma has now been established in at least four different strains, balb/c, C57Bl6, B10D.2 and CBA mice. This represents an excellent platform for the analysis of gene therapy using immunomodulatory approaches; that is, approaches which are ineffective in mice are unlikely to be effective in humans.

Alteration of use of gene-transfected mesothelioma cells to alter immune recognition

Allo MHC class-I molecules were transfected because allo-reactivity induces a vigorous anti-tumour immune response. When the non-immunogenic AC20 line was transfected with an allo class-I molecule (H-2K^b or H-2D^d), the cells were universally rejected, although no protection was demonstrable against the parental cell line. *In vitro* cytotoxicity analysis confirmed induction of allo-reactivity. Thus the vigorous rejection of the allogeneic MHC-expressing tumour did not induce protection against untransfected tumour cells.[20]

Transfection of the co-stimulatory molecules B7-1 (CD80) or B7-2 (CD86) produce different results. B7-1-transfection of CBA lines markedly delayed their outgrowth although eventually tumours formed, contemporaneous with reduction in anti-tumour cytotoxic activity.[21] This appeared to be related to the level of MHC class-II antigen inducibility on those lines. B7-1 transfection of the more immunogenic AB1 line was more effective in inducing protective immunity and some protection against untransfected cells was noted. B7-2 was ineffective, as was transfection of MHC class-II alone.[22]

Gene transfection of mesothelioma cells using cytokines

Mesothelioma cells transfected with either IL-2, IL-4, IL-12 or GM-CSF were all rejected.[23,24] The important experiment, however, was to determine whether or not this rejection was associated with the induction of immune response against the untransfected cell lines (i.e., against the parental line). When injected at a distal site none of these transfectants were able to induce rejection of the parental line, although IL-12 did slow tumour progression and induce a modest T-cell infiltrate.[24] This suggested that cytokine-transfected mesothelioma cells would never be able to be used clinically because of their inability to induce a strong anti-mesothelioma immune response capable of destroying a distal tumour. However, further experiments have been conducted, combining cytokine gene therapy with surgery of mesothelioma. These experiments clearly demonstrate that whereas neither distal gene therapy using cytokine transfectants alone nor surgery alone is capable of inducing 'concomitant' immunity against an unmanipulated distal mesothelioma site, a combination of both approaches is clearly effective at reducing the rate of tumour growth. The two cytokine gene transfectants most effective in this regard were high-level GM-CSF producers and B7-1-expressing mesothelioma cells. IL-4- and IL-2-expressing mesothelioma cells did not exhibit this effect, and combinations of any of the above lines did not augment the effect. These data suggest that cytokine gene therapy of mesothelioma will be most effective when combined with a surgical debulking procedure.

'Combination' gene therapy: tumour vaccines

A Phase I clinical trial combining elements of both the toxic prodrug and genetic immunopotentiation gene therapy approaches is currently underway at the Louisiana State University Medical Center in New Orleans (Table 12.1).[25] This approach involves the intrapleural instillation of an allogeneic, irradiated ovarian carcinoma cell line retrovirally transfected with HSV*tk* (PA1-STK cells), followed by systemic administration of GCV.[25] The rationale behind this trial is that the PA1-STK cells will migrate to areas of intrapleural tumour after instillation, and then facilitate bystander killing of mesothelioma cells after GCV infusion. This bystander killing is theorised to result from passage of toxic GCV metabolites from PA1-STK cells to mesothelioma cells via gap junctions or apoptotic vesicles, as well as the local generation of pro-inflammatory cytokines, such as TNF-α and IL-1, that elicit an influx of cytotoxic lymphocytes producing haemorrhagic tumour necrosis. In experimental models, the combination of intrapleural instillation of HSV*tk* gene-modified cells and systemic GCV infusion alters the tumour microenvironment in mesothelioma from inhibitory to stimulatory, thereby engendering an antitumour immune response.[25-27]

The LSU gene therapy trial is a modified Phase I dose escalation study designed to determine the maximally tolerated dose of intrapleurally delivered PA1-STK cells. Patients are admitted to the hospital after insertion of a small intrapleural catheter and receive an initial dose of lethally irradiated PA1-STK cells combined with intrapleural Bacille Calmette-Guérin (BCG) as an adjuvant. Twenty-four hours after instillation of the HSV*tk* positive cells, a 7-day course of intravenous GCV is started at a dose of 5 mg/kg twice daily. The indwelling pleural catheter remains in place throughout the duration of the protocol, providing an opportunity to monitor the intrapleural immune response to HSV*tk* gene modified cell therapy. Patients are followed clinically for signs of toxicity and radiographically for evidence of response or progression. Serial intradermal challenges with autologous irradiated tumour are performed before, during and after vaccine therapy to assay for anti-tumour delayed-type hypersensitivity reactions.[24-26]

As of November 1998, 6 patients have been treated at two dose levels with a maximal dose of 1×10^8 PA1-STK cells. An additional 3 patients have started a protocol of repeated intrapleural administration of PA1-STK cells followed by courses of systemic GCV. Minimal side effects of treatment have been seen with no documented toxicities greater than National Cancer Institute grade III. The most serious complication to date was an episode of transitory atrial fibrillation precipitated by intrapleural catheter insertion. At the time of the last report, two of the initial six patients were still alive. One patient died secondary to extensive pericardial involvement with tumour with no obvious direct complication of therapy. Pericardial tissue obtained at autopsy proved negative for *tk* DNA via PCR. Immunological evaluation of the initial patients' samples is still ongoing, but preliminary findings have shown significant increases in the percentage of CD8 T lymphocytes in pleural fluid post-instillation of PA1-STK cells.[27] Although all patients underwent skin testing for recall antigens and alloreactivity to PA1-STK cells, only recall reactions to intradermal mumps and *Candida* were observed, with no demonstrable response to the gene-modified tumour cells.[25,26] Pleural fluid was analysed sequentially in patients before and after administration of PA1-STK cells. These results suggest that within 2 hours of administration, GCV is present within the pleural space at concentrations observed to elicit tumour killing in *in vitro* and in *in vivo* models (Schwarzenberger, Cold Spring Harbor Gene Therapy Meeting, September, 1998).

Problems and future approaches

Optimisation of gene delivery remains the major challenge for gene therapy of mesothelioma. Current non-replicating vectors are limited in their ability to transduce all (or most) tumour cells in a localised malignancy and are even less capable of efficiently delivering genes to tumour cells interspersed in a dense, fibrous stroma, as seen in biphasic and sarcomatoid mesotheliomas. One strategy that might be particularly efficient in increasing gene delivery to mesothelioma cells could be the use of replicating viral vectors that have the capability of killing tumours by primary viral lysis and/or via delivery of therapeutic genes to cancer cells.[28] Promising viruses in this regard are replication-competent adenoviruses and mutants of the herpes simplex-1 virus (HSV-1).[29]

Future immunotherapy approaches using gene manipulation

Whilst immunotherapeutic approaches to mesothelioma have a strong scientific basis, and clear evidence of tumour regression in some patients is encouraging, a number of hurdles need to be overcome. Firstly, mesothelioma antigens are yet to be identified. Unlike melanoma, where a vast amount of data has been generated using a number of approaches to tumour antigen discovery, mesothelioma antigen detection is in its infancy. Nevertheless, a number of potential antigens have recently been identified, including topoisomerase-IIb.[30] Further studies in this area are warranted as it is likely that the identification of mesothelioma antigens will enable high doses of such antigens to be used in immunotherapy regimes to increase the 'load' of antigen delivered to the immune system, an essential requirement for the development of a strong immune response. Furthermore, it is likely that multiple antigens will be required, as the immune system will tend to downregulate any anti-self immune response that is induced (i.e. either multiple antigens or sequential antigen stimulation will be required). Secondly, optimum ways of inducing an immune response to these antigens need to be determined. Dendritic cells (DCs) are being widely studied at present, as it is clear that these cells can induce a strong immune response if cultured *in vitro* and then re-injected by adoptive transfer. A number of hurdles remain to be overcome in this regard, however, including a failure of peripheral blood DC maturation in mesothelioma patients (unpublished observations) and uncertainties as to the correct schedule and route and the optimal *in vitro* conditions for DC culture in mesothelioma patients. There is also some evidence that the use of gene therapy vectors on cultured DCs may induce a tolerogenic phenotype in such cells (unpublished observations). Thirdly, one of the major hurdles in tumorotherapy is the targeting of a strong antitumour immune response to the tumour itself. It is not enough to induce a strong cytotoxic T-cell response peripherally – those cells must be able to traffic to the tumour and overcome local immunosuppressive defences to destroy the tumour cell. As tumours consist almost entirely of 'self' tissue, the natural host tolerance mechanisms militate against effective tissue destruction. Whilst this can occur in autoimmune disease, in some cancer patients it will be no small task to generate protocols which effectively target destructive T-cells to a tumour tissue without inducing unacceptable autoimmunity.

Summary

For many years, mesothelioma has been viewed with dread because of its insidious presentation, inexorable progression, and refractoriness to all standard forms of therapy. Over the past decade, advances have been made on several fronts that may improve the quality and quantity of life for patients with mesothelioma. Experimental treatments, such as gene therapy, present a window of hope for all patients with mesothelioma, even if application of these modalities in a routine fashion is years away. The days of therapeutic nihilism by clinicians managing mesothelioma patients may soon be over.

Acknowledgements

We would like to acknowledge the contribution of Dr Larry Kaiser and the many collaborators and colleagues whose work was described here. For the HSV*tk* study this includes past and present members of the Thoracic Oncology Laboratory (Drs Kunjlata Amin, Leslie Litzky, Katherine Molnar-Kimber, Roy Smythe, Harry Hwang, Claude El-Kouri, Ashraf Elshami, John Roberts, John Kucharczuk, Nabil Rizk, Michael Chang, Seth Force, Michael Lanuti, Laura Coonrod), members of the Penn Institute for Human Gene Therapy (Drs Stephen Eck, Joseph Hughes, Nelson Wivel, and James Wilson), Penn Cancer Center (Dr Steven Hahn, Dr Joseph Friedberg, Dr Joseph Treat, Adri Ricio, RN, and Dr John Glick) and Drs Nigel Fraser and Bruce Randazzo at the Wistar Institute. For the immunotherapy/gene therapy studies this includes Drs M. Garlepp, C. Leong, J. Marley, L. Manning, H. Bielefeld-Ohmann, D. Fitzpatrick, B. Scott, A.W. Musk, A. Davidson, T. Christmas, R. Bowman, R. Lake, D. Nelson, and D. Chinn.

References

1. Tiberghien, P. Use of suicide genes in gene therapy. *J Leukoc Biol* 1994; **56**: 203–209.
2. Matthews, T., Boehme, R. Antiviral activity and mechanism of action of ganciclovir. *Rev Infect Dis* 1988; **10**: S490–S494.
3. Elshami, A., Saavedra, A., Zhang, H., Kucharczuk, J.C., Spray, D.C., Fishman, G.I., Amin, K.M., Kaiser, L.R., Albelda, S.M. Gap junctions play a role in the bystander effect of the herpes simplex virus thymidine kinase/ganciclovir system in vitro. *Gene Ther* 1996; **3**: 85–92.
4. Pope, I.M., Poston, G.J., Kinsella, A.R. The role of the bystander effect in suicide gene therapy. *Eur J Cancer* 1997; **33**: 1005–1016.
5. Smythe, W.R., Hwang, H.C., Amin, K.M., Eck, S.L., Davidson, B.L., Wilson, J.M., Kaiser, L.R., Albelda, S.M. Use of recombinant adenovirus to transfer the herpes simplex virus thymidine kinase (HSV*tk*) gene to thoracic neoplasms: an effective in vitro drug sensitization system. *Cancer Res* 1994; **54**: 2055–2059.
6. Smythe, W.R., Kaiser, L.R., Hwang, H.C., Amin, K.M., Pilewski, J.M., Eck, S.J., Wilson, J.M., Albelda, S.M. Successful adenovirus-mediated gene transfer in an in vivo model of human malignant mesothelioma. *Ann Thorac Surg* 1994; **57**: 1395–1401.
7. Esandi, M.C., van Someren, G.D., Vincent, A.J., van Bekkum, D.W., Valerio, D., Bout, A., Noteboom, J.L. Gene therapy of experimental malignant mesothelioma using adenovirus vectors encoding the HSV*tk* gene. *Gene Ther* 1997; **4**: 280–287.

8. Hwang, H.C., Smythe, W.R., Elshami, A.A., Kucharczuk, J.C., Amin, K.M., Williams, J.P., Litzky, L.A., Kaiser, L.R., Albelda, S.M. Gene therapy using adenovirus carrying the herpes simplex-thymidine kinase gene to treat in vivo models of human malignant mesothelioma and lung cancer. *Am J Respir Cell Mol Biol* 1995; **13**: 7–16.

9. Smythe, W.R., Hwang, H.C., Elshami, A.A., Amin, K.M., Eck, S.L., Davidson, B.L., Wilson, J.M., Kaiser, L.R., Albelda, S.M. Treatment of experimental human mesothelioma using adenovirus transfer of the herpes simplex thymidine kinase gene. *Ann Surg* 1995; **222**: 78–86.

10. Treat, J., Kaiser, L.R., Sterman, D.H., Litzky, L., Davis, A., Wilson, J.M., Albelda, S.M. Treatment of advanced mesothelioma with the recombinant adenovirus H5.010RSVTK: a phase I trial (BB-IND 6274). *Hum Gene Ther* 1996; **7**: 2047–57.

11. Sterman, D.H., Treat, J., Litzky, L.A., Amin, K.M., Coonrod, L., Knox, L., Recio, A., Molnar-Kimber, K., Wilson, J.M., Albelda, S.M., Kaiser, L.R. Adenovirus-mediated herpes simplex virus thymidine kinase gene delivery in patients with localized malignancy: results of a phase I clinical trial in malignant mesothelioma. *Hum Gene Ther* 1998; **9**: 1083–1092.

12. Molnar-Kimber, K.L., Sterman, D.H., Chang, M., Elbash, M., Elshami, A., Roberts, J.R., Treat, J., Wilson, J.M., Kaiser, L.R., Albelda, S.M. Humoral and cellular immune responses induced by adenoviral-based gene therapy for localized malignancy: results of a phase I clinical trial for malignant mesothelioma. *Hum Gene Ther* 1998; **9**: 2121–2133.

13. Sterman, D.H., Molnar-Kimber, K., Iyengar, T., Chang, M., Lanuti, M., Amin, K.M., Pierce, B.K., Kang, E., Treat, J., Recio, A., Litzky, L.A., Wilson, J.M., Kaiser, L.R., Albelda, S.M. A Pilot study of systemic corticosteroid administration in conjunction with intrapleural adenoviral vector administration in patients with malignant pleural mesothelioma. *Cancer Gene Ther* 2000; **7**: 1511–1518.

14. Carminschi, I., Venetsanakos, E., Leong, C.C., Garlepp, M.J., Scott, B., Robinson, BWS. Interleukin-12 induces an effective anti-tumour response in malignant mesothelioma. *Am J Respir Cell Mol Biol* 1998; **19**: 738–746.

15. Davidson, J.A., Musk, A.W., Wood Baker, R., Morey, S., Ilton, M., Yu, L.L., Drury, P., Shilkin, K., Robinson, B.W.S. Intralesional cytokine therapy in cancer; a pilot study of GM-SCF infusion in mesothelioma. *J Immunother* 1998; **21**: 389–398.

16. Robinson, B.W., Mukherjee, S.A., Davidson, A., Morey, S., Musk, A.W., Ramshaw, I., Smith, D., Lake, R., Haenel, T., Garlepp, M., Marley, J., Leong, C., Caminischi, I., Scott, B. Cytokine gene therapy or infusion as treatment for solid human cancer. *J Immunother* 1998; 21(3):211–217.

17. Mukherjee, S., Haenel, T., Himbeck, R., Scott, B., Ramshaw, I., Lake, R.A., Harnett, G., Phillips, P., Morey, S., Smith, D., Davidson, J.A., Musk, A.W., Robinson, B.W.S. Replication-restricted vaccinia as a cytokine gene therapy vector in cancer: persistent transgene expression despite antibody generation. *Cancer Gene Ther* 2000; **7**: 663–670.

18. Lukacs, K.V., Oakley, R.E., Pardo, O.E., Steel, R.M., Sorgi, F.S., Huang, L,. Geddes, D.M., Alton, E. Gene therapy for malignant mesothelioma with a heat shock protein gene. *Am J Respir Crit Care Med* 1998; **157**: A741.

19. Davis, M., Manning, L.S., Whitaker, D., Robinson, B.W.S. Establishment of a murine model of malignant mesothelioma. *Int J Cancer* 1992; **52**: 881–886.

20. Leong, C., Robinson, B.W.S., Garlepp, M. Generation of an anti-tumour immune response to a murine mesothelioma cell line by the tranfection of allogeneic MHC genes. *Int J Cancer* 1994; **59**: 212–216.

21. Leong, C., Marley, J.V., Loh, S., Robinson, B.W.S., Garlepp, M.J. Induction and maintenance of T-cell response to a nonimmunogenic murine mesothelioma cell line requires expression of B7-1 and the capacity to upregulate class-II major histocompatibility complex expression. *Cancer Gene Ther* 1996; **3**: 321–330.

22. Leong, C., Marley, J.V., Loh, S., Robinson, B.W.S., Garlepp, M.J. Transfection of the gene for B7-1 but not B7-2 can induce immunity to murine malignant mesothelioma. *Int J Cancer* 1996; **71**: 476–482.

23. Leong, C., Marley, J.V., Loh, S., Robinson, B.W.S., Garlepp MJ. The induction of immune responses to murine malignant mesothelioma by IL-2 gene transfer. *Immunol Cell Biol* 1997; **75**: 356–359.

24. Caminschi, I., Venetsanakos, E., Leong, C., Garlepp, M.J., Robinson, B.W.S., Scott, B. Cytokine gene therapy of mesothelioma: immune and anti-tumor effects of transfected IL12. *Am J Respir Cell Mol Biol* 1999; **21**: 347–356.

25. Schwarzenberger, P., Harrison, L., Weinacker, A., Gaumer, R., Theodossiou, C., Summer, W., Ye, P., Marrogi, A.J., Ramesh, R., Freeman, S., Kolls, J. Gene therapy for malignant mesothelioma: a novel approach for an incurable cancer with increased incidence in Louisiana. *J La State Med Soc* 1998; **150**: 168–174.

26. Schwarzenberger, P., Lei, D., Freeman, S.M., Ye, P., Weinacker, A., Theodossiou, C., Summer, W., Kolls, JK. Antitumor activity with the HSV-tk-gene-modified cell line PA-1-STK in malignant mesothelioma. *Am J Respir Cell Mol Biol* 1998; **19**: 333–337.

27. Kolls, J., Freeman, S., Ramesh, R., Marroqi, A., Weinacker, A., Summer, W., Schwarzenberger, P. The treatment of malignant pleural mesothelioma with gene modified cancer cells: a Phase I study. *Am J Respir Crit Care Med* 1998; **157**: A563.

28. Russell, S. Replicating vectors for gene therapy of cancer: risks, limitations and prospects. *Eur J Cancer* 1994; **30A**: 1165–1175.

29. Kucharczuk, J.C., Randazzo, B., Chang, M.Y., Amin, K.M., Elshami, A.A., Sterman, D.H., Rizk, N.P., Molnar-Kimber, K.L., Brown, S.M., MacLean, A.R., Litzky, L.A., Fraser, N.W., Albelda, S.M., Kaiser, L.R. Use of a 'replication-restricted' herpes virus to treat experimental human malignant mesothelioma. *Cancer Res* 1997; **57**: 466–471.

30. Robinson, C., Callow, M., Lake, R.A. *et al.* Serologic responses in patients with malignant mesothelioma: evidence for both public and private specificities. *Am J Respir Cell Mol Biol* 2000; **22**: 550–556.

=13=

Photodynamic Therapy (PDT) and Pleural Mesothelioma

Harvey I. Pass

Light has been the subject of medical treatments since the ancient Greeks.[1] Raab first prescribed photodynamic therapy (PDT) in 1900 by documenting the death of *Paramecia* with acridine and light,[2] and skin cancer was treated with eosin and light in 1903.[3] Various chemicals have been examined in efforts to optimise the cytotoxic effect of PDT. Hauseman found that **porphyrins**, naturally occurring iron- or-magnesium-free respiratory pigments present in the protoplasm of plant and animal cells, promoted photochemically induced cell death.[4] Studies with the complex porphyrin mixture haematoporphyrin derivative (HPD), revealed that this sensitiser concentrates in tumors,[5] and multiple HPD injections and light exposures were used to treat locally recurrent breast cancer.[6] Ensuing studies by Dougherty and others explored the use of PDT in the treatment of a wide variety of animal and human malignancies.[7-13]

PDT is based on the fact that a basic photochemical reaction occurs when a sensitising drug is exposed to light in the presence of oxygen. Absorbed light energy converts the sensitiser to an excited state, which in turn interacts with molecular oxygen to form singlet oxygen or oxygen free radicals. Singlet oxygen is a powerful oxidising agent which damages plasma membranes and other subcellular organelles. PDT is of no value unless all three components of a photochemical reaction – light, oxygen, and sensitiser – are simultaneously present when treating disease.

Components of PDT

Light

Light is high-velocity energy transmitted in electromagnetic waves which displays particulate characteristics by delivering energy in discrete measurable units called photons. The absorption of photons by a photosensitiser is the first reaction of a photodynamic system, and photochemical reactions can occur only if light is absorbed.[14] The **action spectrum** of a sensitiser defines the rate of a photochemical reaction when the sensitiser is stimulated by a given wavelength of light and usually corresponds to the absorption spectrum of the sensitiser. The **absorption spectrum** of a sensitiser determines the wavelength of light, measured in nanometres (nm), to use to achieve the maximum photodynamic effect, and generally falls within the visible light spectrum between ultraviolet (UV) and infrared (IR) light. Porphyrin sensitisers have an intense absorption band at the UV end of the spectrum called the Soret band,[14] which maximally excites a sensitiser. The energy of light is *inversely related to its wavelength*, with lower wavelengths delivering more energy. However, shorter wavelengths are attenuated by haemoglobin as they pass through tissue, and the depth of tissue penetration by light is also inversely proportional to wavelength. Therefore, light at the *IR* end of the spectrum will penetrate much deeper into a tumour than *UV* light. Although stimulation of a porphyrin sensitiser with blue-violet light may result in more energy production, the tissue penetration of <1 mm is inadequate to treat malignancy. Therefore, PDT with porphyrin-based sensitisers is usually performed with 630 nm red light or higher wavelengths, which give tissue penetration of at least 10 mm.

The **total energy delivered** depends on the **duration** of light delivery and the **dose rate** of light. The dose rate, or power density, of light is usually expressed in mW/cm^2. *In vitro*, higher dose rate delivery to tumour cells at a given total energy results in greater PDT cytotoxicity.[15] The relative inefficiency of PDT at lower dose rates may result from the ability of tumour cells to repair sublethal damage or buffer toxic oxidative stresses. The importance of these potential protective capabilities remains questionable, since *in vivo* studies have yielded contradictory results. Using human mesothelioma allografts in nude mice, Foster demonstrated that decreasing the power density from 200 to 50 mW/cm^2 resulted in lower tumour regrowth rates.[16] Low fluence rates may increase the level of singlet oxygen in areas of low capillary density, resulting in greater tumour cytotoxicity or may prevent quenching of the existing photosensitiser, i.e. photobleaching.

The appropriate method of light delivery for PDT depends on the experimental or clinical situation. An x-ray view box covered with a ruby-red acetate filter can be used for *in vitro* PDT experiments,[15] while an argon pump-dye laser exciting either Kiton red or rhodamine B producing up to 5 W of red light or a less expensive diode laser or LED array will be used as a typical light source for PDT in the clinical environment. The light source is coupled to one or more fibreoptic cables used to convey light with minimal energy loss to the treatment field. The end of the cable is fitted with a tip designed to disperse light in a pattern appropriate for the clinical application. A cleaved tip projects light forward for treating flat surfaces, and a bulbous tip projects light in an isotropic spherical distribution for illuminating large cavities. A tip specially coated with cylindrical scattering material will disperse light perpendicular to the axis of the fibre. This type of tip can be used for intraluminal applications, such as endobronchial or oesophageal PDT.

Oxygen

Although there are a few photodynamic systems which are oxygen-independent, molecular oxygen is required to achieve cytotoxicity with porphyrin-based PDT.[17,18] PDT kills cells by selective destruction of essential molecules through photo-oxidative reactions.[19] Several studies corroborate the importance of oxygen to photochemical systems. Using sodium dithionate to remove oxygen from the system, Lee showed that tumour cytotoxicity correlates directly with oxygen concentration.[18] Mitchell used a customised Petri glass system to demonstrate that cells treated in hypoxic conditions are extremely resistant to PDT.[17] Similar studies have been performed *in vivo*. Gomer found that restricting the blood flow to the hind limbs of albino mice inhibited the photosensitising effects of porphyrin PDT.[20] Although attempts to directly quantitate singlet oxygen *in vivo* have been unsuccessful,[21,22] investigators have used transcutaneous oxygen-detecting electrodes to measure microcirculatory damage after PDT.[23,24] This technology may one day be used to determine the clinical effectiveness of photochemical systems.

Photosensitisers

Several properties determine the clinical effectiveness of a photosensitiser. It is unlikely that a single sensitiser would effectively treat all malignancies or situations relevant to a given malignancy, and a sensitiser's propensity for normal tissue toxicity should be minimised in the treatment port used. For these reasons, the perfect photosensitiser probably does not exist, and there is a plethora of drugs under investigation for various uses. The properties of optimal photosensitisers have been recently discussed by Moan.[25]

The selective uptake or **retention of sensitiser by tumours** increases tumour cytotoxicity while decreasing normal tissue toxicity. Most sensitisers presently used have tumour to tissue ratios of 2–5:1. This appears to be an *in vivo* phenomenon, since *in vitro* studies using dihaematoporphyrin ether (DHE), a purified form of HPD, fail to show differences in either sensitiser uptake or survival between normal and malignant cells. NIH3T3 cells transformed by the *ras* oncogene have similar sensitiser levels and PDT survival curves to the parent NIH3T3 cell line[26] and Perry found no survival differences after PDT between normal lung fibroblasts and a variety of lung cancer cell lines.[27] However, numerous *in vitro* studies have demonstrated differences in sensitiser retention between tumour and normal tissue. Levels of DHE in animal flank tumours remain elevated for 48 hours after intravenous injection while skin and muscle exhibit significantly lower levels for 2–48 hours.[26] The method of delivery appears to play a role in determining levels of sensitiser in tumour cells depending on the type and location of tumour. In an ovarian cancer ascites model, Tochner showed that intraperitoneal injection resulted in maximum sensitiser levels.[28] The direct administration of sensitiser to cancer cells without dependence on vascular delivery probability explains this phenomenon.

The mode of presentation at the cell membrane can affect sensitiser uptake. The hydrophobicity and degree of aggregation of a sensitiser determine its internalisation by the cell. When exposed to sensitisers *in vitro*, cells take up and retain liposomal-bound porphyrins much better than aqueous phase porphyrins.[29] Cells sensitised with these liposomal-bound porphyrins sustain damage to the mitochondria and cytoplasm while porphyrins in aqueous phase target the plasma membrane. *In vitro*, hydrophilic sensitisers localise to the extracellular tissue stroma. These sensitisers are not internalised by specific receptors and therefore deposit at the cell membrane.[30] Lipophilic sensitisers such as DHE are transported to the cell membrane by low-density lipoproteins (LDL). LDL-bound fractions enter the lysosomal compartment by endocytosis, and upon exposure to light, cause release of lysosomal hydrolases into the cytoplasm.[31,32] Studies of different tumour cell lines have revealed that tumours endocytose LDL at a faster rate than normal tissues, possibly accounting for the tumour-selective properties of LDL-bound photosensitisers.

In addition to uptake, hydrophobicity may contribute to sensitiser retention as well. Porphyrins become more water soluble as pH is decreased and would therefore be retained in acidotic tumour cells. Other theories regarding the selective uptake and retention of sensitisers involve tumour cell heterogeneity, tumour neovascularity, abnormal lymphatic drainage, and stromal cell binding.

Lipophilic sensitisers that localise to the intracellular compartment also appear to generate more singlet oxygen when exposed to light than do hydrophilic sensitizers. These first-generation porphyrin sensitisers are not extremely efficient, however, for reasons discussed earlier. Maximal quantum yield of a photochemical system occurs with light wavelengths that correspond to the sensitiser's Soret band, which for porphyrin sensitisers is in the 400 nm region. Since light energy is also indirectly proportional to wavelength, the greatest quantum yield results from exposure to light just above the ultraviolet range. Light wavelengths in this range are impractical for PDT, however, because tissue penetration is directly proportional to wavelength. To balance maximal quantum yield with deepest tissue penetration, PDT is performed at higher wavelengths (> 590 nm) corresponding to minor peaks further along the absorption spectrum of the sensitiser. Under these conditions, PDT sensitisers generate singlet oxygen with quantum yield of 0.2–0.6 with tissue penetration up to 10 mm. Investigators are developing second-generation sensitisers in efforts to increase quantum yield at longer wavelengths.[33]

Another goal in the search for better sensitisers relates to photolability, the deactivation of sensitiser by light. An ideal way to decrease the toxic side effects of PDT would be to use a sensitiser that could be deactivated ('photobleached') in normal tissue but remain cytotoxic in tumour tissue. A dose of sensitiser could be chosen that resulted in sensitiser concentrations high enough in the tumour to cause photodestruction of the tumour. Lower sensitiser concentrations in adjacent normal tissue would result in photodegradation of the sensitiser to non-toxic levels.

Effects of PDT

In vitro cytotoxicity

A wide variety of cell lines show sensitivity to PDT.[2,27,34-42] Comparison of different lung cancer histologies reveals few real differences in the characteristics which influence PDT cytotoxicity[27] and the survival curves for a variety of thoracic malignancies, including adenocarcinoma, squamous cell carcinoma, large-cell carcinoma, small-cell carcinoma and mesothelioma, are quite similar.[27]

The most impressive effect seen *in vitro* soon after cells are treated with PDT is damage to the plasma membrane.[42,43] Membranes are the primary targets of PDT, partly because of the water–lipid partition coefficient of DHE. Porphyrins bind initially to the plasma membrane, followed by migration to intracellular regions. In only a few hours after PDT, normal cellular movement stops and large membrane blebs form on the cell surface.[44] These large balloon-like structures, often as large as the cell itself, indicate severe membrane damage and are the first visible sign of photo-oxidation in the cell.[45,46] This disruption of the integrity of the plasma membrane results in leakage of intracellular contents out of the cell.[47,48] After membrane blebbing occurs, cell division comes to a halt, and cell lysis begins. As alluded to earlier, PDT damages other membranes in addition to the plasma membrane. Because of these effects on cell membranes, PDT may injure the nucleus, lysosomes, Golgi apparatus, endoplasmic reticulum and mitochondria. Mitochondrial damage after PDT may involve inhibition of oxidative phosphorylation and electron transport with subsequent reduction in ATP production.[49,50] One cellular target that appears to escape serious damage by PDT is nuclear DNA. While PDT can induce DNA strand breaks, this does not lead to cell death. PDT does not appear to be mutagenic.[51]

Resistance of cells to PDT may one day determine the clinical efficacy of PDT in cancer treatment. Several investigators have begun to examine the role of the multidrug resistance phenotype (MDR) in PDT resistance. In MDR associated with chemotherapy, a membrane pump actively transports drug out of the cell. Conceivably, this mechanism could transport photosensitiser out of the cell, thereby reducing the photodynamic effect at treatment. This could become a particular problem when treating patients with combined chemotherapy–PDT regimens. Similarly, patients who have previously failed to respond to chemotherapy might likewise develop cross-resistance to PDT. Studies comparing the sensitivities of cells which express MDR versus wild-type cells from the same cell line revealed no cross-resistance to PDT.[52] Using cells made resistant to PDT by repeated exposure to PDT, investigators have shown that this resistance is not due to decreased intracellular levels of sensitiser, the mechanism of action of classic MDR.[5,54] MDR may be associated with cross-resistance to PDT, depending on the sensitiser used.[55] A more plausible explanation for PDT resistance involves the mechanism of action of PDT. Buffering of toxic oxygen radicals by free radical scavengers could explain the induced resistance of cells to PDT. Studies by Ryter have shown that PDT can enhance transcription and translation of oxidative stress genes.[56] Many studies involving chemotherapy resistance have shown that free radical buffering enzymes such as glutathione can protect cells against drugs which produce free radicals. While no one knows how cells become resistant to PDT, mechanisms other than MDR are probably involved.

In vivo cytotoxicity

Flank tumours in mice will regress completely by two days after treatment with PDT. Soon after PDT, blood flow stasis occurs in both arterioles and venules.[57-59] A vascular effect is one of the main components of tumour destruction with many of the presently investigated sensitisers. Vasoconstriction of arterioles, thrombosis of venules, and oedema of perivascular tissues accompany the reduction in blood flow. Ben-Hur *et al.* suggest that PDT induces the endothelium to release vasoconstrictors and clotting factors which cause local coagulation and stasis.[60] This begins a cascade in which local blood flow stasis and endothelial damage retain red blood cells in the treatment field longer, thereby exposing them to higher doses of PDT. Subsequent damage results in red cell agglutination, which further exacerbates the low flow state. The binding of neutrophils and platelets to damaged endothelium with release of prostanglandins and arichidonates which also act on the microvasculature. Other factors such as von Willebrand factor, platelet activating factor, and nitric oxide may also be involved. The photodynamic process itself may lead to alterations in tumour blood flow.[61] A positive feedback cycle of oxygen depletion by the photo-oxidative system, acidosis, increased intratumoral swelling with decreased blood flow, and worsening hypoxia could account for static blood flow followed by tumour necrosis. Nuclear magnetic resonance studies examining tumour energy substrate levels during and after PDT indicate that ATP levels are virtually undetectable by 2–4 hours[62-64] and appear to decline in a dose-dependent fashion.[65]

The anti-tumour effect of PDT may in part be due to modulation of the immune system. Various studies have documented the release of vasoactive agents such as prostaglandins, thromboxane, and histamine from murine peritoneal macrophages and mast cells.[66-68] These mediators could contribute to the vascular and metabolic effects of PDT in mediating tumour necrosis. PDT also induces macrophages to release tumour necrosis factor (TNF) in a dose-dependent fashion[69] and, conversely, PDT may exert a net inhibitory effect on the immune system, however. Contact hypersensitivity remains suppressed 2 weeks after PDT,[70] and this effect is adoptively transferred by macrophages.[71] PDT also inhibits the mitogen-stimulated division of human peripheral blood lymphocytes.[72] Therefore, while PDT can induce non-specific immune cells to produce substances such as TNF, prostaglandins, thromboxanes and histamines that could either directly or indirectly mediate tumour necrosis, the overall effect of PDT on the immune system is unknown.

Increased specificity and sensitivity of PDT resulting in an improved tumour/normal treatment index may result by treating tumours with antibody-sensitiser conjugates. A photosensitising agent could be combined with a monoclonal antibody with idiotypic specificity for a known tumour. Theoretically, this would increase the specificity of the sensitiser for the tumour, resulting in increased tumour cytotoxicity with reduced side effects in normal tissues. Mew *et al.* demonstrated this concept by showing that monoclonal antibody-photosensitiser conjugates effectively mediated tumour regression *in vivo* and killed a variety of cell lines *in vitro*.[73,74] PDT using monoclonal antibody-sensitiser conjugates appears to result in greater tumour specificity, longer remission and less normal tissue toxicity in murine subcutaneous tumours.[75] While similar constructs have demonstrated selective killing of human ovarian carcinoma and melanoma cells,[76,77] work in this area remains highly investigational.

Intrapleural PDT

The management of pleural neoplasms, specifically malignant pleural mesothelioma (MPM), remains difficult. Surgery alone cannot cure patients with MPM, and chemotherapy response rates range from 10% to 20% with few complete responses.[1] The role of radiation therapy, either as definitive therapy or via intraoperative or postoperative techniques, remains undefined.[2] Novel, more aggressive, approaches for managing these malignancies have included intraoperative chemotherapy, surgery and postoperative multimodality therapy, intrapleural or systemic immunotherapy, and intraoperative PDT.[3-10] All of these approaches rely on the idea that at least an effective cytoreduction of the tumour can be accomplished such that the adjuvant therapy may have a chance to affect local control and eventually survival. Certainly the ability to accomplish such a cytoreduction consistently, either by extrapleural pneumonectomy or by pleurectomy is a key issue, and not all mesothelioma surgeons adhere to the same criteria with regard to the completeness of the cytoreduction, or even the role of lymph node dissection in the management of the disease.

There has been keen interest in the use of PDT as an adjuvant intraoperative therapy for pleural malignancies such as mesothelioma. Thoracic malignancies, including mesothelioma, were sensitive to *in vitro* PDT[27,34] and others confirmed its cytotoxicity *in vivo*.[78-80] Large animal studies confirmed the safety of intrapleural PDT to the heart, lungs, oesophagus and diaphragm at doses up to 40 J/cm^2.[81]

A technique to 'uniformly' illuminate the entire chest cavity using light scattering media was investigated. Sensitiser loaded cells which were treated with light while they were in various concentrations of intralipid were found to undergo significantly better PDT cytotoxicity than controls.[82] Such a strategy was used at the National Cancer Institute to treat the pleural space.

Accurate quantitation of 'dose' of the individual components of the PDT package, i.e., sensitiser and light energy, would be necessary to make decisions regarding efficacy and toxicity for such a treatment. A photodiode system was developed to record on line light doses, and tested in a phantom model of the thoracic cavity. Initially using a 4-photodiode system, light measurements were recorded in a phantom model of the chest comparing buffered saline solution to intralipid as light scattering media. Excellent light distribution from a single fibre placed in the center of the intralipid filled model occurred with uniform power densities noted.[83] Maximum light scattering occurred between 0.01% and 0.05% intralipid. The system was upgraded to measure light intensity at a number of sites and to integrate the values in real time to provide the light dose at each, all in a way that was convenient and safe to use in the operating room.[84]

From these studies a feasibility trial in 8 patients was conducted which demonstrated that mechanical delivery of light to the pleura using dye lasers could be accomplished 48 hours after sensitiser delivery safely up to a dose of 15 J/cm^2.[85] A phase I study of PDT in the management of pleural malignancies to define the maximal tolerated dose of PDT that could be delivered to the chest cavity after maximum cytoreductive surgery was then performed from June 1990 to April 1992.[86] The problem of uneven geometry for light distribution was overcome partially by using a light scattering medium which was simply poured into the chest into which the laser fibre was placed. The light scattering medium, low concentration intralipid, minimally absorbed the light and was well tolerated by tissues. Commercially available photodiodes, mounted on transparent lucite bases, gathered light to a custom-designed amplifier box, isolation transformers and computer. Each photodiode gave instantaneous readings of light in J/cm^2 as well as the cumulative dose seen. Such a system allowed treatment of a given area to a prescribed dose. Some 54 patients with isolated hemithorax pleural malignancy were prospectively entered into the trial, which, in cohorts of 3 patients, escalated the intraoperative light dose from 15 to 35 J/cm^2 *48 hours* after intravenous delivery of 2.0 mg/kg Photofrin II and then escalated the light dose from 30 to 32.5 J/cm^2 after a 24 hour sensitiser–operation interval. The tumours of 12 patients could not be debulked to the prerequisite 5 mm residual tumour thickness. The remaining 42 patients (31 mesothelioma, 5 adenocarcinoma, 4 sarcoma, 2 other) received 19 modified pleuropneumonectomies, 5 lobectomy-pleurectomies, and 18 pleurectomies. Intrapleural PDT was delivered using 630 nm light from two argon pump-dye lasers, and real-time as well as cumulative light doses were monitored using 7 uniquely designed, computer-interfaced photodiodes. One patient (1.9%) died <30 days after surgery, from intraoperative haemorrhage. Operation duration was 6.5 ± 0.3 hours, median intensive care unit stay was 4.9 ± 0.3 days, and patients were discharged 12.4 ± 1.0 days after surgery. Arrhythmia (11/42; 26%) was the most common complication, and 59% of patients were complication-free. In the 48 hour sensitiser-operation group (n=33), possible PDT-related complications included an empyema with late haemorrhage in 1 of 3 patients at 17.5 J/cm^2, and a bronchopleural fistula at 35 J/cm^2. At each of these light doses, 3 additional patients were treated without complication. Two patients with 24 hour sensitiser dosing and 32.5 J/cm^2 developed oesophageal perforations after pleuropneumonectomy at identical sites. These patients were treated with open thoracostomy, jejunostomy, and gastro-oesophageal junction stapling. Subsequent left colon oesophagogastric interposition reestablished normal swallowing in both. The MTD was declared as *30 J/cm^2 light with a 24 hour dosing interval* when none of the six patients (3 original, 3 repeat) at that level developed toxicity. Consistent patient-to-patient light measurements were substantiated by analysis of the dosimetry system which revealed a 0.99 correlation of the laser treatment time with patient body surface area, projected light dose, and available power.

In a subsequent phase III study, 63 patients with localised MPM were randomly assigned to either *PDT* or no *PDT* groups between July 1993 and June 1996. Patients were considered for the trial if, on review of the chest computed tomogram, it was felt that the disease was amenable to a subtotal extirpation such that the maximum thickness after debulking at any intrathoracic site was 5 mm or less. There could be multiple discontinuous sites of disease or one large plaque-like area of residual disease; in all cases, however, by gross examination the residual disease was felt to be of 5 mm thickness or less. Either pleurectomy decortication alone, or in combination with anatomic or non-anatomic resection, as well as extrapleural pneumonectomy, was performed. The extrapleural pneumonectomy could be modified to include or not include portions of the pericardium or diaphragm. Postoperative staging was defined by the International Mesothelioma Interest Group Staging System.[87]

All patients were required to understand and sign informed consent for entry into the trial, which was approved by the Institutional Review Board of the National Cancer Institute, as well as by the Cancer Therapy Evaluation Programme. Patients who were registered for randomisation were stratified by mesothelioma histology (epithelial, biphasic or sarcomatoid), age and sex. The randomisation determined whether the patient would receive or not receive intraoperative PDT at the time of maximal cytoreduction. All patients fulfilling criteria for cytoreduction received postoperative immunochemotherapy (see later).

Intraoperative PDT

Sensitiser

All patients randomised to intraoperative PDT received 2 mg/kg intravenous dihaematoporphyrin ethers (Photofrin II [PII], courtesy of Quadra Logic Technologies, Vancouver, Canada) 24 hours before the planned cytoreduction. All patients receiving photosensitiser received specific instructions to avoid sun exposure for a minimum of 6 weeks to prevent skin photosensitivity reactions.

Light source and dosimetry

Light delivery (630 nm) was achieved with two Coherent pump-dye lasers using Kiton red as the dye or with a specially designed 50 W laser (Laserionics, Tampa, FL). The Coherent lasers (Model PRT 100 Coherent, Inc., Palo Alto, CA and Innova 200-25, Model CR 599, Coherent, Inc., Palo Alto, CA) could each deliver 25 W from the argon tube and 5 W[88] at 630 nm from the dye table, and the Laserionics instrument could deliver 9–11 W at 630 nm. The system of light delivery using optical fibers housed in sterile endotracheal tubes has been previously described. Briefly, the fibreoptic system is assembled from 600 micron diameter fused silica optical fibre (Quartz Products Corporation, Plainfield, NJ) and fibre connectors (Radiall Corporation, Stratford, CT) or purchased with specialty terminations to produce spherical or cylindrical light distributions (Laser Therapeutics, Inc., Buellton, CA). These fibres were used directly by attachment to the laser or indirectly by an attachment delivery fibre. The transmission characteristics of fused silica are excellent in this wavelength range. The fibres enable 85% of the laser power to be delivered 65 metres to the operating suite from the laser site including coupling losses. Total power delivered into the optical fibres ranged from 4.8 to 10 W.

Light dosimetry was accomplished with a specially designed system to measure light intensity at a number of sites and integrate the values on real time to provide the light dose at each site. The system consisted of an amplifier box, isolation transformers, photodiodes and a computer. A custom-designed amplifier box provided individual current to voltage converters for 12 photodiodes. Signals were transmitted to a Compaq Model 4 portable computer (Houston, TX) with the appropriate software for photodiode calibration, and the location of each photodiode was recorded as well as real-time and cumulative dose in J/cm^2. The patented photodiodes (Model VTB 4051, Vactec, St. Louis, MO) were mounted on transparent methyl-methacrylate (lucite) bases, and were placed in 7 strategic areas: apex, pericardial or epicardial, anteromedial chest wall, posterolateral chest wall, posterior mediastinal (perioesophageal), anterior diaphragmatic gutter, and posterior diaphragmatic gutter. The cumulative light dose at each diode site for each patient was 30 J/cm^2.

Immunochemotherapy with Cisplatin, Interferon alpha and Tamoxifen

Patients whose tumours were cytoreduced to 5 mm thickness were to receive 2 cycles of immunochemotherapy 4–6 weeks after surgery. Tamoxifen, 20 mg by mouth twice daily, was given every day for 35 days and interferon-α 2B (5 mU/m^2) was delivered 3 times a week by subcutaneous injection. Cisplatin (CDDP), 25 mg/m^2, was delivered in 250 cc of normal saline with prehydration, and it induced diuresis on days 8, 15, 22 and 29 at least 30 minutes after interferon delivery. Prophylactic antiemetic therapy with ondansetron (0.15 mg/kg) was given one-half hour before CDDP and 2 hours after the CDDP. Each patient was monitored prospectively for clinically adverse reactions resulting from the interaction of cisplatin, interferon and tamoxifen with history and physical examination, and complete blood count, blood urea nitrogen, creatinine and serum magnesium levels were obtained on days 0, 8, 15, 22, 29 and 36. Serum electrolytes as well as hepatic and mineral panels were performed on days 0, 15 and 29. Toxicities were graded according to the Common Toxicity Criteria for Cancer Clinical Treatment Trials, and dose modifications were specified for dose-limiting myelosuppression, nephrotoxicity, interferon-related fatigue, or elevation of liver enzymes.

Chest and abdominopelvic computed tomograms were performed every 3 months after cessation of therapy for 2 years and then every 6 months and progression/recurrence of disease was documented histologically if possible.

There were 18 females and 45 females. Of these, 15 patients (3 females and 12 males) were taken off study due to inability to debulk to the prerequisite 5 mm (8 patients, 4 PDT; 4 non-PDT), progressed prior to operative intervention (6), or withdrew prior to resection (1).

The two groups of patients were similar with regard to preoperative characteristics including sex, age, symptoms, and interval from diagnosis to treatment. All patients were ECOG performance status I, and the majority had a history of asbestos exposure. Pulmonary function tests were comparable between the groups and there were no significant differences between the two groups with regard to the preoperative tumour burden, as determined by preoperative quantitative computerised volumetrics (294± 63 vs 247± 85 cc, PDT vs no PDT, mean + standard error of the mean). The residual solid tumour volume as estimated by CT volumetrics prior to the inception of immunochemotherapy was also comparable (28 ± 10 vs 44± 21 cc, PDT vs no PDT, mean + standard error of the mean).

The extent of resection to accomplish the 5 mm residual disease cytoreduction, as well as the postoperative histology and stage, was very similar between the two groups. The photodynamic therapy added an additional 137 minutes to the resection, of which a mean of 64 minutes was laser-on time. Laser power at 630 nm ranged from 6.2 to 9.2 W.

There were no differences in the number or severity of surgical or immunochemotherapeutic complications comparing PDT to no PDT. There were 11 postoperative complications in 10 patients, including medically reversible arrhythmia in 4 patients, bronchopleural fistula in 4 patients, cardiac herniation requiring pericardial patching in 1 patient, postoperative bleeding requiring reexploration in 1 patient, and postoperative pancreatitis in one patient. There were two bronchopleural fistulae in each group, all occurring more than 30 days after the pleuropneumonectomy. All were treated with open thoracostomy with drainage. One patient has had her fistula closed 18 months after the extrapleural pneumectomy (EPP), and another patient whose thoracostomy remains open is alive with disease 34 months after his operation. There was one operative death in a PDT patient whose inferior vena cava avulsed after a right-sided pleuropneumonectomy at the termination of anaesthesia.

Immunochemotherapy was started at a similar interval from surgery in both arms (1.4 months post-operative-PDT vs 1.2 months post-operative-no PDT). The majority of patients received 2 full cycles (21-PDT, 17-no PDT). Patients who did not receive both cycles of CIT either progressed after one cycle or refused further therapy.

In order to verify whether the light detection was stable from patient to patient, it was theorised that the amount of time to deliver the prescribed light dose should be directly proportional to: (1) size of the patient's chest (which would be in proportion to the patient's body surface area); and (2) the prescribed dose of light. An inverse relationship, however, should exist between the laser treatment time and the amount of wattage (power) available from the lasers on that given day. When such a proportion was calculated, there was a 95% correlation between these parameters and laser 'on' time, revealing consistency of the diode measuring system from patient to patient.

The median potential follow-up (time from treatment to either last known follow-up for survivors or time to death for non-survivors) for the entire group of 63 patients was 23.1 months at the time of the report. The median survival for the 48 PDT and no PDT groups was 14.4. months, and there was no significant difference between the two groups (PDT: 14.1 months, no PDT: 14.4 months. The median survival for the 15 patients whose tumour could not be surgically cytoreduced was 7.2 months. The median recurrence-free survival was 8.0 months for the entire group (PDT:8.5 months, no PDT:7.7 months). Once a recurrence was diagnosed, the median time to death was 5.1 months.

This study represented one of the few prospective randomised trials incorporating surgery for the management of MPM. The lack of a uniform management strategy, the small number of cases, and the futility in dealing with this disease as expressed by both surgeons and medical oncologists has contributed to the inability to conduct innovative and aggressive approaches for MPM. Most recently, however, there has been an increasing interest in the management of MPM, as well as the exploration of novel approaches including gene therapy and immunotherapeutic strategies.

At least 5 other centres have had an interest in the management of pleural mesothelioma with photodynamic therapy (Table 13.1).[89-92] In reviewing the data, most of which is only presented in abstract form, it can be appreciated that the studies represent a tremendous amount of labour. Nevertheless, the PDT delivery is heterogeneous with regard to sensitiser used and dose of light used, and the staging of the patients treated is very unclear. It is far too early to draw conclusions regarding efficacy from these phase I/II trials, but they reinforce the position of the NCI group that the delivery is feasible, and can be performed safely. Moreover, the operative mortalities are low in all the studies.

Analysis of the two groups studied in this randomised trial reveals that they are quite comparable with regard to extent of disease at the time of randomisation. This is

Table 13.1. International PDT trials for pleural mesothelioma.

Group	N	Sensitiser/dose	Light dose	Technique	Comments
Roswell Park, Buffalo, NY	40	2 mg/kg PII	20–30 J/cm^2	Preoperative simulation; multiple fibers intraoperative; no online dosimetry	45% complications: 3 deaths; non-uniform debulking
Orebro, Sweden	1	2 mg/kg PII	20 J/cm^2	Preoperative simulation; thoracoscopic delivery; no online dosimetry	6 hours of treatment; no recurrence at 10 months
Bern, Switzerland	8	0.3 mg/kg mTHPC	10 J/cm^2	2 'thoracoscopic': 2 intraoperative; no online dosimetry	1 death; only 3 month follow-up available
Amsterdam, Netherlands	8	0.1 mg/kg mTHPC	10–15 J/cm^2	intraoperative; no online dosimetry	Myocardial infarction (1); 25% complication rate
University of Pennsylvania, PA	9	0.1–ongoing phase I	5 J/cm^2 – ongoing phase I	Intraoperative online dosimetry	1 death (ARDS), 6/9 NED 2-9 months postoperative
Melbourne, Australia	25	5 mg/kg HPD	NA	Direct surface illumination; no online dosimetry	Median survival 713 days compared to 250 days in non-matched controls
Oslo, Norway	9	2 mg/kg PII	15–30 J/cm^2	'cooled spherical diffusing fibre' intraoperative; no online dosimetry	6 patients had local recurrence 4–14 months postoperatively

PII: Photofrin II; mTHPC: *m*-tetrahydroxyphenylchlorin; HPD; haematoporphyrin derivative.

confirmed by the measurement of T status using the CT volumetrics, as well as by the postoperative distribution of IMIG stages, including the number with involved lymph nodes. Moreover, there were no obvious differences in the number of cycles of postoperative adjuvant immunochemotherapy delivered, or in the toxicity from the regimens.

The failure to detect any difference in the two groups with regard to time to recurrence, recurrence patterns, or the median survival strongly implies that first generation intrapleural PDT is not beneficial to patients with MPM. Moreover, the anticipated accrual of 44 patients per arm was not reached for logistical reasons; however, the impact of decreased sample size, considering the identical nature of the survival and recurrence curves, was probably minimal. As with any new therapeutic intervention which does not succeed in its first attempt, it would be foolish to simply claim that PDT is unsuited for intrapleural cancer control and should be condemned to historical interest. There are obvious aspects of the treatment which can be improved, and at the very least, this study confirms the ability to (1) perform the cytoreduction safely and (2) deliver safe doses of intrapleural PDT after describing the maximal tolerated dose in phase I trials. Newer trials can be constructed, based on the evolving interest in the development of longer wavelength sensitisers, as well as a redesigning of light delivery techniques.

References

1. Daniell, M.D., Hill, J.S. A history of photodynamic therapy. *Aust N Z J Surg* 1991; **61**: 340–348.
2. Raab, O. Über die Wirkung fluoreszierenden Stoffen. *Infusoria Z Biol* 1900; **39**: 524.
3. Jesionek, A., Tappeiner, V.H. Zur Behandlung der hautcarcinomit mit fluorescierenden Stoffen. *Munch Med Wochenschr* 1903; **47**: 2042.
5. Gregorie, H.G., Horger, E.O., Ward, J.L. *et al.* Hematoporphyrin-derivative fluorescence in malignant neoplasms. *Ann Surg* 1968; **167**: 820–828.
4. Hausman, W. Die sensibilisierende Wirkung des Hematoporphyrins. *Biochem Z* 1911; **30**: 276–286.
6. Lipson, R.L., Gray, M.J., Baldes, E.J. Hematoporphyrin derivative for detection and management of cancer. *Proc 9th Int Cancer Cong.* Tokyo, Japan, 1966; 393.
7. Dougherty, T.J. Activated dyes vs anti-tumor agents. *J Natl Cancer Inst* 1974; **51**: 1333–1336.
8. Dougherty, T.J., Grindley, G.E., Fiel, R., *et al.* Photoradiation therapy II. Cure of animal tumors with hematoporphyrin and light. *J Natl Cancer Inst* 1975; **55**: 115–121.
9. Dougherty, T.J., Kaufman, J.E., Goldfarb, A., *et al.* Photoradiation therapy for the treatment of malignant tumors. *Cancer Res* 1978; **38**: 2628–2635.
10. Dougherty, T.J. Photoradiation therapy. *Urology* 1984; Suppl, **23**: 61–61.
11. Mang, T.S., Dougherty, T.J., Potter, W.R., *et al.* Photobleaching of porphyrins used in photodynamic therapy and implications for therapy. *Photochem Photobiol* 1987; **45**: 501–506.
12. Dougherty, T.J. Photosensitizers: therapy and detection of malignant tumors. *Photochem Photobiol* 1987; **45**: 879–889.
13. Kelly, J.F., Snell, N.E., Berenbaum, M.C. Photodynamic destruction of human bladder carcinoma. *Br J Cancer* 1975; **31**: 237–244.
14. Spikes, J.D. Photobiology of porphyrins. In: D.R. Doiron, C.J. Gomer (eds.), *Porphyrin Localization and Treatment of Tumors*. New York: Alan R. Liss, 1984.
15. Matthews, W., Cook, J., Pass, H.I. *In vitro* photodynamic therapy of human lung cancer: investigation of dose-rate effects. *Cancer Res* 1989; **49**: 1718–1721.

16. Foster, T.H., Gibson, S.L., Gao, L., Hilf, R. Analysis of photochemical oxygen consumption effects on photodynamic therapy. Proceedings of Optical Methods for Tumor Treatment and Detection: Mechanisms and techniques in photodynamic therapy. *International Society for Optical Engineering* 1992; **45**: 104–114.

17. Mitchell, J.B., McPherson, S., DeGraff, W., *et al.* Oxygen dependence of hematoporphyrin derivative-induced photoinactivation of Chinese hamster cells. *Cancer Res* 1985; **45**: 2008–2011.

18. Lee See, K., Forbes, I.J., Betts, W.H. Oxygen dependency of phototoxicity with haematoporphyrin derivative. *Photochem Photobiol* 1984; **39**: 631–634.

19. Gorden, P., Comi, R.J., Maton, P.N., Go, V.L.W. Somatostatin and somatostatin analogue (SMS 201–995) in treatment of hormone-secreting tumors of the pituitary and gastrointestinal tract and non-neoplastic diseases of the gut. *Ann Intern Med* 1989; **110**: 35–50.

20. Gomer, C.J., Razum, N.J. Acute skin response in albino mice following porphyrin photosensitization under oxic and anoxic conditions. *Photochem Photobiol* 1984; **40**: 435–439.

21. Gomer, C.J. Preclinical examination of first and second generation photosensitizers used in photodynamic therapy. *Photochem Photobiol* 1991; **54**: 1093–1107.

22. Patterson, M.S., Madsen, S.J., Wilson, B.C. Experimental tests of the feasibility of singlet oxygen luminescence and monitoring *in vivo* during photodynamic therapy. *J Photochem Photobiol* 1990; **5**: 69–84.

23. Tromberg, B.J., Orenstein, A., Kimel, S., *et al.* In vivo tumor oxygen tension measurements for the evaluation of the efficiency of photodynamic therapy delivery. *Photochem Photobiol* 1990; **52**: 375–385.

24. Reed, M.W., Mullens, A.P., Anderson, G.L., Miller, F.N., Wieman, T.J. The effect of photodynamic therapy on tumor oxygenation. *Surgery* 1989; **106**: 94–99.

25. Moan, J. Properties for optimal PDT sensitizers. *J Photochem Photobiol* 1990; **5**: 521–524.

26. Pass, H.I., Evans, S., Matthews, W.A., Perry, R., Venzon, D., Roth, J.A., Smith, P. Photodynamic therapy of oncogene-transformed cells. *J Thorac Cardiovasc Surg* 1991; **101**: 795–799.

27. Perry, R.R., Matthews, W., Pass, H.I., *et al.* Sensitivity of different human lung cancer histologies to photodynamic therapy. *Cancer Res* 1990; **50**: 4272–4276.

28. Tochner, Z., Mitchell, J.B., Smith, P., *et al.* Photodynamic therapy of ascites tumours within the peritoneal cavity. *Br J Cancer* 1986; **53**: 733–736.

29. Jori, G., Tomio, L., Reddi, E., Corti, L., Zorat, L., Calzavara, F. Preferential delivery of liposome-incorporated prophyrins to neoplastic cells in tumor-bearing rats. *Br J Cancer* 1983; **48**: 307–309.

30. Peng, Q., Moan, J., Farrants, G., Danielson, H.E., Rimington, C. Localization of potent photosensitizers in human tumor LOX by means of laser scanning microscopy. *Cancer Lett* 1990; **53**: 129–139.

31. Miller, D.L. Arteriography and venous sampling for the localization of endocrine tumors. In: J.M. Taveras (ed.), *Radiology: Diagnosis-Imaging-Intervention*. Philadelphia: J.B.Lippincott Co., 1992; 1–10.

32. Mazière, J.C., Morlière, P., Santus, R. The role of the low density lipoprotein receptor pathway in the delivery of lipophilic photosensitizers in the photodynamic therapy of tumors. *J Photochem Photobiol* 1991; **8**: 351–360.

33. Kreimer-Birnbaum, M. Modified porphyrins, chlorins, pthalocyanines, and purpurins: second-generation photosensitizers for photodynamic therapy. *Sem Hematol* 1989; **26**: 157–173.

34. Keller, S.M., Taylor, P.D., Weese, J.L. *In vitro* killing of human malignant mesothelioma by photodynamic therapy. *J Surg Res* 1990; **48**: 337–340.

35. Roberts, W.G., Berns, M.W. *In vitro* photosensitization I. Cellular uptake and subcellular localization of MONO-ʟ-aspartyl chlorin e6, chloro-aluminum sulfonated phthalocyanine, and Photofrin II. *Lasers Surg Med* 1989; **9**: 90–101.
36. Matthews, E.K., Cui, Z.J. Photodynamic action of sulfonated aluminum phthalocyanines (SALPCS) on AR4-2J cells, a carcinoma cell line of rat exocrine pancreas. *Br J Cancer* 1990; **61**: 695–701.
37. Sery, T.W., Shield, J.A., Augsburger, J.J., *et al.* Photodynamic therapy of human ocular cancer. *Ophthalmic Surg* 1987; **18**: 413–418.
38. Pope, A.J., Masters, W., MacRobert, A.J. The photodynamic effect of a pulsed dye laser on human bladder carcinoma cells *in vitro*. *Urol Res* 1990; **18**: 267–270.
39. Jamieson, C.H., McDonald, W.N., Levy, J.G. Preferential uptake of benzoporphyrin derivative by leukemia versus normal cells. *Leuk Res* 1990; **14**: 209–219.
40. Rogers, D.W., Lanzafame, R.J., Hinshaw, J.R. Effect of argon laser and Photofrin II on murine neuroblastoma cells. *J Surg Res* 1991; **50**: 255–271.
41. West, C.M.L. Size-dependent resistance of human tumor spheroids to photodynamic treatment. *Br J Cancer* 1989; **59**: 510–514.
42. Kessel, D. Sites of photosensitization by derivatives of hematoporphyrin. *Photochem Photobiol* 1986; **44**: 489–493.
43. Volden, G., Christensen, T., Moan, J. Photodynamic membrane damage of hematoporphyrin derivative-treated NHIK 3025 cells in vitro. *Photochem Photobiophys* 1981; **3**: 105.
44. Jewell, S.A., Bellomo, G., Thor, H. *et al.* Bleb formation in hepatocytes during drug metabolism is caused by disturbances in thiol and calcium ion homeostatis. *Science* 1982; **217**: 1257–1259.
45. Borrelli, M.J., Wong, R.S.L., Dewey, W.C. A direct correlation between hyperthermia-induced blebbing and survival in synchronous G₁ CHO cells. *J Cell Physiol* 1986; **126**: 181–190.
46. Dubbelman, T.M.A.R., Smeets, M., Boegheim, J.P.J. Cell models. In: G. Moreno, R.H. Potter T.G. Truscott (eds.), *Photosensitization: Molecular and Medical Aspects*. 1988.
47. Sonoda, M., Murali-Krishna, C., Riesz, P. The role of singlet oxygen in the photohemolysis of red blood cells sensitized by phthalocyanine sulfonates. *Photochem Photobiol* 1987; **46**: 625–31.
48. Hilf, R., Murant, R.S., Narayanan, U., Gibson, S.L. Hematoporphyrin derivative-induced photosensitivity of mitochondrial succinate dehydrogenase and selected cytosolic enzymes of R3230AC mammary adenocarcinomas of rats. *Cancer Res* 1984; **44**:1483–1488.
49. Hilf, R., Murant, R.S., Narayanan, U., Gibson, S.L. Relationship of mitochondrial function and cellular adenosine triphosphate levels to hematoporphyrin derivative-induced photosensitization in R3230AC mammary tumors. *Cancer Res* 1986; **46**: 211–217.
50. Gomer, C.J. DNA damage and repair in CHO cells following hematoporphyrin photoradiation. *Cancer Lett* 1980; **11**: 161–161.
51. Ben-Hur, E., Fujihara, T., Suzuki, F., Elkind, M.M. Genetic toxicology of the photosensitization of Chinese hamster cells by phthalocyanines. *Photochem Photobiol* 1987; **45**: 227–230.
52. Kessel, D., Erickson, C. Porphyrin photosensitization of multi-drug resistant cell types. *Photochem Photobiol* 1992; **55**: 397–399.
53. Singh, G., Wilson, B.C., Sharkey, S.M., Browman, G.P., Deschamps, P. Resistance to photodynamic therapy in radiation induced fibrosarcoma. *Photochem Photobiol* 1991; **54**: 307–312.
54. Luna, M.C., Gomer, C.J. Isolation and initial characterization of mouse tumor cells resistant to porphyrin-mediated photodynamic therapy. *Cancer Res* 1991; **15**: 4243–4249.
55. Diddens, H. Role of multidrug resistance in photodynamic therapy. Proceeding of Optical Methods for Tumor Treatment Detection. Mechanisms and techniques in photodynamic therapy. *International Society for Optical Engineering* 1992; **45**: 115–123.

56. Ryter, S.W., Gomer, C.S., Ferrario, A., *et al.* Cellular stress responses following photodynamic therapy. In: B.W. Henderson, T.J. Dougherty (eds.), *Photodynamic Therapy: Basic Principles and Clinical Applications.* New York: Marcel Dekker, Inc., 1992; 55–62.

57. Reed, W.P., Newman, K.A. An improved technique for the insertion of Hickman catheters in patients with thrombocytopenia and granulocytopenia. *Surg Gynecol Obstet* 1983; **156**: 355–358.

58. Stern, S.J., Flock, S., Small, S., Thomsen, S., Jacques, S. Chloraluminum sulphonated phthalocyanine versus dihematoporphyrin ether: Early vascular events in the rat window chamber. *Laryngoscope* 1991; **101**: 1219–1225.

59. Wieman, T.J., Mang, T.S., Fingar, V.S., *et al.* Effect of photodynamic therapy on blood flow in normal and tumor vessels. *Surgery* 1988; **104**: 512–517.

60. Ben-Hur, E., Orenstein, A. The endothelium and red blood cells as potential targets in PDT- induced vascular stases. *Int J Radiat Biol* 1991; **60**: 293–301.

61. Bellnier, D.A., Henderson, B.W. Determinants for photodynamic tissue destruction. In: B.W. Henderson and T.J. Dougherty (eds.), *Photodynamic Therapy.* New York: Marcel Dekker, 1992; 117–127.

62. Dodd, N.J.F., Moore, J.V., Poppitt, G., Wood, B. *In vivo* magnetic resonance imaging of the effects of photodynamic therapy. *Br J Cancer* 1989; **60**: 164–167.

63. Moore, J.V., Dodd, N.J.F., Wood, B. Proton nuclear magnetic resonance imaging as a predictor of the outcome of photodynamic therapy of tumors. *Br J Radiol* 1989; **62**: 869–870.

64. Mattiello, J., Evelhoch, J.L., Brown, E., Schaap, A.P. Effect of photodynamic therapy on RIF-1 tumor metabolism and blood flow examined by 31P and 2H NMR spectoscopy. *NMR Biomed* 1990; **3**: 64–70.

65. Chopp, M., Hetzel, F.W., Jiang, Q. Dose dependent metabolic response of mammary carcinoma to photodynamic therapy. *Radiat Res* 1990; **121**: 288–294.

66. Henderson, B.W., Donovan, J.M. Release of prostaglandin E2 from cells by photodynamic treatment in vitro. *Cancer Res* 1989; **49**: 6896–6900.

67. Fingar, V.H., Wieman, T.J., Doak, K.W. Role of thromboxane and prostacycline release on photodynamic therapy-induced tumor destruction. *Cancer Res* 1990; **50**: 2599–2603.

68. Ortner, M.J., Abhold, R.H., Chignell, C.F. The effect of protoporphyrin on histamine secretion by rat peritoneal mast cells: a dual phototoxic reaction. *Photochem Photobiol* 1981; **33**: 355–360.

69. Evans, S., Matthews, W., Perry, R., Fraker, D.L., Norton, J.A., Pass, H.I. Effect of photodynamic therapy on tumor necrosis factor production by murine macrophages. *J Natl Cancer Inst* 1990; **82**: 34–39.

70. Elmets, C.A. Bowen, K.D. Immunological suppression in mice treated with hematoporphyrin derivative photoradiation. *Cancer Res* 1986; **46**: 1608–1611.

71. Lynch, D.H., Haddad, S., King, V.J., Ott, M.J., Straight, R.C., Jolles, C.J. Systemic immunosuppression induced by photodynamic therapy (PDT) is adoptively transferred by macrophages. *Photochem Photobiol* 1989; **49**: 453–458.

72. Kol, R., Ben Hur, E., Marko, R., Rosenthal, I. Inhibition of human lymphocyte stimulation by visible light and phthalocyanine sensitization: nitrogen and wavelength dependency. *Int J Radiat Biol* 1989; **55**: 1015–1022.

73. Mew, D., Wat, C.-K., Levy, J.G. Photoimmunotherapy: treatment of animal tumors with tumor-specific monoclonal antibody–hematoporphyrin conjugates. *J Immunol* 1993; **130**: 1473–1477.

74. Mew, D., Lum, C.K., Wat, G.H., *et al.* Ability of specific monoclonal antibodies and conventional antisera conjugated to hematoporphyrin to label and kill selective cell lines subsequent to light activation. *Cancer Res* 1985; **45**: 4380–4386.

75. Pogrebniak, H.W., Matthews, W., Black, C., Russo, A., Mitchell, J.B., Smith, P., Roth, J.A., Pass, H.I. Targetted phototherapy with sensitizer-monoclonal antibody conjugate and light. *Surg Oncol* 1993; **2**: 31–42.

76. White, E.A., Schambelan, M., Rost, C.R., *et al.* Use of computed tomography in diagnosing the cause of primary aldosteronism. *N Engl J Med* 1980; **303**: 1503–1507.

77. Thibonnier, M., Sassano, P., Joseph, A., *et al.* Diagnostic value of a single dose of captopril in renin-and aldosterone-dependent, surgically curable hypertension. *Cardiovasc Rev Rep* 1982; **3**: 1659.

78. Pelton, J.J., Kowalyshyn, M.J., Keller, S.M. Intrathoracic organ injury associated with photodynamic therapy. *J Thorac Cardiovasc Surg* 1992; **103**: 1218–1223.

79. Feins, R.H., Hilf, R., Ross, A., Gibson, S.L. Photodynamic therapy for human malignant mesothelioma in the nude mouse. *J Surg Res* 1991; **49**: 337–340.

80. Ris, H.-B., Altermatt, H.J., Nachbur, B., *et al.* Photodynamic therapy with *m*-tetrahydroxyphenylchlorin in vivo: optimization of the therapeutic index. *Int J Cancer* 1993; **53**: 141–146.

81. Tochner, Z., Pass, H., Smith, P., *et al.* Intrathoracic photodynamic therapy: A canine normal tissue tolerance study and early clinical experience. *Lasers Surg Med* 1994; **14**: 118–123.

82. Perry, R.R., Evans, S., Matthews, W., Rizzoni, W., Russo, A., Pass, H.I. Potentiation of phototherapy cytotoxicity with light scattering media. *J Surg Res* 1989; **46**: 386–390.

83. Pass, H.I., Delaney, T. Innovative photodynamic therapy at the National Cancer Institute: intraoperative, intracavitary treatment. In: B.W. Henderson, T.J. Dougherty (eds.), *Photodynamic Therapy: Basic Principles and Clinical Applications*. New York: Marcel Dekker, 1992; 287–301.

84. Friauf, W.S., Smith, P.E., Russo, A., DeLaney, T.F., Pass, H.I., Cole, J.W., Gibson, C.C., Sindelar, W.F., Thomas, G. Light monitoring in photo-dynamic therapy. In: H.T. Nagle, W.J. Tompkins (eds.), *Case Studies in Medical Instrument Design*. New York: The Institute of Electrical and Electronics Engineers, Inc., 1992; 127–138.

85. Pass, H.I., Delaney, T., Russo, A., Mitchell, J., Smith, P., Friauf, W., Thomas, G. Feasibility of intrapleural photodynamic therapy: the first eight patients. Proceedings of Optical Methods for Tumor Treatment and Detection: Mechanisms and techniques in photodynamic therapy. *International Society for Optical Engineering* 1992; **45**: 2–9.

86. Pass, H.I., DeLaney, T.F., Tochner, Z., *et al.* Intrapleural photodynamic therapy: results of a Phase I trial. *Ann Surg Oncol* 1994; **1**: 28–37.

87. Rusch, V.W. A proposed new international TNM staging system for malignant pleural mesothelioma. *Chest* 1995; **108**: 1122–1129.

88. Pass, H.I., Tochner, Z., Delaney, T., Smith, P., Friauf, W., Glatstein, E., Travis, W. Intraoperative photodynamic therapy for malignant mesothelioma [letter; comment]. *Ann Thorac Surg* 1990; **50**: 687–688.

89. Ris, H.B., Altermatt, H.J., Nachbur, B., Stewart, C.M., Wang, Q., Lim, C.K., Bonnett, R., Althaus, U. Intraoperative photodynamic therapy with *m*-tetrahydroxyphenylchlorin for chest malignancies. *Lasers Surg Med* 1996; **18**: 39–45.

90. Baas, P., Murrer, L., Zoetmulder, F.A., Stewart, F.A., Ris, H.B., Van Zandwijk, N., Peterse, J.L., Rutgers, E.J. Photodynamic therapy as adjuvant therapy in surgically treated pleural malignancies. *Br J Cancer* 1997; **76**: 819–826.

91. Moskal, T.L., Dougherty, T.J., Urschel, J.D., Antkowiak, J.G., Regal, A.M., Driscoll, D.L., Takita, H. Operation and photodynamic therapy for pleural mesothelioma: 6-year follow-up. *Ann Thorac Surg* 1998; **66**: 1128–1133.

92. Lofgren, L., Larsson, M., Thaning, L., Hallgren, S. Transthoracic endoscopic photodynamic treatment of malignant mesothelioma [letter]. *Lancet* 1991; **337**: 359.

=14=

Doctors in the Courtroom: Medico-Legal Aspects of Mesothelioma in Australia

John Gordon

Claims for damages by persons with mesothelioma have been pursued in Australian courts now for over 20 years. This chapter reviews the history of the litigation and the medico-legal issues that have been tried and determined, and discusses some current controversies.

History of asbestos-disease litigation in Australia

Because of the misfortune of having the Wittenoom mine located in its far north, Western Australia (WA) has one of the highest per capita rates of mesothelioma in the world. It is not surprising to find that the first claims for damages for contracting mesothelioma were brought in that State.

We now know, from files of internal documents from CSR Ltd, the operators of the mine, that were given to an Australian journalist in 1988, that CSR was well aware in the 1970s of the impending risk of litigation.[1] Accordingly, it was no surprise but still a matter of great consternation for CSR when Cornelius Maas, a former Wittenoom worker, recently diagnosed with mesothelioma, filed a suit against CSR's operating subsidiary in June 1977.[2]

Maas died less than a month after issuing the writ and the claim was not pursued at that time by his dependants.

Then, in 1978, a woman who had worked in an office near the mine at Wittenoom, Joan Joosten, contracted mesothelioma and issued a writ against the CSR subsidiary Midalco Pty Ltd.[3] Her claim occupied about four days in court. The judge ruled that the company, in Mrs Joosten's case at least, had not been negligent. Mrs Joosten's lawyers advised her to appeal the decision and the appeal was listed to be heard before the Full Court of the Western Australian Supreme Court. However, on the morning the appeal was to be heard, Mrs Joosten succumbed to the illness and the pressure, and died uncompensated.

It was clear that the greatest enemy of people wishing to litigate damages actions for asbestos-related diseases was time, with the average period between diagnosis of mesothelioma and death being nine months. Another difficulty was the statute of limitations,[4] which limited the right to bring an action to a period of 6 years from the cause of the action being complete.

Discouraged by the result in *Joosten*, the asbestos victims, and the Perth legal community, did not pursue the issue for a number of years. However, after the Asbestos Diseases Society of Australia made submissions to the WA government, changes to the Limitation Act resulted, enabling claims to be brought forward. As a consequence of Asbestos Diseases Society pressure, the government also released Mines Department and Health Department records, which had been thought long destroyed, relating to Wittenoom and the James Hardie company, Australia's largest asbestos product manufacturer. These records told a completely different story to that which had emerged in the Joosten trial and the Asbestos Diseases Society began pressing for another test case.

The law firm Slater & Gordon first became involved in the area of asbestos litigation in the 1985 Victorian action of *Pilmer v McPhersons Ltd*.[5] Mr Pilmer suffered from malignant mesothelioma as a consequence of his asbestos exposure at work in a hardware store. He was successful in the Supreme Court of Victoria in his claim for damages.

The case of Pilmer was the first successful claim in negligence in Australia in relation to mesothelioma and he received damages of $270 000. It was the first time in Australia that any worker had received common law damages for asbestos-related disease and it demonstrated that such cases could be won, even though the exposures which caused the disease had occurred 30–40 years earlier.

The Asbestos Diseases Society then approached Slater & Gordon and they combined resources in order to bring test cases before the courts in Western Australia, where the numbers of persons contracting asbestosis and mesothelioma continued to escalate dramatically.

The first of these, the case of *Simpson v Midalco*[6] came before the courts and ran for more than 40 days. At the end of the case the judge ruled that Mr Simpson did not have asbestosis as he claimed. With two cases having run and lost, there was enormous pressure – financial and legal – to abandon the fight for justice.

However, the fight was not abandoned and Slater & Gordon and the Asbestos Diseases Society brought on two more cases on behalf of two more mesothelioma sufferers, Peter Heys and Tim Barrow. Both had worked at Wittenoom in the 1950s and each sued both CSR's subsidiary Midalco and CSR itself. CSR devoted enormous resources to defending the case, and it ran for more than 130 sitting days over eight months in Western Australia's Supreme Court.[7]

It was one of the longest civil trials in Australian court history. Peter Heys did not survive until the end of the trial, but his family continued his claim. On 4 August 1988, in the Supreme Court of Western Australia, Justice Rowland ruled both cases successful and ordered CSR and its subsidiary to pay damages.

Slater & Gordon had, by this time, also run another Wittenoom case, that of *Rabenalt v Midalco* in the Supreme Court of Victoria.[8] For the first time ever in an Australian industrial accident case, the plaintiff was awarded not just compensatory damages ($426 000), but punitive damages of $250 000 against CSR's subsidiary. The appeal court, upholding the award, said there was a clear case of 'continuing, conscious and contumelious disregard' by CSR's subsidiary for Mr Rabenalt's right to be free of the risk of injury and disease.[9]

Whilst the Heys and Barrow action was proceeding the case of *Watson v State of Western Australia*[10] was commenced. Mr Watson claimed damages against the State for his asbestosis, which arose as a result of his exposure to Wittenoom-mined asbestos whilst working at the port at Point Samson in northern Western Australia where the asbestos was shipped to the State's major port of Fremantle for on-shipment throughout Australia and the world. The court ruled in favour of Mr Watson and awarded him over $400 000 in damages. The State of Western Australia appealed but the Appeal Court dismissed the appeal and increased the damages payable to Colin Watson to $600 000.[11]

Slater & Gordon and the Asbestos Diseases Society then pressed CSR to settle the 200 cases of former Wittenoom workers that were then proceeding in the courts. Eventually an out of court settlement involving in excess of 20 million dollars to settle the claims of 200 former Wittenoom workers or their families was agreed. Included in those claims were the families of Cornelius Maas and Joan Joosten. After a successful appeal, Wally Simpson's case was also settled by CSR[12]

In December 1994 the New South Wales Dust Diseases Tribunal found in favour of a claim by Vivien Olson, 34-year-old mother of two, who had contracted malignant mesothelioma. Mrs Olson's exposure to asbestos occurred as a child when she was living in Wittenoom where her father worked for CSR's subsidiary.[13] Judge O'Meally found that CSR Ltd and Midalco Pty Ltd owed Mrs Olson a duty of care even though she was not one of their employees. Judge O'Meally awarded Mrs Olson $823 594 in damages.

An appeal against the judgment brought by CSR failed.[14]

In relation to claims by persons with lung cancer the decision of the High Court in the case of *Culkin v CSR Ltd* is significant.[15] In April 1995 the High Court refused leave to CSR to appeal against a verdict[16] that the development of the deceased's lung cancer had been contributed to by his asbestos exposure and that it was not necessary to show an underlying condition of asbestosis for the causal link to be established.

In the action of *Sangston v Fire Fighting Enterprises*[17] a jury in the Victorian Supreme Court found that while Daniel Sangston's substantial asbestos exposure had been only for a period of some four months in the mid-1940s it had played a significant role in the development of his lung cancer, despite his lifetime history of smoking cigarettes. In December 1992 the jury awarded Mr Sangston $360 000 in damages and applied a discount of 60% to take account of his smoking.

Subsequent cases tried, or settled, have confirmed the legal position in Australia to be that persons suffering from lung cancer who were negligently exposed to asbestos, do not need to establish the presence of asbestosis before being entitled to an award of damages against the party responsible for exposing them to that asbestos, regardless of their smoking history.[18]

In March 1994 the matter of *Bodsworth v City of Nunawading* was tried before a jury in the Supreme Court of Victoria. Mr Bodsworth was successful in his claim that his exposure to asbestos whilst sitting at his desk under an asbestos-sprayed ceiling in the course of his employment with the defendant was the cause of his mesothelioma and that such exposure was as a consequence of his employer's negligence.

In August 1993 Gerald Cashman received almost $300 000 in damages for his oesophageal cancer when he settled his action against his previous employer, Tomlinson Steel. Mr Cashman had issued proceedings in the Supreme Court of Victoria alleging negligence on the part of his employer in exposing him to asbestos in the course of his job as a boiler engineer in the 1970s.

Another landmark case from late 1994 was the case of *Napolitano v CSR Ltd*.[19] The case concerned a former Wittenoom worker who was awarded more than $200 000 damages after contracting mesothelioma – and a further $25 000 compensation for the five years of misery and suffering leading up to the diagnosis confirming his condition. This is believed to be the first time damages have been awarded for suffering apprehension of illness.

One of the last remaining issues of asbestos liability was finally resolved in the High Court of Australia on 10 November 1999, in the case of *Crimmins v Stevedoring Industry Finance Committee*, i.e., (1999)200 CLR1. From the 1930s to the 1980s stevedores and wharf labourers at all Australian ports had been exposed to asbestos, often heavily, in loading and unloading asbestos imported from Canada and South Africa, and, of course, Wittenoom blue. Unlike at Point Samson where Colin Watson worked for the State, the position in the major ports was that waterside workers were employed casually by the stevedoring companies on a boat by boat basis. Identifying which employer exposed a worker to the asbestos which resulted in mesothelioma 40 years later had proven impossible. However, Brian Crimmins, who had suffered significant asbestos exposure at the Port of Melbourne in the early 1960s, decided to sue the Commonwealth statutory authority which ran and oversaw the waterside labour schemes at all major Australian ports, alleging it failed to use its powers to enforce basic health and safety regimes when workers were working with asbestos cargoes. He was successful and he was awarded $833 000 in damages (subject to appeal). The Victorian Court of Appeal, however, overturned the decision, before the High Court reinstated the verdict, finally opening the way for other waterside workers, similarly afflicted, to bring damages claims.

Medico-legal issues

It can now be asserted with some confidence that most of the medico-legal issues that have attended asbestos diseases litigation in Australia have been resolved as a result of the 20 years of litigation referred to above.

An earlier review[20] detailed a number of controversies which had arisen in the asbestos cases, most of which have now been settled by court judgment or verdict, or concession that the medical science has resolved a debate one way or the other. In New South Wales, legislation by the government, based upon, and giving effect to such courtroom resolutions, has significantly reduced the potential for further legal argument[21]

The most contentious and important of these issues are reviewed here, with the current position summarised.

Causation

The issue which has most vexed asbestos litigation is, undoubtedly, that of causation.

There are three contexts in which the issue of cause potentially arises in asbestos disease claims:

1. Has a particular asbestos exposure 'caused' the disease suffered by the claimant?
2. Which one or more of a number of exposures to asbestos give rise to legal culpability for the disease suffered by a claimant?
3. Has the disease for which legal culpability exists caused the loss and damage suffered by the claimant with the disease?

These causation issues arise both in statutory workers' compensation claims where the issue of fault in exposing the worker to asbestos is irrelevant (and so the causation issue becomes – subject to statutory abrogation – has the work exposure caused the disease?), and in common law damages claims (where the issue is usually) has the breach of a duty to take care (i.e. fault or breach of a duty imposed by a statute) caused the disease?

Although a good deal of court time has been occupied by physicians, pathologists, epidemiologists, medical scientists, and lawyers in arguing this issue, it would seem that its resolution has been achieved by the application of legal principles of reasonably long standing and is encapsulated in two judgments by Australia's foremost jurist and most highly regarded judge, Sir Owen Dixon, former Chief Justice of the High Court.

Where medical science cannot definitively resolve an issue in litigation – either because the issue has not been resolved by medical scientists or because medical experts have different views in a particular case – Justice Dixon said:

> Upon a question of fact of a medical or scientific description a Court can only say that the burden of proof has not been discharged [by a claimant] where, upon the evidence, it appears that the present state of knowledge does not admit of an affirmative answer and that competent and trustworthy expert opinion regards an affirmative answer as lacking justification, either as a probable inference or as an accepted hypothesis. . . . Whether an inference can or should be drawn . . . seems to me to depend upon the answer first given to the pathological question whether there is any natural connection [between the alleged precipitating factor and the disease]. Tempting, as it always is, particularly in matters of bodily health, to argue from a sequence of external events, such reasoning is justified only when positive knowledge or common experience supplies some adequate ground for believing that the events are naturally associated.[22]

This judgment, which has been relied upon often by courts in Australia (and elsewhere) in the resolution of causation issues,[23] essentially means that where there is no convincing opposing evidence, a claimant may succeed, not simply because there has been a work-related event or a breach of a duty, and a subsequent illness, but because competent and trustworthy medical experts opine that there is, or even that there could be, a connection between the two events, and the court accepts the probable inference or hypothesis. A similar decision was reached by Britain's highest court in another case where medical science could not explain the relationship between exposure to coal dust mixed with sweat and resultant dermatitis in *McGhee v National Coal Board* [1973 1 WLR 1]. In that case, the House of Lords held that there was no difference in law between a material increase in the risk of an injury (caused by a breach of a duty to take care), and material contribution to the injury.

This then leaves the more difficult cases where there is no controversy about the theoretical connection between the two events – e.g., asbestos exposure and mesothelioma – and the question becomes whether, in the *particular* case, the facts justify the attribution of cause. In other words, what must a claimant establish to make out cause and effect in a legal sense, in such a case.

Again, in the words of Justice Sir Owen Dixon:

> Breach of duty coupled with an accident of the kind that might thereby be caused is enough to justify an inference, in the absence of any sufficient reason to the contrary, that in fact the accident did occur owing to the act or omission amounting to the breach.[24]

In that case, Justice Dixon was deciding whether the breach of duty led to the accident in which the injuries suffered by the plaintiff undoubtedly were sustained, which involves the same reasoning as the question of whether the breach of duty (which in effect *is* the accident – e.g., the exposure to dangerous levels of asbestos) caused the injury.

In cases where a positive act by the defendant constitutes a breach of duty of care, few problems arise in determining the question of cause; e.g., a car proceeds through a red traffic light (breach of duty) and crashes into a car proceeding correctly into the intersection, injuring its driver. The breach of duty is the cause of the injury – they are one and the same.

Although cases of omission, where a failure to act constitutes the breach of duty of care, sometimes occasion more difficulty in observing the breach/cause dynamic – perhaps because, as with asbestos disease, the omissions constituting the breach – e.g., failure to warn of the risks of inhalation of asbestos or failure to provide appropriate mitigating measures or respiratory protection – are not contemporaneous events. However, the principle enunciated by Dixon is still applicable – and note that His Honour specifically includes the word 'omission' in his definition.

Justice Gaudron of the High Court of Australia referred to that definition by J. Dixon in Her Honour's judgment in the recent case of *Bennett v Minister of Community Welfare*[25] and commented:

> In practice it is not always necessary to inquire what would have happened in the circumstances under consideration had a positive duty been performed. . . . And although it is sometimes necessary for a plaintiff to lead evidence as to what would or would not have happened if a particular common law duty had been performed, generally speaking, if an injury occurs within an area of foreseeable risk, then in the absence of evidence that the breach had no effect, or that the injury would have occurred even if the duty had been performed, it will be taken that the breach of common law duty caused or materially contributed to the injury.

Thus, putting these principles into an asbestos disease context, if a worker was exposed to circumstances where he probably inhaled asbestos in the course of his work, and the worker's employer should have warned of the danger of inhalation, and/or should have prevented or reduced the worker's risk of inhalation of the asbestos, and/or should have provided the worker with appropriate respiratory protection – all omissions which therefore constitute a breach of a duty of care owed by the employer to the worker – and if the worker subsequently develops a disease which is caused by inhalation of asbestos, then 'in the absence of evidence that the breach had no effect, or that the injury would have occurred even if the duty had been performed, it will be taken that the breach of common law [or statutory] duty caused or materially contributed to the injury'.[26]

In a case of mesothelioma, of course, it would be virtually impossible for a defendant employer to bring himself within either of the two exceptions mentioned – 'no effect' or 'inevitable anyway' – and liability would therefore be established by proof of the breach of duty and the diagnosis of an injury that the duty existed to prevent.

These principles have evolved for both legal and policy reasons. The law has always been far more concerned with common sense notions of cause[27] rather than 'philosophical or scientific notions',[28] 'logic or philosophy',[29] or even 'percentages of occurrence or percentages of increase in risk'.[30] It differs even from John Stuart Mills' definition of cause as the sum of the conditions which are jointly sufficient to produce the effect.[31]

This principle operates, for example, to obviate the need for the worker exposed to asbestos in the above example to adduce evidence of the precise cellular or genetic changes which might have been induced by the asbestos exposure and which have led to the development of the presently diagnosed mesothelioma, for that clearly is an impossibility which, as a matter of policy, should not stand in the way of an otherwise established entitlement to damages.

The tobacco industry, for example, wrongly assumes that it is protected from successful suit by lung cancer sufferers because the relationship between smoking and lung cancer is 'statistical only' and that the precise chain of cellular or genetic causation in an individual between the smoking and the cancer cannot be shown. As we have seen from the above,[32] such an argument on causation would not, on its own, save the tobacco manufacturer if it could be shown that there was a breach of duty of care.

This 'policy consideration' was explained by the House of Lords (Britain's highest court) in *McGhee v National Coal Board.* [3]

> First, it is a sound principle that where a person has, by breach of a duty of care, created a risk, and injury occurs within the area of that risk, that loss should be borne by him unless he shows that it had some other cause. Secondly, from the evidential point of view, one may ask, Why should a man who is able to show that his employer should have taken certain precautions, because without them there is a risk or an added risk, of injury or disease, have to assume the burden of proving more; namely that it was the addition to the risk, caused by the breach of duty which caused, or materially contributed to the injury? In many cases of which the present is typical, this is impossible to prove, just because honest medical opinion cannot segregate the causes of an illness between compound causes. And if one asks which of the parties, the workman or the employers should suffer from this inherent evidential difficulty, the answer as a matter in policy or justice should be that it is the creator of the risk, who, ex hypothesi, must be taken to have foreseen the possibility of damage, who should bear its consequences.

The Australian High Court has endorsed this approach to causation in cases of breach of duty by omission, or where there is some other difficulty in establishing each link in the chain of causation, in resolving two cases of medical malpractice. They are *Chappel v Hart* (1998) 156 ALR 517 and *Naxakis v Western General Hospital* (1999) 162

ALR 540 wherein a clear majority of the High Court concurred that the relevant test for establishing causation in such cases was that:

> If a wrongful act or omission results in an increased risk of injury to the plaintiff and that risk eventuates, the defendant's conduct has materially contributed to the injury that the plaintiff suffers whether or not other factors also contributed to that injury occurring. And in that situation, the trier of fact is entitled to conclude that the act or omission caused the injury in question unless the defendant establishes that the conduct had no effect at all or that the risk would have eventuated and resulted in the damage in question in any event (per Gaudron J in *Naxakis* at 547).

The Supreme Court of Canada seems to take a similar view, but is prepared to go further and accept that in some circumstances where the defendant's own actions have created the difficulty in proof, or where there is a serious imbalance in knowledge of the possible causative connection between the breach of duty and the injury (such as in some medical malpractice cases), then the plaintiff might be relieved of the burden of establishing the causal connection at all, with the onus shifting to the defendants to prove that their acts or omissions had no relevant causal effect; *Cook v Lewis* (1951) SCR 830; *Snell v Farrell* (1990) 72 DLR (4th) 289; *Hollis v Dow Corning Corp* (1995) 4 SCR 634.

Causation – multiple possible causes

The question then naturally arises as to whether a defendant can defeat a claim by demonstrating either:

1. that only some of the asbestos exposure occasioned to the worker was the result of a breach of duty (either common law or statutory); or
2. that the worker had other asbestos exposure, either occasioned by a breach of duty by some other person or not. A subsidiary question is whether a party can escape liability because some third party also owed a duty to the worker, breach of which caused the same exposure for which that defendant is being pursued – e.g. where an employer and an asbestos product manufacturer both failed to warn a worker of the risks of asbestos inhalation, in breach of their respective duties to the worker as employer and product supplier.

The answer in the case of scenarios (1) and (2) above is 'no', liability cannot be escaped in those circumstances, provided it is established that the defendant, regardless of other circumstances or contributory factors, by his own default or breach, materially increased the risk of the disease that has been suffered. A material increase in risk has been defined as a risk that is 'more than minimal'.[34]

Accordingly in scenario (1) where only some of the exposure to asbestos was in breach of the duty, that part that was in breach must be considered to determine if it 'materially' (more than minimally) increased the risk of contracting the disease. In the case of mesothelioma, it will therefore be only the most fleeting or transitory exposure, or alternatively low exposure of such short latency before the manifestation of the disease that might fall into this category, and thus be exculpated.

Similarly in scenario (2) the same considerations apply having regard to the other exposures, in order to determine whether the particular breach/exposure sued upon, has made a material increase to the risk of disease, and consequently, in law, made a material contribution to the disease. Again, in the case of mesothelioma, there would be few circumstances where a breach of a duty resulting in the risk of a worker inhaling asbestos would not give rise to liability.

It should be noted that the onus of introducing evidence of such exculpatory circumstances lies upon the party seeking to avoid liability, and if that evidence is acceptable, the court must then decide whether the plaintiff has proved his or her case having regard to the whole of the evidence – the matters for and against the attribution of causation consequent upon the established breach of duty.

Without such evidence negating a material contribution to the injury, or demonstrating that the breach has made minimal, or no, contribution to the risk (or that there was minimal, or no exposure and therefore no breach), it is likely that a plaintiff will succeed simply by having established that there was a breach of duty and he or she has suffered a disease of the type that the duty existed to prevent.

The resolution of the subsidiary scenario – where two (or more) parties are responsible for the same culpable exposure in breach of their respective duties – is dependent upon the parties asking the court to apportion responsibility between them in accordance with their relative culpability. If they do not request such apportionment, each will be liable to the plaintiff (if sued) for the full extent of the damages awarded, although, of course, the plaintiff is entitled to only one award of damages and may elect against whom enforcement of the judgment is pursued.

Whether or not a given defendant is found to be in breach of a duty of care to a given plaintiff will be, in part, determined by the concept of 'foreseeability'.

Foreseeability

An employer will owe an employee a duty of care if there exists a 'foreseeable risk of injury' in the event that the employer fails to discharge the duty. Similarly the manufacturer of a product owes the user of that product a duty of care, if there is a foreseeable risk of injury in the use of the product, or if dangers, of which the manufacturer is aware, are not advised to the product user.

Thus, in order to establish that a duty exists, the employee or product user must show that there was, at the time of the alleged breach, a foreseeable risk of injury occurring as a result of that breach. Furthermore, the employee or product user, in order to claim damages as a result of the breach of duty, must show that the injury or disease that they have suffered was an injury that is the same type as that which should have been foreseen (as well as, as we have seen above, that the injury was caused or materially contributed to, by the breach of duty).

The concept of foreseeability is, therefore, important in two contexts in mesothelioma damages claims. Firstly to establish a duty of care, and secondly, to establish that the injury suffered was one that the duty existed to prevent, and is thus compensable.

Foreseeability and duty

A party will not be liable for a disease or injury caused to a person unless the disease was 'foreseeable' in the event that a duty were breached.

A disease may be foreseeable even if its occurrence is unlikely, provided its occurrence was at the time of the alleged breach, not far-fetched or fanciful.[35]

Moreover, foreseeability does not require the precise way in which the injury might occur, or even the precise type of injury that might be suffered, to be anticipated. It would seem, from recent decisions in Australia and Britain, that all that must be foreseen is a risk of physical injury (or disease) if the duty of care is breached.

In one recent mesothelioma case the court (Beazley JA; Mason P and Stein JA agreeing in the NSW Court of Appeal) put it this way in dealing with an argument put by an asbestos corporation that the onus on the plaintiff was to establish that at the time of his being exposed in the course of his employment to chrysotile asbestos, the employer knew or should have known that chrysotile could cause mesothelioma:

> It was not necessary in my opinion, for the respondent (worker) to establish that it was foreseeable that exposure to a particular type of asbestos could cause injury. At the relevant time, it was known that asbestos, as a generic substance, was hazardous. Nor was it necessary for Mr Barnes to prove that it was foreseeable that he could contract the particular injury of mesothelioma. It was sufficient that the inhalation of asbestos could cause an injury of the kind which he suffered.[36]

Thus, although there may have been an exposure to chrysotile, in the 1940s (i.e. before the publication of the work of Wagner *et al.* in the *British Journal of Industrial Medicine* in 1960) and the only disease which a reasonable employer at the time might associate with exposure to chrysotile is asbestosis, or, perhaps lung cancer, foreseeability will have been established by an employee who has contracted mesothelioma in the 1990s, as the employer was, or should have been aware of a risk of injury in the 1940s if the employee was exposed to asbestos.

This would apply even if the exposure was at seemingly low levels, not normally associated at the time with disease or injury, because, as we have seen above, foreseeability is established even if a disease (or any disease) is unlikely to occur provided the risk is not far-fetched or fanciful. In a given case the evidence of levels of asbestos exposure will often be estimated, at best, and in any event, the exposure 'standards' of the time (e.g. the so-called Dreesen standard of 5 000 000 pcf) were tentative only, related to whole dust exposure (of which asbestos may only have been a small constituent) and, if dust were visible, were probably breached.[37] Thus there would be few cases where there was an exposure to asbestos where it could be concluded on the balance of probabilities that the objective risk of injury occurring must be held to have been fanciful.

The only other restriction that applies is that the physical injury must be of the same class, type or character as that for which the risk existed.

One recent case involved a woman whose only known exposure to asbestos was to that brought home on her husband's work clothes, subsequently washed by her in the years 1962–65. Although this is arguably not a 'low exposure'[38] (whatever that might mean in the context of a substance as inherently dangerous as asbestos) and although even some of the cases reported by Wagner *et al.* must have involved comparatively little risk of inhalation,[39] the trial judge and the Queensland Court of Appeal both dismissed the woman's claim on the ground that during her period of exposure 'there was no published material which identified dosages as low as that inhaled by Mrs Bale with the contraction of harmful disease'.[40]

Mrs Bale sought leave to appeal to the High Court. In the application for leave heard on 2 December 1996, the three High Court judges made their views clearly known on this issue of the foreseeable risk of harm. Justice Gaudron wondered whether the Court of Appeal had asked the right question: 'They seem to have focused on knowledge of the possibility of the illness which this unfortunate lady has eventually suffered, rather than the risk of some harm.'[41] Later Her Honour asked: 'But why are we looking in any event at mesothelioma rather than personal injury in the broad; a risk of personal injury?'[42]

Kirby J went further:[43]

If you look at Justice McPherson in the Court of Appeal ... it says 'the defendant could not reasonably have foreseen that she might contract that disease'. This is the point that Justice Gaudron put ... that His Honour (in the Court of Appeal) is focusing on the particular consequence, whereas the test merely requires focusing on some harm with the detail to work its way out ... so one of the two foundations for your judgment is really erroneous with respect.

And Justice McHugh also questioned the Court of Appeal's approach to the foreseeability issue:

In the context of this case, surely what one was looking at was whether or not there was some sort of risk ... what the risk was, one was not certain about, but if there was, then simple precautions were available to eliminate it.[44]

Justice McHugh even wondered whether in a case like that one, the traditional approach was appropriate:

The problem is more about the uncertainty of the effects of asbestos dust. May not the correct test be, having regard to the uncertain knowledge as to the effects of asbestos dust and what degree of exposure was required, was it reasonable for the defendant to carry on its operations in the way it did?[45]

Leave to appeal was granted to Mrs Bale, but, not surprisingly, in light of the observations of the High Court Justices, the defendant settled the claim before the appeal was heard.

In a similar vein was a claim brought by a woman who had been born in 1959 in the notorious town of Wittenoom – the company town that serviced the blue asbestos mine and mill operated by CSR Limited. As a child, Vivian Olson was exposed to asbestos tailings spread around her home and the town until she left in December 1961. She developed mesothelioma in 1994 and claimed damages from CSR on the grounds that CSR had owed her a duty of care to warn those responsible for her of the dangers of asbestos inhalation and/or to alleviate that risk (e.g. by ceasing the spreading of tailings in the town etc.).[46] CSR argued, as Seltsam had done in Mrs Bale's case, that they did not owe Mrs Olson a duty of care, because they could not have foreseen a risk of mesothelioma from 'low dose township exposure before she left Wittenoom in 1962'. The trial judge and the majority of the NSW Court of Appeal rejected this argument, having considered, *inter alia*, the High Court's special leave application in *Bale v Seltsam*, the dissenting judgment in the Court of Appeal in that case by Fitzgerald P, the English Court of Appeal decision in *Margereson v JW Roberts Ltd*,[47] *Bendix Mintex v*

Barnes[48] and *Barrow & Heys v CSR Ltd*,[49] concluding that, having regard to the known risks of asbestos exposure, and given the uncertain state of knowledge, CSR should have foreseen that there might be harm.[50]

The British Court of Appeal had come to a similar conclusion in relation to a claim which probably involved a greater exposure to asbestos, but at a much earlier time in the development of knowledge.[51]

In the 1930s, Arthur Margereson as a child, lived and played near the Turner & Newall-owned J W Roberts asbestos factory at Armley in Leeds, England. Asbestos dust was emitted from the factory into the surrounding streets, and the children played in and with it. In particular, they played around the factory where conditions were not materially different from conditions within the factory, in which Roberts undoubtedly owed a duty to its employees to protect them.

The defendants argued that no duty of care was owed, however, to the children, who were 'unknown individuals in a wide and ill-defined catchment area'.[52] The trial judge rejected this argument, but focused attention on the evidence that the children were exposed to the same conditions outside that obtained inside the factory and thus the company, from at least 1933 – being two years after the promulgation of the UK Asbestos Regulations in 1931[53] and three after the seminal Merewether and Price report of 1930[54] – must have been aware of the potential of harm to those exposed to such conditions, including those outside.

On appeal by Roberts against this finding, the Court of Appeal went further, defining the test more broadly.

The Court of Appeal referred to the important decision of the House of Lords in *Page v Smith*,[55] in which it was argued that psychiatric injury was not a foreseeable risk of a potential breach of duty that would undoubtedly, and admittedly, cause physical injury. The House of Lords had rejected that distinction:

> The test in every case ought to be whether the defendant can reasonably foresee that his conduct will expose the plaintiff to risk of personal injury. If so, he comes under a duty of care to that plaintiff. If a working definition of 'personal injury' is needed, it can be found in section 38(1) of the Limitation Act 1980; ('personal injury' includes any disease and any impairment of a person's physical or mental condition).[56]

The Court of Appeal in *Margereson* endorsed this approach, although, curiously, inserting a qualification that the injury required to be foreseen was 'some pulmonary injury not necessarily mesothelioma'.[57]

If this were the applicable test, it is somewhat narrower than 'injury' or 'harm', and is difficult to reconcile with *Page v Smith* and other cases where persons exposed to asbestos have suffered psychiatric injury (see discussion below) or been permitted to pursue claims where the injury, ostensibly caused by asbestos exposure, was not necessarily a pulmonary injury.[58,59]

The Court of Appeal then considered when it was that J W Roberts ought to have knowledge of pulmonary injury, that is, the date at which information was available to establish that asbestos exposure was likely to be harmful to the lungs. They concluded that this was long before 1933:

The information which should have operated on the defendant's corporate mind was in existence long before Mr Margereson's birthdate (1925)[60].

Such knowledge therefore was available from the turn of the century.[61]

In Australia, the Commonwealth Government included asbestos on a list of health hazards in industry, and named asbestos work as a hazardous occupation in 1922.[62]

Foreseeability of injury suffered

It follows from what has been said about foreseeability as a constituent element in the establishment of a duty of care, that the same criteria apply in establishing that the injury with which the plaintiff presents, and for which he or she claims, must be of the kind that the duty existed to prevent. If the test is 'foreseeability of personal injury', as the House of Lords put it, or, as Judges of the High Court of Australia suggest, 'risk of harm', then any type of injury caused or materially contributed to by the asbestos exposure (see discussion on causation above) will suffice, be it a physical non-pulmonary injury – e.g. chronic lymphatic leukemia[63] or oesophageal cancer; or a pulmonary injury – asbestosis, mesothelioma, pleural disease, pulmonary cancer; or a psychiatric injury. The particular arguments relating to bronchopulmonary cancer, non-pulmonary cancer and psychiatric injury are discussed further below.

For the purposes of foreseeability, it is beyond argument at least that asbestosis, benign pleural disease, pleural and peritoneal mesothelioma, and bronchopulmonary carcinoma are diseases of like type, class or character, and fine distinctions relating to the aetiology, organs affected, or fatal outcomes have been consistently rejected.[64]

Bronchopulmonary carcinoma

There has raged, for a decade or more, a medico-legal debate about the attribution for damages or compensation-liability purposes, of bronchopulmonary carcinoma to asbestos exposure.

This debate, the outcome of which, admittedly, will cost or save asbestos mining and manufacturing companies billions of dollars, has been marked by considerable vehemence of views on each side.

In Australia at least, it would now seem, partly as a result of the resolution of causation and foreseeability issues (see above), and partly as a result of the advance of the science on the subject, that the issue is substantially resolved.

Put in simple terms which belie the ambit of the controversy, the debate involved the question of whether a plaintiff who had contracted lung cancer, having been exposed to asbestos, ought be entitled to damages or compensation from the party responsible for the exposure (assuming other aspects of liability had been made out), if the cancer sufferer did not have asbestosis present on chest radiograph, and even more problematically, if the person had been a cigarette smoker.

That there was a controversy regarding this at all seems to have been a result of the publication of work done by Professor Hans Weill and Dr Janet Hughes on a cohort of Johns Manville factory workers in New Orleans.[65] Their work appeared to show, in the population studied, that there was only a statistically significant increase in lung cancer incidence in the subgroup of workers who also showed clearly demonstrable evidence of asbestosis on chest radiograph. The numbers involved were small (450) and the group with radiographic abnormality were also the workers with the heaviest time × exposure, which meant that the results were also interpretable simply as a factor of dose rather than consequent x-ray abnormality. There remained also the question of the biological or genetic process that might explain the necessity for pre-existing asbestosis (and only asbestosis at a level sufficient to show clear abnormality on radiograph) in order to give rise to a cancer, and, at an arguably 'distant' site.

Given such concerns, it would have been difficult to argue that this study led to any definitive conclusions, and indeed, the authors did not so argue. They concluded:

> This study is the latest in an emerging body of evidence supporting the view that asbestos is a lung carcinogen because of its ability to cause lung fibrosis. Further results in support of these findings are necessary before a firm conclusion concerning such a mechanism can be reached.

No such studies appear to have emerged and this study, with its tentative conclusions, appears to be the high water mark of the science in support of the hypothesis.

Nonetheless, its results were seized upon by asbestos corporations, virtually under siege in courts the world over, to argue that it would be reasonable to attribute causation to the asbestos exposure only where there was radiographic evidence of asbestosis, especially if the person had smoked. This argument found favour with a number of legislatures for the purposes of statutory workers compensation (e.g. Britain) and with a number of courts at first instance in Britain and Australia.

But soon, medical and legal advances and some difficult cases put an end to the acceptance of the theory to deny compensation to asbestos-exposed individuals. Legally, the courts increasingly accepted and applied the causation principles referred to above, which inevitably meant that the evidence of a material increase in the risk of asbestosis, mesothelioma and lung cancer in an asbestos-exposed individual, and the inarguable proposition that the asbestos exposure multiplied that risk manyfold, would require a finding of attribution of the cancer to the exposure, unless the exposure was insignificant or minimal (i.e. not material as a factor contributing to the risk).

Medically, many pathologists were increasingly troubled by the undiscerning requirement to attribute only cancers where there was radiological evidence of fibrosis. What was to be made of findings on dissected lung tissue *in vivo* or post-mortem of fibrosis, especially accompanied by asbestos bodies or massive numbers of fibres? What of the cases where there had been significant occupational exposure with or without confirmation by body or fibre counting, and what if the worker (admittedly uncommon in the 1950s and 1960s) had not been a smoker, or had given up many years before contracting the carcinoma?

Then, as more research emerged, it became clear that other cohorts, including cohorts with much greater numbers enabling greater confidence in the data produced, were showing significant increases in risk in both those workers with asbestosis and those with significant exposure but without asbestosis.[66] The obvious conclusion was that the cancer risk was dose-related without the necessity of prior-occurring asbestosis, which thus accorded with the legal position on increasing risk and causation.

A number of test cases brought by plaintiffs succeeded,[67] and it thus appears that the present preponderance of authority in Australia does not require the presence of asbestosis prior to attribution of a bronchopulmonary cancer to an asbestos exposure in breach of a duty of care, provided the exposure is not insignificant. In the case of most of the statutory workers' compensation schemes, a prior occupational exposure and a subsequent bronchopulmonary cancer will suffice to claim the statutory benefits.

In either type of claim, however, prior smoking by the claimant will not disentitle a claimant, as smoking is only an alternative contributory factor, and indeed one that multiplies the risk of cancer occasioned by the culpable asbestos exposure. In some cases, a court may reduce the damages otherwise payable, if satisfied that the claimant has negligently contributed to his or her own injury by continuing to smoke after (if it be the case) learning of the risks involved.

Other cancers of the respiratory system and the gastrointestinal tract

The law continues to reflect the uncertainty in the medical community regarding such tumours occurring after asbestos exposure. Claims have successfully been pursued to verdict on behalf of persons with oesophageal cancer.[68] There have not been such significant numbers of cases to posit any concluded views about potential liability, but applying the principles of causation and foreseeability referred to above, it is likely that other cases of this type will succeed where there has been a prior significant asbestos exposure.

Psychiatric injury

In Australia, persons who suffer psychiatric injury as a result of contracting a serious or terminal illness are entitled (subject to otherwise establishing liability) to damages for that psychiatric injury[69] as part of the overall award for the injuries caused.

Further, damages for purely psychiatric injury have been allowed where a party's negligence has caused horrific injuries which are witnessed by another who is shocked by what is observed.[70]

A developing question is whether damages are to be awarded for psychiatric injury caused by communication of the person's diagnosis of a serious illness such as mesothelioma. Similarly the courts are grappling with the question of whether a person, previously exposed to asbestos, but as yet without physical symptoms, who develops a morbid fear of contracting a severe or fatal illness might be compensated for such psychiatric illness.

In the first class of (communication) cases, it would seem that damages would be payable if negligence was shown. The psychiatric injury is still consequential upon the physical injury and is a foreseeable consequence of negligently exposing an individual to unsafe levels of asbestos.

The second class of cases, the so-called cancer phobia cases, is perhaps more problematic. Three recent decisions in Australia suggest that courts might be willing to entertain these types of claims in appropriate cases.

Firstly in *Napolitano v CSR Ltd*,[71] a worker developed a morbid fear of contracting mesothelioma after seeing so many of the friends he had come with to Australia, to work at Wittenoom, dying of asbestos diseases. The condition developed into what psychiatrists termed 'a major depressive illness' and a claim for damages was commenced on his behalf. Unfortunately, while the claim was in progress, the plaintiff's worst fears were realised and he was diagnosed with mesothelioma. The further claim was added, and in giving judgment, Justice Seaman of the WA Supreme Court, recognising both injuries, awarded $100 000 general damages for the cancer and a further $25 000 for the psychiatric illness.

In the case of *Mosley v BHP*[72] a former shipyard worker exposed to asbestos developed a fear that he had contracted a fatal asbestos-related injury, to the point where it became a diagnosable psychiatric condition. As it turned out, the plaintiff had some diffuse benign pleural disease. The court awarded significant damages for both injuries. A similar claim was allowed in New Zealand in the case of *Bryan v Phillips (NZ) Ltd.*[73]

APQ v Commonwealth Serum Laboratories Ltd[74] was not a case of asbestos disease but a claim by a woman who had received hormone treatment which, it was later recognised, could result in her contracting the fatal degenerative brain disease Creutzfeldt-Jakob disease (CJD).

The plaintiff developed a psychiatric illness, as a result, it is alleged, of learning of this risk and the constant fear and worry associated with it, and sued the defendant, who had rendered the treatment.

The defendants applied to strike out the claim, saying it was hopeless and not known to the law in Australia. Harper J in the Supreme Court of Victoria,[75] whose decision was upheld by the Victorian Court of Appeal,[76] refused to strike out the claim:

> In my opinion, it cannot be said that the plaintiff's claim has no prospects of success. On the contrary it seems to me that a person who suffers psychiatric illness when informed that medical treatment undergone by her may leave her with a horrible and terminal disease, probably has a good cause of action against the manufacturer of a drug used in the plaintiff's treatment, where its manufacture (and subsequent distribution) was conducted negligently, and where that negligence exposed the plaintiff to that risk. Any other conclusion could only be reached were psychiatric injury to be placed in a quite different category to other kinds of harm to one's body or mind.[77]

Such reasoning would equally apply if the product were an asbestos product and, *a fortiori*, where the exposure was an incident of the plaintiff's employment.

Conclusion

Whenever claims for damages or compensation are made consequent upon exposure to asbestos, physicians, pathologists, epidemiologists, general practitioners and psychiatrists will be called upon by attornies to express their views and appear in court. Many medical practitioners tend to disdain this work or regard it with apprehension. I would venture to suggest, however, that it is one of the greatest virtues of their calling. Not only does it render a very real service to their patients, at a time when they are scared and vulnerable, but it is a forum for the exchange of views by experts in relevant fields which may well advance the scientific debate to the benefit of many. It is an honourable duty not to be discharged lightly.

The author is an Australian lawyer with experience in asbestos litigation over 20 years including in the conduct of the Wittenoom test cases. He and his former firm, Slater & Gordon, have acted in several hundred such claims for plaintiffs. He has also conducted other important environmental and product liability litigation.

References

1. Vojakovic R and Gordon J. The Victim's Perspective. In: Peters & Peters *Sourcebook on Asbestos Disease* Vol **13** pp 373–410.
2. Maas v Midalco Pty Ltd; Supreme Court of WA 1997
3. Joosten v Midalco Pty Ltd (1989) AILR 499
4. Limitation Act (WA) section 38.
5. Supreme Court of Victoria, Pilmer v McPherson Ltd 18 September 1985
6. Supreme Court of WA, Simpson v Midalco, 20 November 1987
7. Supreme Court of WA No. 1147 of 1987, Barrow v CSR Ltd and Midalco Pty Ltd and Supreme Court No. 1161 of 1987 Heys v CSR Ltd and Midalco Pty Ltd
8. Rabenalt v Midalco Ltd, Supreme Court of Victoria, 24 May 1988
9. 'Having a regard to the weight of uncontradicted evidence of information concerning the risks to which its employees were exposed in the mill and mine . . . I consider that a strong case supporting the finding of recklessness – indeed of continuing, conscious and contumelious disregard by the defendant for the plaintiff's right to be free from the risk of injury or disease – was made out' per Kaye J.
   Midalco Pty Ltd v Rabenalt, Supreme Court of Victoria, the Full Court (1989) VR 461 at 467
10. Supreme Court of WA; Watson v Western Australia
11. Western Australia v Watson [1990] WAR 248 Full Court
12. Simpson v Midalco Pty Ltd Supreme court of WA, Full Court 7 December 1988
13. Olson v CSR Ltd and Midalco Pty Ltd Dust Diseases Tribunal (NSW) No. 74 of 1994
14. NSW Court of Appeal No. 40037 of 1995, del. 25 February 1998
15. CSR Ltd v Culkin, Supreme Court of WA, Full Court, del. 19 October 1995
16. CSR Ltd v Culkin, High Court, Application for Special Leave 20 April 1995
17. Supreme Court of Victoria, December 1992
18. Pizzini v Dust Diseases Board, NSW Compensation Court, Duck J, 23 December 1994
    Cavanough v Dust Diseases Board, NSW Compensation Court, (1998) 16 NSNCCR 626
    Dhue v CSR Ltd, Supreme Court of WA, settled 4 June 1998
19. Napolitano v CSR Ltd, Supreme Court of WA, 1450 of 1994, 30 August 1994
20. Gordon J R C. Medico-legal issues in Mesothelioma and Asbestos Disease Litigation. In: Henderson *et al. Malignant Mesothelioma*. Hemisphere, 1992.
21. NSW Workers Compensation Legislation Amendment/Dust Diseases and other matters) Act 1998
22. per Dixon J in Adelaide Stevedoring Co. Ltd v Forst (1940) 64 CLR 538 AT 569–70.
23. Tubemakers of Australia Ltd v Fernandez [1976] ALJR 720 (High Court); EMI (Aust) Ltd v BES [1970] 2 NSWR 238 (NSW Court of Appeal); Dahl v Grice [1981] VR 513 (Victorian Full Supreme Court); ABA Ltd v Rees, 9 October 1981 (WA Full Supreme Court); Chance

v Alcoa Ltd (1990) Aust Torts Rep 67,719 (WA Full Supreme Court); Drakos v Woolworths Ltd [1991] 56 SASR 431 (SA Full Supreme Court)

24. Dixon J in Betts v Whittingslowe, (1945) 71 CLR 637 at 649
25. [1992] 176 CLR 408 at 420
26. per Gaudron J *op. cit.*
27. see Adelaide Stevedoring v Forst op cit; March v Stramare (E&MH) Pty Ltd (1991) 171 CLR 506 at 515; Stapley v Gypsum Mines Ltd [1953] AC 633 at 681
28. per Mason CJ in March v Stramare (E&MH) Pty Ltd (1991) 171 CLR 506 at 509
29. per Lord Reid in McGhee v National Coal Board [1973] 1 WLR 1 at 5
30. per Lord Salmon in McGhee v National Coal Board at 12
31. per Mason CJ in March v Stramare at 509
32. McGhee v National Coal Board, supra, Bennett v Minister of Community Welfare, supra
33. per Lord Wilberforce at 6
34. Bonnington Castings Ltd v Wardlaw [1958] AC 613 at 621; Nicholson v Atlas Steel Foundry [1957] 1 WLR 613 at 616 per Viscount Simons; at 622 per Lord Cohen; McGhee v National Coal Board per Lord Reid at 5; per Lord Simon at 8; per Lord Kilbrandon at 10; per Lord Salmon at 11-12
35. Wyong Shire Council v Shirt (1980) 146 CLR 40 at 48; Nagle v Rottnest Island Authority (1993) 177 CLR 423
36. Bendix Mintex Pty Ltd v Barnes (1997) 42 NSWLR 307
37. Cook WA. The Occupational Disease Hazard. *Industrial Medicine* 1942; **11**:193–198.
38. Handsley E. The asbestos worker's wife; excluded by science. (1997) 5 *Torts Law Journal* 154 at 170
39. Wagner JC, Sleggs CS, Marchant P. Diffuse Pleural Mesothelioma and Asbestos Exposure in the North-Western Cape Province. *British Journal of Industrial Medicine* 1960; **17**:260–271.
40. Bale v Seltsam Pty Ltd, unreported Supreme Court of Queensland judgment 14 December 1996 per White J at p.61
41. *ibid*
42. *ibid*
43. *ibid*
44. *ibid*
45. *ibid*
46. Olson v CSR Ltd (unreported) DDT NSW judgment 24 December 1994; on appeal CSR Ltd v Young (unreported) NSW Court of Appeal - judgment 25 February 1998
47. Margereson v JW Roberts Ltd (Holland J) (unreported) 27 October 1995; Court of Appeal *op cit supra* 2 April 1996; summarised at 1996 (TLR) 238 (17 April 1996)
48. *op cit supra*
49. *op cit supra*
50. per Giles AJA at 16
51. Margereson v JW Roberts Ltd *op cit*
52. *op cit* p.54
53. Asbestos Industry Regulations (UK) 1931 SI 1931 No. 1140
54. Merewether ERA, Price CW. *Report on Effects of Asbestos Dust on the Lungs and Dust Suppression in the Asbestos Industry.* London: HMSO, 1930.
55. (1996) 1 AC 155
56. *ibid* per Lloyd at p190
57. *op cit* per Russell LJ at p6

58. eg. chronic lymphatic leukaemia - Kasczmarek v CSR Ltd (unreported) Supreme Court of Victoria per Brooking J 15 December 1986

59. see generally; Steele J and Wikely N. Dust on the Streets and Liability for Environmental Cancers. (1997) **60** *Modern Law Review* 265 at 272

60. *op cit* per Russell J at p9

61. *Chief Inspector of Factories and Workshops Annual Report for 1898* (HMSO) 1900; and see Greenberg. Knowledge of the Health Hazards of Asbestos prior to the Merewether Price Report. *Social History of Medicine* 1994; **7**:493.

62. Robertson DG. *An Index to Health Hazards in Industry.* Commonwealth of Australia Department of Health, 1922

63. see note 58 above

64. see Barrow & Heys v CSR *op cit* at 150-151; CSR Ltd v Young *op cit* at 15-16 per Giles AJA; Bendix Mintex Ltd v Barnes *op cit* at 334, 344

65. Weill H, Hughes J; 'Asbestosis as a Precursor of Asbestos-Related Lung-Cancer; Results of a Prospective Mortality Study' *British Journal of Industrial Medicine* **48** 229-233, 1991

66. De Klerk N, Musk AW, Glancy J. Crocidolite, Radiographic Asbestosis and Subsequent Lung Cancer. *Annals of Occupational Hygiene* 1997; **41**: Supp 1 (Inhaled Particles viii) 134–136. Finkelstein M. Radiographic Asbestosis is not a pre-requisite for Asbestos-associated Lung Cancer in Ontario Asbestos Cement Workers. *American Journal of Industrial Medicine* 1997; **32**: 341–348. Case B, Dufresne A. Asbestos, Asbestosis and Lung Cancer: Observations in Quebec Chrysotile Workers. *Environmental Health Perspectives*, Vol. **106** Supplement 5, September 1997; Wilkinson P, Janssens J, Rudd R, Reubens M, Taylor A, Newman, Hansell D, McDonald JC. Is lung cancer associated with asbestos exposure when there are no small opacities on the chest radiograph? *Lancet* 1995; **345**(April 29): 1074–1078

67. *op cit* see note 18

68. Haar v Uneedus Scaffolding Pty Ltd (unreported) Supreme Court of Victoria; Cashman v Tomlinson Steel (unreported) Supreme Court of Victoria, August 1993

69. Jaensch v Coffey (1983-84) 155 CLR 549 per Brennan J at 565

70. Mt Isa Mines Ltd v Pusey (1970) 125 CLR 383, Jaensch v Coffey per Brennan J at 565

71. Napolitano v CSR Ltd (unreported) Supreme Court of WA del. 30 August 1994

72. (1998) 196 LSJS 99

73. (1995) 1NZLR 632

74. (unreported) Supreme Court of Victoria per Harper J del. 2 February 1995

75. *ibid*

76. (unreported) Vic Court of Appeal 28 April 1995

77. *op cit* at p3

=15=

Asbestos Fibres and their Interaction with Mesothelial Cells *in vitro* and *in vivo*

V. Courtney Broaddus and Marie-Claude Jaurand

The mesothelial cell appears to be a major target of the asbestos fibre (Figure 15.1). This cell is the likely progenitor of the tumour, mesothelioma, a tumour strongly associated with asbestos exposure. In addition, the mesothelial cell may play a role in other asbestos-induced pathology, including pleural plaques, benign asbestos pleurisy and pleural fibrosis.

After much study of the asbestos fibre and its interaction with the mesothelial cell *in vitro*, it is still unclear what determines asbestos-induced pleural disease. On the one hand, the uniqueness of this pleural pathology may be dependent on the tendency of asbestos fibres to accumulate in the pleural space by their lodging in the parietal pleura around the draining lymphatic stomata. In fact, with decreases in occupational exposure to asbestos fibres, lung disease is waning in incidence, but pleural disease is rising.[1] One explanation is that, with a lower burden of fibres in the lung, the lung can avoid injury as the fibres gradually clear to the pleural space where they accumulate, thereby shifting disease from lung to pleura. This may in part explain how the risk of mesothelioma can be enhanced by only low exposure to asbestos.[2] On the other hand, the pleural pathology may arise from the unique features of the mesothelial cell, a lining cell neither epithelial nor endothelial but derived from the mesoderm. Indeed, the mesothelial cell is unusual in several respects: it coexpresses different intermediate filaments, it alters their expression during the cell cycle and it has a sensitivity to a wide array of growth factors. There is some evidence that mesothelial cells *in vitro* are more sensitive to the toxic effects of asbestos than other cells,[3,4] although the cell appears to be no more sensitive than other cells to oxidant-induced DNA damage.[5,6]

Asbestos is both a fibrogenic and carcinogenic fibre, and presents a challenge to those who would understand its mechanism of action. Clearly some of its biological toxicity relates to its fibrous shape, and yet other fibres of a similar shape are not harmful. Understanding how the shape, surface structure and chemical composition interact to produce such a biologically harmful agent is important to understanding the mechanisms of toxicity and for avoiding other harmful fibrous materials in the future.

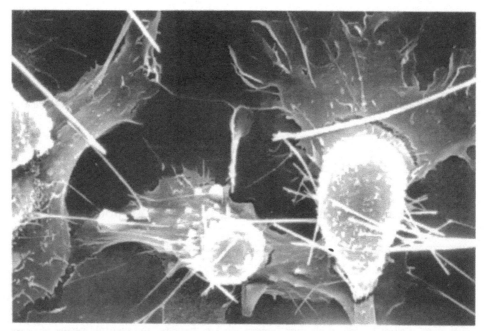

Figure 15.1. *A scanning electron micrograph of two rabbit pleural mesothelial cells exposed to crocidolite asbestos. The cell on the left appears shrunken, with surface blebs characteristic of apoptotic changes (2200X magnification; white bar, 10 µm).*

The lungs and pleura are the major sites of asbestos-related disease. Inhaled into the body, the fibres reach distal bronchi and lodge there, later to migrate to other areas of lung and to enter the pleural space. Over many years, asbestos fibres can induce lung diseases such as pulmonary fibrosis and lung cancer and a wide array of pleural diseases including pleural plaques, pleural effusions, pleural fibrosis, and the tumour mesothelioma.[1] No relationship has been recognised between other asbestos-induced diseases and mesothelioma. Although asbestos acts together with tobacco smoke to produce lung cancer, asbestos is a complete carcinogen for the tumour mesothelioma.

It is not known what features of asbestos are pathological and which of them account for the pleiotropic changes in the body. In particular, the tumour mesothelioma raises interesting issues because of its unusual nature and its close association with asbestos. The cytogenetic and molecular changes in malignant mesothelioma may be assumed to be due to cellular interactions with asbestos (see below). While SV-40 DNA sequences have been found recently in some human mesotheliomas, suggesting a viral contribution in the development of this disease, this may not be a unique feature of malignant mesothelioma.[7]

Asbestos fibres

The asbestos fibre types more frequently used in industry belong to 2 groups of minerals: serpentine and amphibole.[8] The major difference between each fibre type lies in the nature of the cations present in the particles. The chemical differences lead to differences in the overall shape of the fibres. Some physical and physico-chemical properties are important to explain the toxicity of the fibre, predominantly the shape, surface reactivity and chemical composition.

Shape and dimensions

The long thin shape of asbestos may enhance its entry deep into the lung, its migration within the lung and its toxicity upon interaction with lung cells. Following inhalation, fibres of several micrometres' length can enter the distal respiratory airways, whereas other particles of greater than 5 micrometres of mean aerodynamical diameter could not penetrate. In the lung, the long fibres may avoid macrophage clearance and, with their needle-like shape, fibres may more easily migrate along tissue planes, along lymphatic channels and into the sub-pleural and pleural space. Once in the pleural space, the long fibres may not be able to manoeuvre through the lymphatic stomata that clear liquid and protein from the pleural space, and thus may accumulate around the stoma in the parietal pleura.[9] Finally, both *in vivo* and *in vitro* studies have shown that long thin fibres have a greater intrinsic cytotoxicity than short fibres, as will be discussed below.

Shape has been considered a primary characteristic determining asbestos toxicity, particularly its carcinogenicity, since Stanton recognized length and width as major determinants of the ability to induce mesothelioma in animals.[10,11] The importance of shape can be illustrated in two ways. First, other materials with the same shape but different chemical composition share the ability to produce mesothelioma in animal studies. When implanted into the pleural space, for example, long thin glass fibres can also induce mesothelioma.[12] Similarly, the long thin shape is important for the production of lung cancer in inhalational studies.[13] In *in vitro* studies, the long thin asbestos fibres are more able to induce chromosomal abnormalities and to induce transformation than are shorter fibres.[14,15] Secondly, materials with the same chemical composition but a different shape do not share the same toxic profile or activity. Riebekite, a non-fibrous particle with the same chemical composition as crocidolite, is generally nontoxic,[16] as are samples of a shorter mean length or long thin fibres when ground to a shorter shape.[17] Such arguments have led to consideration of asbestos as a physical carcinogen, in which chemical composition plays little or no role in toxicity.[11,18]

Although shape plays a prominent role in the toxicity of asbestos, other features of the fibres must be important. Within the similarly shaped types of asbestos and asbestiform fibres, one finds differences between their apparent toxicity. For example, erionite, a long, thin zeolite fibre similar to amphibole asbestos, is the most toxic and carcinogenic fibre in *in vitro* and *in vivo* studies, suggesting a role of its different surface properties.[19,20] Also, differences in toxicity for production of mesothelioma appear to exist between crocidolite and chrysotile fibres, perhaps due to their different persistence in the tissues.[13,18]

Surface activity

Fibre surface properties appear to be an important parameter of toxicity for several reasons. For one, asbestos fibres, in large part due to the catalytic effect of the iron on the surface of the fibre, can generate toxic oxygen species even in acellular systems.[21] The same iron may catalyse toxic oxygen production during phagocytosis, due to exposure to peroxides within phagolysosomes. For another, the fibre surface is adsorptive. Fibres have been shown to absorb proteins, phospholipids or DNA.[22-24] Thus, they can interact with macromolecules present in the biological environment, affecting their ability to interact with cell surfaces. When exposed to serum, for example, crocidolite fibres adsorb vitronectin, an adhesive protein that preferentially adsorbs to glass[25] (Figure 15.2). This protein then allows the fibre to interact with the cell surface integrin, a vitronectin-receptor $\alpha v \beta 5$, an interaction that increases fibre uptake by the cell. The adsorptive surface may also capture chemical carcinogenic molecules or compounds of cigarette smoke. The surface of the asbestos also contains a charge; at physiological pH, crocidolite displays a negative charge while chrysotile displays a positive charge.[26] These differently charged surfaces may explain some of the different adsorptive characteristics of the two fibres.[22] The positive charge of chrysotile also is responsible for the ability of this fibre to induce haemolysis in cells, by concentrating sialic acid moieties on the cell surface.[26,27] Finally, the surface of fibres may be an active site for chemical reactions.

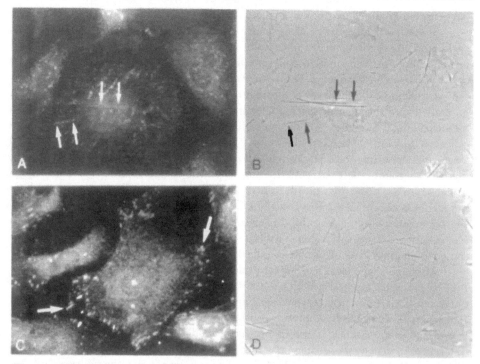

Figure 15.2. Biologically modified asbestos fibres can react with specific cell receptors. Crocidolite asbestos fibres have been incubated with vitronectin, washed and added to rabbit pleural mesothelial cells for 4 hours. By immunocytochemistry, two integrins that are receptors for vitronectin are identified, $\alpha v \beta 5$ **(A)** and $\alpha v \beta 3$ **(C)**. By comparing the fluorescence with the accompanying phase micrograph, vitronectin-coated crocidolite fibres can be seen to colocalize with $\alpha v \beta 5$ **(A, B**; double arrows), but not with $\alpha v \beta 3$ **(C, D)**.

Asbestos bodies, found in asbestos-exposed subjects, are composed of a centre fibre surrounded by added iron and proteins, and appear to result from the interaction of macrophages with long, incompletely phagocytosed fibres.[28] These structures emphasise the complex reactions with the biological milieu arising at the fibre surface.

Chemical composition

The composition of the fibres determines their resistance to dissolution and their persistence in the tissues. The persistence of asbestos generally may explain why asbestos fibres are biologically more harmful than other fibres, even when *in vitro* studies show similar responses to the different fibres. In *in vivo* exposure studies, the initial inflammatory effects of asbestos and other non-asbestos fibres may be similar, while the long-term effects correlate with the persistence of fibres.[29,30] Fibres that demonstrate toxicity in animals have not always shown toxicity in humans, perhaps because the fibres may not persist in the longer-lived humans to the extent necessary to produce disease with a long latency.[18] Even among asbestos fibres, differences in persistence may account for a different toxic profile in people. Crocidolite has been identified as a more resistant fibre than chrysotile, and appears to persist longer in the body. In long-term inhalation studies in rats, despite an equivalent likelihood of inducing lung cancer, crocidolite was 3 times more likely to induce mesothelioma than was chrysotile.[13] Even in short-term inhalational studies in rats, crocidolite was retained at a higher fibre burden and induced more pleural mesothelial proliferation than chrysotile.[31] While amphibole asbestos persists in the body basically unchanged for decades, chrysotile dissolves,[18] with *in vivo* radioisotope studies showing as much as 35% of the structural magnesium leached away in 1 month.[32] Longer persistence could account for the close association of crocidolite fibres with mesothelioma, a tumour with a 3–4 decade latency. So far, however, it has been difficult to establish the link between long-term biopersistence and carcinogenicity. It is worth remembering that chemical carcinogens or radiation does not need to persist in the lung to produce cancer and, therefore, persistence of a carcinogen may not always be necessary to induce cancer.[33]

The mesothelial cell

The mesothelial cells line the serosal cavities of the body, the pleural, peritoneal and pericardial spaces. Geographically, across the serosal surfaces, mesothelial cells can be seen to have a variety of morphologies between flat or cuboidal and showing few or a dense forest of microvilli.[34] Although their important *in vivo* functions have not been identified, they have the potential to regulate cell traffic, the balance between coagulation and fibrinolysis, cell proliferation, and fibrogenesis within and around the pleural space. They likely represent the progenitor cell for mesothelioma.

In *in vitro* studies, the mesothelial cell demonstrates a multitude of abilities. Mesothelial cells can produce most of the components of the submesothelial matrix, at amounts comparable to that of fibroblasts.[35] They can also release growth factors such as TGF-beta and insulin-like growth factor I.[36,37] The cells may regulate the fibrinolytic and procoagulant activities on their cell surface and in the pleural space.[38,39] They express the urokinase plasminogen activator receptor, which may regulate local fibrinolysis as well as cell proliferation.[40] They produce a number of chemotactic factors, including IL-8 and MCP-1, that may help regulate influx of neutrophils and monocytes to the pleural space.[41-43] They express adhesion molecules including ICAM-1, VCAM-1 and PECAM-1 that could function to assist cell movement into the pleural space,[41,44,45] and integrins that participate in phagocytosis of material, including asbestos.[25] Mesothelial cells bind to each other by means that do not produce a tight barrier to movement of liquid or protein;[46] this leaky barrier, which allows successful dialysis across the peritoneal mesothelium, may also allow movement of cytokines, of cells and perhaps of asbestos itself into the pleural space.

When compared to other cells, mesothelial cells have some unique features. Their cytoskeleton, particularly their expression of intermediate filaments, appears to be unlike other cells. While epithelial cells express mostly cytokeratins and no vimentin, and fibroblastic cells express vimentin, mesothelial cells can express both. This coexpression can be used to identify mesothelial cells. It is also unusual that the expression of cytokeratin varies greatly. From quiescence to growth, the cell alternates its morphology from epithelial to fibroblastic. As cells proliferate, they greatly reduce the expression of the keratins, often to undetectable levels, a striking feature compared to epithelial cells which maintain a fairly steady amount of cytokeratins even during growth.[47] These differences suggest a unique and plastic cytoskeletal arrangement. Mesothelial cells also appear to have a responsiveness to a broader array of growth factors than do other cells.[48] For example, human mesothelial cells respond to typically epithelial-type mitogens, like EGF, and also to non-epithelial mitogens, such as TGF-beta and PDGF; TGF-beta, for example, may actually inhibit epithelial cell proliferation.[49] Since the mesothelial cell can produce some of these same growth factors such as TGF-beta, the potential for autocrine growth stimulation is present.[50] Mesothelial cells have a relative lack of antigens specific to their cell type. For example, most immunohistochemical tests diagnose mesothelioma with negative staining, that is, with tests that are negative for mesothelioma while positive for other tumours. However, some antigens may be used as markers in mesothelial cells such as the Wilms' tumour antigen WT-1 and a 40 kDa glycoprotein, called mesothelin.[51,52] Another diagnostic feature that appears to be unique to mesothelial cells is their long, branching microvilli. Which of these unique features may have relevance to the development of asbestos-related pleural pathology is not known.

Interaction of mesothelial cells and asbestos *in vitro*

Effects of asbestos on the mesothelial cells *in vitro* appear to be wide ranging, encompassing activation of an adaptive response to oxidative stress, production of many inflammatory and fibrogenic factors, activation of an adaptive response to DNA damage, and finally death by apoptosis or necrosis. The initial interaction between the asbestos fibre and the mesothelial cell takes place on the cell surface, at which time the fibre either becomes adherent or is phagocytosed.

Fibres are phagocytosed by the mesothelial cells, as early as 15 minutes after exposure, and may be seen within membrane-bound structures including phagolysosomes.[53] In large newt epithelial cells, fibre motion within the cell can be observed. In these cells, fibres are carried to the nucleus, with fibres less than 5 microns in length demonstrating a saltatory motion characteristic of microtubular transport of endosomes.[54] By electron microscopy, the fibres are seen to be enveloped in a membrane layer at least for weeks after phagocytosis, although it is not known whether all fibres are taken up or remain in membrane-bound structures and whether the presence of a membrane affects the toxicity of the fibres. Asbestos later appears to be enmeshed in and closely entangled with the cytokeratin surrounding the nucleus and in close contact with the nuclear membrane.[55] In transmission electron micrographs, asbestos fibres can be found near or actually touching chromosomes in metaphase cells.[56,57]

Although the exact role of phagocytosis in toxicity is not known, phagocytosis of fibres may be necessary for many aspects of toxicity, especially of carcinogenicity, to become manifest. This point has been difficult to establish, in part because of the difficulty of identifying phagocytosis and distinguishing it from adherence to these extremely thin cells. Even confocal microscopy cannot easily distinguish intracellular from extracellular fibres, unless combined with a lipid marker to show the membrane coat around the fibre that identifies the fibre as intracellular[25] (Figure 15.3). Using such an approach, Boylan *et al.* found that coating crocidolite fibres with vitronectin, a protein that enhanced fibre internalisation in rabbit pleural mesothelial cells, enhanced cytopathic features.[25] Most

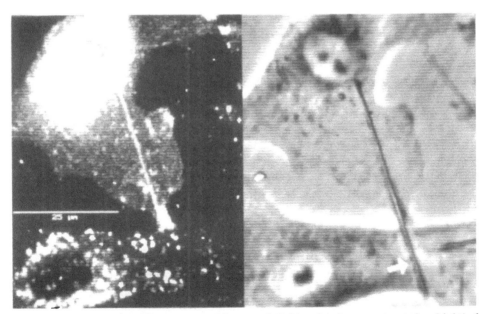

Figure 15.3. *A confocal fluorescence micrograph (left) and a phase contrast view (right) of rabbit pleural mesothelial cells and a crocidolite asbestos fibre. The cell membranes have been labelled with a lipid-permeable fluoroprobe. The fibre with the upper cell is seen to fluoresce, indicating that it is surrounded by a membrane and thus intracellular. The fibre with the lower cell does not fluoresce, indicating that it is extracellular (size bar = 25 μm).*

studies of the role of phagocytosis in cytotoxicity have been carried out with other cell types, using electron microscopy to quantitate uptake and discriminate it from adherence of fibres. In a promyelocytic cell line, Takeuchi and Morimoto observed that inhibition of crocidolite fibre uptake with cytochalasin B inhibited the increase in the DNA adduct 8-hydroxy guanine, but not the production of reactive oxygen species.[58] They concluded that the increase in DNA adducts was correlated more closely with fibre internalisation than with overall reactive oxygen species generation. In other cell systems, the importance of phagocytosis was reported with the use of metal particulates. As demonstrated by morphological transformation assays in Syrian hamster embryo cells, phagocytosed nickel particulates were more toxic than soluble nickel compounds.[59] de Vries et al. concluded that phagocytosis of lead particles was necessary to produce cytopathic changes in rabbit alveolar macrophages.[60] There is also evidence in Syrian hamster embryo cells that long glass fibres are preferentially phagocytosed compared to shorter fibres; long fibres were inherently more able to produce transformation and cytogenetic abnormalities but the preferential uptake may enhance the already greater toxicity of the long compared with the short fibres.[61] The lack of phagocytosis of asbestos by bacteria may explain why asbestos has failed to induce mutations in various bacterial assays.[62] Phagocytosis is likely to play an important role in toxicity of a physical carcinogen such as asbestos.

The role of phagocytosis in asbestos-induced toxicity for mesothelial cells has recently been examined directly in two studies.[63,64] By both increasing fibre uptake using vitronectin-coating of fibres and decreasing it using integrin blockade or an actin poison, the number of internalised fibres could be altered without altering the total number of fibres added to the mesothelial cells. With this approach, fibre uptake was shown to be necessary for fibre-induced intracellular oxidation, DNA damage and apoptosis. Of note, when uptake was blocked, the fibres lying on the surface of the cells caused no detectable DNA damage or apoptosis over the duration of these experiments (4–8 hours).[63]

Another interesting feature was that vitronectin adsorption, known to be important for negatively charged crocidolite asbestos and glass, was also shown to be important for chrysotile asbestos, a positively charged fibre not expected to adsorb vitronectin. The importance of phagocytosis in these studies supports the importance of an intracellular location of fibres for mesothelial cell toxicity.

With the fibres either adherent or ingested by the cells, the cells are exposed to an oxidant stress that appears to stimulate various signalling cascades, including NF-κB, AP-1, protein kinase C and mitogen-activated protein pathways. Rat pleural mesothelial cells respond to asbestos by a persistent enhancement of c-fos and c-jun mRNA expression and AP-1 binding activity.[65] This enhancement is reduced when cells are pretreated with protein kinase C inhibitors, suggesting the involvement of protein kinase C in asbestos-induced signal transduction pathways.[66] Janssen et al. reported activation of NF-κB in crocidolite-treated rat pleural mesothelial cells that was not observed in riebeckite-treated cells.[67] It is known that NF-κB and AP-1 are early responding transcription factors, sensitive to redox conditions prevalent in the cell by virtue of their several cysteine residues that modulate DNA binding, depending on their reduced or oxidized states. Other pathways stimulated by asbestos include the mitogen-activated protein (MAP) kinase pathway, which may be related to asbestos-induced phosphorylation and activation of the epidermal growth factor (EGF) receptor.[68]

In response to the asbestos and its oxidant stimulation, the mesothelial cell also produces and releases various agents, either inflammatory, fibrogenic or clastogenic. Mesothelial cells exposed to asbestos have been shown to produce fibronectin, a chemotactic factor for fibroblasts,[69] and interleukin-8, a chemotactic factor for neutrophils.[43] In the presence of interleukin-1, mesothelial cells exposed to asbestos produce reactive nitrogen species and thus may account for some of the reactive nitrogen species found in the lung and pleura after inhalation of asbestos.[70] Such nitrogen species may also constitute clastogenic factors that injure DNA of neighbouring cells. Mesothelial cells exposed to asbestos also increase their expression of urokinase plasminogen activator receptor, known to provide mitogenic signals to the mesothelial cell.[40,71]

In addition to a stimulatory effect of asbestos, there is a clearly toxic effect. Often this is recognised by a decrease in clonal efficiency, the ability of single cells to produce clones of mesothelial cells. In fact, mesothelial cells may be more sensitive to the toxic effects of asbestos than are other cells. In a few studies in which mesothelial cells have been compared with other cells, the mesothelial cell shows a selective sensitivity to asbestos-induced cytotoxicity. When compared to normal human bronchial epithelial cells or fibroblasts, mesothelial cells were 10–100 times more sensitive to the toxic effects of amosite asbestos.[3] When mesothelial cells and fibroblasts were exposed to a variety of different particulates, mesothelial cells showed a 20–100 times higher sensitivity to asbestos and asbestos-shaped glass fibres, but no difference in sensitivity to many other fibrous (ceramic, glass wool, mineral wool), non-fibrous (aluminium oxide, nickel subsulphide) or soluble (hydrogen peroxide, sodium azide) agents.[1] Transmission electron microscopy showed the number of intracellular fibres to be equivalent, suggesting that differences in sensitivity were not due to differences in phagocytosis. The similarity of response to hydrogen peroxide also suggests that the differences in sensitivity were not due to different antioxidant defences. Indeed, in later studies, mesothelial cells have shown a similar sensitivity to oxidant-induced DNA injury as bronchial epithelial cells, when measured by the comet assay[5,6] and by intracellular nucleotide depletion.[6] These data suggest that any heightened sensitivity of mesothelial cells to asbestos is not due to sensitivity to oxidant-induced DNA injury.

While cytotoxicity appears to be dependent on reactive oxygen species (ROS) production in different cell systems such as macrophages, the role of oxidative damage in mesothelial cells has been less clear. In amosite-exposed mesothelial cells, for example, no reactive oxygen species were demonstrated in the mesothelial cells[72] and no direct oxidant-type injury could be attributed to the amosite in either primary human cells or transformed MeT 5A cells.[72,73] Until recently, only indirect evidence of the involvement of ROS had been shown. Janssen *et al.* demonstrated an increase in the antioxidant enzyme, manganese superoxide dismutase, in human pleural mesothelial cells in response to asbestos.[16] At the same time, Dong *et al.* reported that antioxidant enzymes (superoxide dismutase and catalase) partly protected rat pleural mesothelial cells against the toxic effect of asbestos.[74]

In recent studies, however, intracellular oxidation has been measured directly in mesothelial cells exposed to asbestos.[63,64] After exposure to asbestos fibres, hydrogen

Table 15.1. *Studies of DNA damage in asbestos-treated pleural mesothelial cells.*

Effects on DNA		Mesothelial cell types	Fibre types	References
DNA adducts:				
• oxidised guanine bases	+	MeT 5A*	crocidolite	(Chen *et al.*, 1996)[80]
• 8-OHdG†	+	rat	crocidolite	(Fung *et al.*, 1997)[81]
	–	MeT 5A	crocidolite	(Fung *et al.*, 1997)[81]
DNA breakage:				
• alkaline elution	0	human	amosite	(Gabrielson *et al.*,1986)[72]
• alkaline unwinding	0	MeT 5A	amosite	(Kinnula *et al.*, 1994)[73]
• Comet assay	+	meT5A	crocidolite	(Ollikainen, 1999)[82]
	+	rat	croc/chrys	(Levresse, 2000)[83]
DNA repair:				
• unscheduled DNA synthesis	+	rat	croc/chrys‡	(Renier *et al.*, 1990)[75]
	+	rat	croc/chrys	(Dong *et al.*, 1994)[74]
• activation of PARP	+	rat	croc/chrys	(Dong *et al.*, 1995)[76]
• AP endonuclease gene expression	+	rat	crocidolite	(Fung *et al.*, 1998)[78]

*MeT 5A, human pleural mesothelial cells immortalised by transformation with SV40 large T antigen.
† 8-OHdG, 8-hydroxydeoxyguanosine, an oxidative lesion in DNA.
‡ Croc/chrys refers to both crocidolite and chrysotile.
Comet assay refers to single cell gel electrophoresis.
Symbols mean: + an increase; –, a decrease; 0, no change.

peroxide or glass beads, mesothelial cells were loaded with an intracellular oxidation-sensitive fluorescent dye and analysed for the fluorescence shift of the dye signifying intracellular oxidation. Asbestos fibres induced a shift as did hydrogen peroxide, indicating oxidative stress. Oxidation did not apparently arise from the process of phagocytosis itself, because phagocytosis of glass beads did not induce an oxidative shift, although it should be noted that phagocytosis of fibres and of non-fibrous particles may differ. Compared to professional phagocytes such as macrophages, non-professional phagocytes such as mesothelial cells may not generate ROS with phagocytosis.[75] For the mesothelial cell, it is the intracellular fibre itself that appears to generate the ROS and, by fibre translocation, to bring those toxic products close to the nucleus.

After some hours of exposure to asbestos, mesothelial cells begin to show an adaptive response to genotoxic damage. Adaptive responses induced by asbestos in mesothelial cells include cell cycle arrest, the activation of DNA repair (unscheduled DNA synthesis)[76] and the activation of poly(ADP)ribose polymerase, an enzyme activated by single-strand breaks.[77] In mesothelial cells, fibre exposure has been shown to

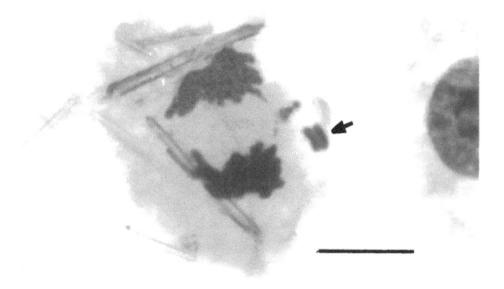

Figure 15.4. *Abnormal anaphase in a rat pleural mesothelial cell treated with crocidolite fibres. Lagging chromatin (arrow) can be seen at the periphery of the cell (size bar = 10 μm). (Photomicrograph courtesy of Dr Michel Yegles.)*

induce AP-endonuclease, an enzyme nicking DNA at apurinic sites for repair of DNA base hydroxylation.[78] Fibre exposure also increases expression of p53, a transcription factor strongly activated by DNA damage.[79] This complex adaptive response provides compelling but indirect evidence of the existence of DNA damage.

There is also some direct evidence of DNA damage produced by asbestos in mesothelial cells (Table 15.1). DNA adducts such as oxidised guanine residues are found in asbestos-exposed mesothelial cells.[80,81] These base oxidation products are commonly produced DNA modifications that may be related to the induction of ROS such as the hydroxyl radical (OH) or the more stable peroxynitrates and lipid peroxidation products. Some ROS, especially the highly reactive OH⁻, may have short half-lives and distances over which they are active. Thus, internalised fibres near the nucleus are in a much better position to injure nuclear DNA than extracellular or adherent fibres. Oddly enough, despite evidence of oxidation in mesothelial cells and of oxidative DNA damage, two studies have failed to find evidence of DNA strand breaks in amosite-exposed mesothelial cells.[72,73] In two more recent studies using single cell gel electrophoresis, however, mesothelial cells exposed to chrysotile or crocidolite asbestos have been shown to suffer DNA damage.[82,83]

In addition to DNA damage, many chromosomal and mitotic abnormalities are generated by asbestos (Table 15.2). Of interest, these abnormalities resemble those found in mesothelioma cells.[84] Asbestos fibres may induce either structural abnormalities of the chromosomes or abnormalities in chromosome number. In mesothelial cells, such

Table 15.2. Studies of chromosomal damage in asbestos-treated pleural mesothelial cells.

Chromosome/mitotic abnormalities	Mesothelial cell types	Fibre types	References
Structural abnormalities[*]	human human	croc/chrys/amos[¶] amosite	(Olofsson & Mark, 1989)[84] (Pelin et al., 1995)[86]
Numerical chromosome changes[†]	human rat human	amosite chrysotile croc/chrys	(Lechner et al., 1985)[3] (Jaurand et al., 1986)[86] (Pelin et al., 1995)[86]
Anaphase/telophase abnormalities[‡]	rat	croc/chrys	(Yegles et al., 1993;[88] Yegles et al., 1995)[15]
G2/M delay[§]	rat	croc/chrys	(Levresse et al., 1997)[79]

[*] Structural abnormalities included deletions, reciprocal translocations, and acentric chromosome fragments. [†]Numerical chromosome changes included aneuploidy, polyploidy and binuclei. [‡]Anaphase/ telophase abnormalities included lagging chromatin, bridging chromatin, or asymmetric segregation of chromosomes. [§]G2/M delay indicates an increased percentage of cells in this cell cycle phase. [¶]Croc, crocidolite; chrys, chrysotile; amos, amosite.

structural abnormalities include acentric fragments, deletions, and translocations.[84–86] Chromosome segregation abnormalities commonly result in the formation of aneuploid as well as polyploid and binucleated cells.[3,86] In human and rat mesothelial cells in anaphase/telophase, asbestos has been shown to induce lagging chromatin and bridges as evidence of chromosomal segregation abnormalities during mitosis[15,87] (Figure 15.4). In the case of rat mesothelial cells, mitosis alteration was confirmed in a cell cycle study demonstrating cell accumulation in the G2/M compartment, corresponding to an increase in observed binucleated cells.[79] Such a block or delay in this phase of the cell cycle may be an indication of a checkpoint function of the cell in response to DNA damage. Chromosome abnormalities may be due to the mechanical effects of internalised fibres, in which the fibres either interact directly with chromosomes themselves[56] or interfere with the movement of the chromosomes.[54] The length of fibres may determine their ability to penetrate the spindle apparatus and physically interfere with chromosomes. In studies with mesothelial cells, Yegles et al. found that the production of abnormal anaphases/telophases depended on the presence of long thin fibres, the same Stanton fibres with a propensity to cause mesothelioma.[11,88] In studies with other mammalian cells, Hesterberg and Barrett found the ability of asbestos to transform the cells depended on the presence of the long, thin fibres.[14]

The frequency of deletions and loss of chromosomes found in these in vitro studies as well as in mesothelioma itself suggests a role for loss of tumour suppressors in the formation of mesothelioma.[33,89] Recurrent loss of genetic material involves chromosome arms 1p, 3p, 6q, 9p, 15q and 22q.[89] Candidate tumour suppressors have been found that lie on 9p (p16/CDKN2A) and on 22q12 (neurofibromatosis type 2).[90] In particular, the neurofibromatosis type 2 (NF2) gene has been shown to have multiple abnormalities, both in structure and expression,[91,92] which may be specific to mesothelioma.[93] Interestingly, there appears to be no obvious abnormalities in other likely genes or their products, including p53, retinoblastoma protein, Wilms' tumour antigen, and Bcl-2.[94,95] It is likely that other gene abnormalities tied to the loss of chromosomes are yet to be identified.

If the asbestos-induced injury is too severe for cellular adaptation or repair, asbestos-exposed mesothelial cells may die by necrosis or by apoptosis. The necrotic response, shown *in vitro* and *in vivo* by the early loss of membrane integrity and release of intracellular enzymes such as lactate dehydrogenase, is presumably due to overwhelming damage to the cells.[9] Apoptosis, a type of death that requires a complex sequence of signals initiating protease activation, may predominate if the damage is less severe, allowing time for the apoptotic signal cascade to proceed. DNA damage and oxidative stress, both well known apoptotic stimuli, may play an important role in asbestos-induced mesothelial cell apoptosis.[96] Persistent c-*fos* activation, shown to be a pro-apoptotic condition, as well as oxidant-induced signalling via the extracellular signal-regulated protein kinases of the MAP pathway, have been described in mesothelial cells exposed to asbestos.[65,97] Apoptosis may exist in concert with proliferation, either stimulated by the loss of cells and their cell–cell contact or stimulated directly by the asbestos.[98] Apoptosis may be the major mechanism by which the organism deletes cells with a damaged genome. If so, then loss of the apoptotic response could be an important step in the process of malignant progression.[99] Although not demonstrated yet *in vivo*, apoptosis could be an important response to asbestos over the years of exposure. Indeed, mesothelioma cell lines show a resistance to apoptosis that is not yet explained by abnormalities in known apoptotic regulating proteins such as p53 or Bcl-2.[95] Nonetheless, loss of normal checkpoints to cell-cycle control and apoptosis, such as by loss of functional p53, increases sensitivity to asbestos-induced toxicity and increases susceptibility to develop mesothelioma.[88,100,101]

Interaction of mesothelial cells and asbestos *in vivo*

Asbestos fibres continually clear from the lung toward the pleura and lymphatics.[102] Short fibres may make this translocation more readily, but long fibres also move from the lung.[103] The rapidity of fibre translocation can be surprising. In rats, after intratracheal injection of chrysotile asbestos, fibres could be found in the pleura within 7 days[104] and, in 1 of 3 rats after inhalation of asbestos, fibres could be found in the pleural space 1 week after a 2-week exposure.[105] Free fibres or those within macrophages likely move with pleural liquid toward the lymphatic stomata, where liquid and protein are removed from the pleural space.[106] Here, it appears fibres cannot be completely removed and many of the longer ones accumulate and become concentrated in these discrete areas. After inhalation of asbestos in animals, asbestos fibres can be found adjacent to mesothelial cells, in the submesothelial space and occasionally within mesothelial cells themselves.[107] In human subjects exposed to asbestos in whom several different tissues were analysed, the concentration of asbestos fibres in pleural plaques or lymph nodes consistently exceeded that in the lung.[103] Indeed, fibre counts from the pleura may have been underestimated in the past, when the pleura was analysed as a whole. It is now recognised that fibres in the pleura are not distributed homogeneously, but are found at high concentrations in certain areas. In asbestos-exposed patients undergoing diagnostic thoracoscopy, samples of tissue obtained from anthracotic areas (black spots) in the parietal pleura had high concentrations of fibres, whereas tissue from nearby pleura had almost no fibres.[108] In some cases, the fibres, which included many long, thin fibres, were found at higher concentrations in the anthracotic regions of pleura than in the lung parenchyma.

Fibres also reach the peritoneum, possibly by direct translocation across the gut wall after ingestion of fibres into the gastrointestinal tract. Free fibres in the peritoneal space are cleared toward the diaphragm where they can lodge in the stomata on the undersurface of the diaphragm.[9] Compared to ingestion, however, inhalation of asbestos appears to be a more potent means of distributing fibres throughout the body.[18]

Asbestos fibres can affect the mesothelium indirectly via its effects on the lung. Following a single intratracheal instillation of asbestos in mice or rats, mesothelial proliferation was noted to increase from a baseline of 0.3% to a peak of 3% a week after instillation,[109,110] and to taper off by 4 weeks.[109] The mesothelial response was seen without evidence of fibres reaching the pleural surface and was associated with long fibres, not short fibres.[109,111] A recent study has attributed this early mesothelial proliferation to keratinocyte growth factor.[112] Interestingly, a similar temporal pattern of mesothelial proliferation was noted after other non-asbestos-induced lung injury, suggesting a nonspecific effect of inflammatory cytokines on the mesothelium.[110] Whether due to a specific or nonspecific effect of asbestos, a proliferative stimulus to the mesothelium that persists over many years may contribute to asbestos-induced mesothelial pathology.

Asbestos that reaches the serosal spaces may interact with the mesothelium and other cells such as neutrophils and macrophages. The fibres, either free or within phagocytes, move with the serosal liquid to the lymphatic clearance stomata. In the pleural space, these stomata lie on the parietal pleura; in the peritoneal space, stomata lie on the undersurface of the diaphragm. When long crocidolite asbestos (greater than 2 microns) was injected into the peritoneal space of mice, the diaphragm showed evidence of mesothelial injury as early as 3 hours after injection, followed by inflammatory cell infiltration and mesothelial regeneration over the next 2–3 weeks. Short fibres (90% less than 2 microns), on the other hand, had little effect on the mesothelium and appeared to clear via the lymphatics without accumulating in the diaphragm. As late as 6 months after the one injection, fibres could be seen in clusters, lying underneath regenerating mesothelium and surrounded by macrophages. Fibres instilled into the pleural space of mice have also been shown to induce apoptosis of mesothelial cells.[113]Mesothelial cell damage may be due to effects of the asbestos itself or of the phagocytes responding to the asbestos with the release of toxic free radicals.[109]

Mesothelioma in animals can be generated by *in vivo* implantation or instillation of fibres in the pleural or peritoneal spaces[10] or, in a smaller percentage of animals, by inhalation.[13] Direct injection of fibres into the serosal spaces bypasses physiological barriers to inhaled fibres. Inhaled fibres must migrate over weeks to years in tissues to reach the pleural space. Differences in relative carcinogenic potencies of fibres when given by different routes of delivery demonstrate the potential importance of biopersistence or migration to the ability of fibres to induce mesothelioma. Thus, by direct pleural injection, certain long thin fibres can be found to be carcinogenic whereas upon inhalation, many of these long thin fibres may not be as dangerous presumably because of dissolution.[18,114,115] The ability to reproduce mesothelioma by direct injection suggests that a direct interaction between fibres and pleural cells is sufficient to produce mesothelioma.

Summary

Fibres that are readily dispersed in air and respirable deep in the lung lodge in the bifurcation of the airways. There they first interact with the biological environment, adsorbing materials, activating proteins, attracting macrophages. The inflammatory and fibrogenic activity set in motion by the fibre–cell interactions within the lung release mitogens and other cytokines that appear to stimulate the mesothelium.

The fibres also begin dispersing in the lung and those that are less persistent begin to fragment into smaller fibres and dissolve. The fibres that persist migrate along lymphatics to the mediastinal lymph nodes or along pressure gradients to the subpleural and then to the pleural space. To enter the pleural space, the fibres may have to move across the mesothelium or between mesothelial cells. There fibres may be taken up by mesothelial cells. Other fibres, if free or within macrophages, may move in the pleural liquid flow to the lymphatic stomata where longer fibres may accumulate by mechanical means.

There, fibres induce a local inflammation and injury. Over the ensuing years of contact between the cells and fibres, a complex pathologic response is set in motion. Normally a nonproliferative tissue, the mesothelium is stimulated by proliferative signals generated by other asbestos-exposed cells in the lung and the pleura and perhaps by the stimulation of asbestos directly on the mesothelial cells. Reactive oxygen and reactive nitrogen species are generated from inflammatory cells, from the phagocytotic process of the asbestos-exposed cell or from the fibre itself.

Mesothelial cells may be stimulated as well as injured by these asbestos-induced direct and indirect stresses. The cell may initially respond by initiation of signalling cascades and of antioxidant cell defences. Additional responses may include release of inflammatory, mitogenic and clastogenic products. The cell may sustain DNA damage in two major ways, either from oxidant attack on DNA or from mechanical disruption of chromosomes. In the inflammatory environment, mesothelial cells that are stimulated to grow may be most susceptible to the genotoxic effects of fibres, either via oxidant effects on replicating DNA or via mechanical effects on segregating chromosomes. In response to DNA or chromosomal damage, the cell initiates a DNA damage response, arresting the cell cycle, upregulating repair enzymes, and excising/repairing DNA. If the cell stress is great or if the DNA is too severely damaged, the cell may die by necrosis or apoptosis. If cells fail to initiate the apoptotic pathway due to abnormalities in that pathway or to environmental survival signals, then damaged cells may survive with genetic abnormalities and thus initiate a multistep process toward malignancy.

The necessary characteristics of asbestos fibres and of mesothelial cells that leads to their carcinogenic interactions are still not understood. The fibrous shape and dimension of the fibres are clearly important parameters that determine damage. It also appears that the mesothelial cell is more susceptible to the toxic and genotoxic effects of asbestos than are other cells. The mesothelial cell remains poorly understood and, despite years of experimental studies, many mysteries still exist about the nature of the interaction of mesothelial cells with asbestos fibres that leads to mesothelioma.

Acknowledgements

We thank Dr Françoise Levy for her continuous support. This work was supported by NIH R01ES6331 and ES8985 and by INSERM funding.

References

1. Nishimura S.L. and V.C. Broaddus. Asbestos-induced pleural disease. *Clin Chest Med* 1998; **19**: 311–329.
2. Iwatsubo Y., J. C. Pairon, C. Boutin, O. Ménard, N. Massin, D. Caillaud, E. Orlowski, F. Galateau-Salle, J. Bignon and P. Brochard. Pleural mesothelioma: dose-response relation at low levels of asbestos exposure in a French population-based case-control study. *Am J Epidemiol* 1998; **148**: 133–142.
3. Lechner J. F., T. Tokiwa, M. LaVeck, W. F. Benedict, S. Banks-Schlegel, H. Yeager Jr., A. Banerjee and C. C. Harris. Asbestos-associated chromosomal changes in human mesothelial cells. *Proc Natl Acad Sci U S A* 1985; **82**: 3884–3888.
4. Gabrielson E. W., J. F. Lechner, B. I. Gerwin and C. C. Harris. Cultured human mesothelial cells are selectively sensitive to cell killing by asbestos and related fibres: a potential in vitro assay for carcinogenicity. In: *Mechanisms in Fibre Carcinogenesis*. J. A. H. R.C. Brown, N.F. Johnson, eds. New York, NY: Plenum Press, 1991; **223**: 505–511.
5. Churg A., B. Keeling, B. Gilks, S. Porter and P. Olive. Rat mesothelial and tracheal epithelial cells show equal DNA sensitivity to hydrogen peroxide-induced oxidant injury. *Am J Physiol* 1995; **268**: L832–L838.
6. Ollikainen T. R., K. I. Linnainmaa, K. O. Raivio and V. L. Kinnula. DNA single strand breaks and adenine nucleotide depletion as indices of oxidant effects on human lung cells. *Free Radic Biol Med* 1998; **24**: 1088–1096.
7. Galateau-Salle F., P. Bidet, Y. Iwatsubo, E. Gennetay, A. Renier, M. Letourneux, J. C. Pairon, S. Moritz, P. Brochard, M. C. Jaurand and F. Freymuth. SV40-like DNA sequences in pleural mesothelioma, bronchopulmonary carcinoma, and non-malignant pulmonary diseases. *J Pathol* 1998; **184**: 252–257.
8. Pooley F. D. Mineralogy of asbestos: the physical and chemical properties of the dusts they form. *Semin Oncol* 1981; **8**: 243–249.
9. Moalli P. A., J. L. MacDonald, L. A. Goodglick and A. B. Kane. Acute injury and regeneration of the mesothelium in response to asbestos fibres. *Am J Pathol* 1987; **128**: 426–445.
10. Stanton M. F. and C. Wrench. Mechanisms of mesothelioma induction with asbestos and fibrous glass. *J Natl Cancer Inst* 1972; **48**: 797–821.
11. Stanton F., M. Layard, A. Tegeris, E. Miller, M. May, E. Morgan and A. Smith. Relation of particle dimension to carcinogenicity in amphibole asbestos and other fibrous minerals. *J Natl Cancer Inst* 1981; **67**: 965–975.
12. Stanton M. F., M. Layard, A. Tegeris, E. Miller, M. May and E. Kent. Carcinogenicity of fibrous glass: pleural response in the rat in relation to fibre dimension. *J Natl Cancer Inst* 1977; **58**: 587–603.

13. Berman, D. W., K. S. Crump, E. J. Chatfield, J. M. Davis and A. D. Jones. The sizes, shapes and mineralogy of asbestos structures that induce lung tumors or mesothelioma in AF/HAN rats following inhalation. *Risk Anal* 1995; **15**: 181–195.

14. Hesterberg T. W. and J. C. Barrett. Dependence of asbestos- and mineral dust-induced transformation of mammalian cells in culture on fibre dimension. *Cancer Res* 1984; **44**: 2170–2180.

15. Yegles M., X. Janson, H. Y. Dong, A. Renier and M. C. Jaurand. Role of fibre characteristics on cytotoxicity and induction of anaphase/telophase aberrations in rat pleural mesothelial cells in vitro: correlations with in vivo animal findings. *Carcinogenesis* 1995; **16**: 2751–2758.

16. Janssen Y. M., J. P. Marsh, M. P. Absher, E. Gabrielson, P. J. Borm, K. Driscoll and B. T. Mossman. Oxidant stress responses in human pleural mesothelial cells exposed to asbestos. *Am J Respir Crit Care Med* 1994; **149**: 795–802.

17. Brown, R. C., J. A. Hoskins, K. Miller and B. T. Mossman. Pathogenetic mechanisms of asbestos and other mineral fibres. *Mol Aspects Med* 1990; **11**: 325–349.

18. Davis J.M. Mineral fibre carcinogenesis: experimental data relating to the importance of fibre type, size, deposition, dissolution and migration. *IARC Sci Publ* 1989; **90**: 33–45.

19. Wagner J. C., J. W. Skidmore, R. T. Hill and D. M. Griffiths. Erionite exposure and mesothelioma in rats. *Br J Cancer* 1985; **51**: 727–730.

20. Timblin C. R., G. D. Guthrie, Y. M. Janssen, E. S. Walsh, P. Vacek and B. T. Mossman. Patterns of c-fos and c-jun proto-oncogene expression, apoptosis, and proliferation in rat pleural mesothelial cells exposed to erionite or asbestos fibres. *Toxicol Appl Pharmacol* 1998; **151**: 88–97.

21. Hardy J. A. and A. E. Aust. Iron in asbestos chemistry and carcinogenicity. *Chem Rev* 1995; **95**: 97–118.

22. Desai R. and R. J. Richards. The adsorption of biological macromolecules by mineral dusts. *Environ Res* 1978; **16**: 449–464.

23. Jaurand M.-C., P. Baillif, J.-H. Thomassin, L. Magne and J.-C. Touray. X-ray photoelectron spectroscopy and chemical study of the adsorption of biological molecules on chrysotile asbestos surface. *J Colloid Interface Sci* 1983; **95**: 1–9.

24. Gan L., E. F. Savransky, T. M. Fasy and E. M. Johnson. Transfection of human mesothelial cells mediated by different asbestos fibre types. *Environ Res* 1993; **62**: 28–42.

25. Boylan, A. M., D. A. Sanan, D. Sheppard and V. C. Broaddus. Vitronectin enhances internalization of crocidolite asbestos by rabbit pleural mesothelial cells via the integrin $\alpha v \beta 5$. *J Clin Invest* 1995; **96**: 1987–2001.

26. Light W. G. and E. T. Wei. Surface charge and hemolytic activity of asbestos. *Environ Res* 1977; **13**: 135–145.

27. Brody, A. R., G. George and L. H. Hill. Interactions of chrysotile and crocidolite asbestos with red blood cell membranes: chrysotile binds to sialic acid. *Lab Invest* 1983; **49**: 468–475.

28. Koerten H. K., J. D. de Bruign and W. T. Daems. The formation of asbestos bodies by mouse peritoneal macrophages. *Am J Pathol* 1990; **137**: 121–134.

29. Warheit D. B., M. A. Hartsky and S. R. Frame. Pulmonary effects in rats inhaling size-separated chrysotile asbestos fibres or p-aramide fibrils: differences in cellular proliferative responses. *Toxicol Lett* 1996; **88**: 287–292.

30. Macdonald J. and A. Kane. Mesothelial cell proliferation and biopersistence of wollastonite and crocidolite asbestos fibres. *Fundam Appl Toxicol* 1997; **38**: 173–183.

31. BeruBe K. A., T. R. Quinlan, G. Moulton, D. Hemenway, P. O'Shaughnessy, P. Vacek and B. T. Mossman. Comparative proliferative and histopathologic changes in rat lungs after inhalation of chrysotile or crocidolite asbestos. *Toxicol Appl Pharmacol* 1996; **137**: 67–74.

32. Morgan A., A. Holmes and C. Gold. Studies of the solubility of constituents of chrysotile asbestos in vivo using radioactive tracer techniques. *Environ Res* 1971; **4**: 558–570.
33. Barrett J. C. Cellular and molecular mechanisms of asbestos carcinogenicity: implications for biopersistence. *Environ Health Perspect* 1994; **102** Suppl 5: 19–23.
34. Wang N.-S. Anatomy of the pleura. In: *Diseases of the Pleura.* V. B. Antony. Philadelphia, W.B. Saunders, 1998; **19**: 229–240.
35. Rennard S. I., M.-C. Jaurand, J. Bignon, O. Kawanami, V. J. Ferrans, J. Davidson and R. G. Crystal. Role of pleural mesothelial cells in the production of the submesothelial connective tissue matrix of lung. *Am Rev Respir Dis* 1984; **130**: 267–274.
36. Gerwin B. I., J. F. Lechner, R. R. Reddel, A. B. Roberts, K. C. Robbins, E. W. Gabrielson and C. C. Harris. Comparison of production of transforming growth factor-beta and platelet-derived growth factor by normal human mesothelial cells and mesothelioma cell lines. *Cancer Res* 1987; **47**: 6180–6184.
37. Lee T. C., Y. Zhang, C. Aston, R. Hintz, J. Jagirdar, M. A. Perle, M. Burt and W. N. Rom. Normal human mesothelial cells and mesothelioma cell lines express insulin-like growth factor I and associated molecules. *Cancer Res* 1993; **53**: 2858–2864.
38. Idell S., C. Zwieb, A. Kuman, K. B. Koenig and A. R. Johnson. Pathways of fibrin turnover of human pleural mesothelial cells in vitro. *Am J Respir Cell Mol Biol* 1992; **7**: 414–426.
39. Kumar A., K. B. Koenig, A. R. Johnson and S. Idell. Expression and assembly of procoagulant complexes by human pleural mesothelial cells. *Thromb Haemost* 1994; **71**: 587–592.
40. Shetty S., A. Kumar, A. R. Johnson and S. Idell. Regulation of mesothelial cell mitogenesis by antisense oligonucleotides for the urokinase receptor. *Antisense Res Dev* 1995; **5**: 307–314.
41. Jonjic N., G. Peri, S. Bernasconi, F. L. Sciacca, F. Colotta, P. G. Pelicci, L. Lanfrancone and A. Mantovani. Expression of adhesion molecules and chemotactic cytokines in cultured human mesothelial cells. *J Exp Med* 1992; **176**: 1165–1174.
42. Boylan, A. M., C. Rüegg, K. J. Kim, C. A. Hébert, J. M. Hoeffel, R. Pytela, D. Sheppard, I. M. Goldstein and V. C. Broaddus. Evidence of a role for mesothelial cell-derived interleukin-8 in the pathogenesis of asbestos-induced pleurisy in rabbits. *J Clin Invest* 1992; **89**: 1257–1267.
43. Antony, V. B., J. W. Hott, S. L. Kunkel, S. W. Godbey, M. D. Burdick and R. M. Strieter. Pleural mesothelial cell expression of C-C (monocyte chemotactic peptide) and C-X-C (interleukin-8) chemokines. *Am J Respir Cell Mol Biol* 1995; **12**: 581–588.
44. Yamada T., J. Jiping, R. Endo, M. Gotoh, Y. Shimosato and S. Hirohashi. Molecular cloning of a cell-surface glycoprotein that can potentially discriminate mesothelium from epithelium: its identification as vascular cell adhesion molecule 1. *Br J Cancer* 1995; **71**: 562–570.
45. Bittinger, F., C. L. Klein, C. Skarke, C. Brochhausen, S. Walgenbach, O. Rohrig, H. Kohler and C. J. Kirkpatrick. PECAM-1 expression in human mesothelial cells: an in vitro study. *Pathobiology* 1996; **64**: 320–327.
46. Simionescu M. and N. Simionescu. Organization of cell junctions in the peritoneal mesothelium. *J Cell Biol* 1977; **74**: 98–110.
47. Connell N. D. and J. G. Rheinwald. Regulation of the cytoskeleton in mesothelial cells: reversible loss of keratin and increase in vimentin during rapid growth in culture. *Cell* 1983; **34**: 245–253.
48. Laveck M. A., A. N. A. Somers, L. L. Moore, B. I. Gerwin and J. F. Lechner. Dissimilar peptide growth factors can induce normal human mesothelial cell multiplication. *In Vitro Cell Dev Biol* 1988; **24**: 1077–1084.
49. Gabrielson E. W., B. I. Gerwin, C. C. Harris, A. B. Roberts, M. B. Sporn and J. F. Lechner. Stimulation of DNA synthesis in cultured primary human mesothelial cells by specific growth factors. *FASEB J* 1988; **2**: 2717–2721.

50. Walker C., J. Everitt, P. C. Ferriola, W. Stewart, J. Mangum and E. Bermudez. Autocrine growth stimulation by transforming growth factor alpha in asbestos-transformed rat mesothelial cells. *Cancer Res* 1995; **55**: 530–536.

51. Amin, K. M., L. A. Litzky, W. R. Smythe, A. M. Mooney, J. M. Morris, D. J. Y. Mews, H. I. Pass, C. Kari, U. Rodeck, F. J. I. Rauscher, L. R. Kaiser and S. M. Albelda. Wilms' tumor 1 susceptibility (WT1) gene products are selectively expressed in malignant mesothelioma. *Am J Pathol* 1995; **146**: 344–356.

52. Chang K. and I. Pastan. Molecular cloning of mesothelin, a differentiation antigen present on mesothelium, mesotheliomas, and ovarian cancers. *Proc Nat Acad Sci U S A* 1996; **93**: 136–140.

53. Jaurand M.-C., H. Kaplan, J. Thiollet, M.-C. Pinchon, J.-F. Bernaudin and J. Bignon. Phagocytosis of chrysotile fibres by pleural mesothelial cells in culture. *Am J Pathol* 1979; **94**: 529–538.

54. Cole R. W., J. G. Ault, J. H. Hayden and C. L. Rieder. Crocidolite asbestos fibres undergo size-dependent microtubule-mediated transport after endocytosis in vertebrate lung epithelial cells. *Cancer Res* 1991; **51**: 4942–4947.

55. Rüttner J. R., A. B. Lang, D. R. Gut and M. U. Wydler. Morphological aspects of interactions between asbestos fibres and human mesothelial cell cytoskeleton. *Exp Cell Biol* 1987; **55**: 285–294.

56. Wang N. S., M. C. Jaurand, L. Magne, L. Kheuang, M. C. Pinchon and J. Bignon. The interactions between asbestos fibres and metaphase chromosomes of rat pleural mesothelial cells in culture: a scanning and transmission electron microscopic study. *Am J Pathol* 1987; **126**: 343–349.

57. Jaurand M. C. Mechanisms of action of fibres. *Carcinogenesis in Asbestos-related Cancer.* M. Sluyser, ed. New York, Ellis Horwood: 1991; 42–60.

58. Takeuchi T. and K. Morimoto. Crocidolite asbestos increased 8-hydroxyguanosine levels in cellular DNA of a human promyelocytic leukemia cell line, HL60. *Carcinogenesis* 1994; **15**: 635–639.

59. Costa M., J. Simmons-Hansen, C. W. Bedrossian, J. Bonura and R. M. Caprioli. Phagocytosis, cellular distribution, and carcinogenic activity of particulate nickel compounds in tissue culture. *Cancer Res* 1981; **41**: 2868–2876.

60. de Vries C. R., P. Ingram, S. R. Walker, R. W. Linton, W. F. Gutknecht and J. D. Shelburne. Acute toxicity of lead particulates on pulmonary alveolar macrophages. Ultrastructural and microanalytical studies. *Lab Invest* 1983; **48**: 35–44.

61. Hesterberg R. W., C. J. Butterick, M. Oshimura, A. R. Brody and J. C. Barrett. Role of phagocytosis in Syrian hamster cell transformation and cytogenetic effects induced by asbestos and short and long glass fibres. *Cancer Res* 1986; **46**: 5795–5802.

62. Chamberlain, M. and E. M. Tarmy Asbestos and glass fibres in bacterial mutation tests. *Mutat Res* 1977; **43**: 159–164.

63. Liu W., Ernst J. D. and Broaddus V. C. Phagocytosis of crocidolite asbestos induces oxidative stress, DNA damage and apoptosis in mesothelial cells. *Am J Respir Cell Mol Biol* 2000; **23**: 371–378.

64. Wu J., Liu W, Koenig K., Idell S. I. and Broaddus V. C. Vitronectin adsorption to chrysotile asbestos increases phagocytosis and toxicity for mesothelial cells. *Am J Physiol Lung Cell Mol Physiol* 2000; **279**: L916–L923.

65. Heintz N. H., Y. M. Janssen and B. T. Mossman. Persistent induction of c-fos and c-jun expression by asbestos. *Proc Natl Acad Sci U S A* 1993; **90**: 3299–3303.

66. Fung H., T. R. Quinlan, Y. M. Janssen, C. R. Timblin, J. P. Marsh, N. H. Heintz, D. J. Taatjes, P. Vacek, S. Jaken and B. T. Mossman. Inhibition of protein kinase C prevents asbestos-induced c-fos and c-jun proto-oncogene expression in mesothelial cells. *Cancer Res* 1997; **57**: 3101–3105.

67. Janssen Y. M., K. E. Driscoll, B. Howard, T. R. Quinlan, M. Treadwell, A. Barchowsky and B. T. Mossman. Asbestos causes translocation of p65 protein and increases NF-κB DNA-binding activity in rat lung epithelial and pleural mesothelial cells. *Am J Pathol* 1997; **151**: 389–401.

68. Zanella C. L., J. Posada, T. R. Tritton and B. T. Mossman. Asbestos causes stimulation of the extracellular signal-regulated kinase 1 mitogen-activated protein kinase cascade after phosphorylation of the epidermal growth factor receptor. *Cancer Res* 1996; **56**: 5334–5338.

69. Kuwahara M., M. Kuwahara, K. E. Bijwaard, D. M. Gersten, C. A. Diglio and E. Kagan. Mesothelial cells produce a chemoattractant for lung fibroblasts: role of fibronectin. *Am J Respir Cell Mol Biol* 1991; **5**: 256–264.

70. Tanaka S., N. Choe, D. R. Hemenway, S. Zhu, S. Matalon and E. Kagan. Asbestos inhalation induces reactive nitrogen species and nitrotyrosine formation in the lungs and pleura of the rat. *J Clin Invest* 1998; **102**: 445–454.

71. Perkins R. C., V. C. Broaddus, S. Shetty, S. Hamilton and S. Idell. Asbestos upregulates expression of the urokinase-type plasminogen activator receptor on mesothelial cells. *Am J Respir Cell Mol Biol* 1999; **21**: 637–646.

72. Gabrielson E. W., G. M. Rosen, R. C. Grafstrom, K. E. Strauss and C. C. Harris. Studies on the role of oxygen radicals in asbestos induced cytopathology of cultured human lung mesothelial cells. *Carcinogenesis* 1986; **7**: 1161–1164.

73. Kinnula V. L., K. Aalto, K. O. Raivo, S. Walles and K. Linnainmaa. Cytotoxicity of oxidants and asbestos fibres in cultured human mesothelial cells. *Free Radic Biol Med* 1994; **16**: 169–176.

74. Dong H. Y., A. Buard, A. Renier, F. Lévy, L. Saint-Etienne and M.-C. Jaurand. Role of oxygen derivatives in the cytotoxicity and DNA damage produced by asbestos on rat pleural mesothelial cells in vitro. *Carcinogenesis* 1994; **15**: 1251–1255.

75. Rabinovitch M. Professional and non-professional phagocytes: an introduction. *Trends Cell Biol* 1995; **5**: 85–87.

76. Renier A., F. Lévy, F. Pilliere and M. C. Jaurand. Unscheduled DNA synthesis in rat pleural mesothelial cells treated with mineral fibres. *Mutat Res* 1990; **241**: 361–367.

77. Dong H. Y., A. Buard, F. Levy, A. Renier, F. Laval and M. C. Jaurand. Synthesis of poly(ADP-ribose) in asbestos treated rat pleural mesothelial cells in culture. *Mutat Res* 1995; **331**: 197–204.

78. Fung H., Y. W. Kow, B. Van Houten, D. J. Taatjes, Z. Hatahet, Y. M. W. Janssen, P. Vacek, S. P. Faux and B. T. Mossman. Asbestos increases mammalian AP-endonuclease gene expression, protein levels and enzyme activity in mesothelial cells. *Cancer Res* 1998; **58**: 189–194.

79. Levresse V., A. Renier, J. Fleury-Feith, F. Levy, S. Moritz, C. Vivo, Y. Pilatte and M. C. Jaurand. Analysis of cell cycle disruptions in cultures of rat pleural mesothelial cells exposed to asbestos fibres. *Am J Respir Cell Mol Biol* 1997; **17**: 660–671.

80. Chen Q., J. Marsh, B. Ames and B. Mossman. Detection of 8-oxo-2'-deoxyguanosine, a marker of oxidative DNA damage, in culture medium from human mesothelial cells exposed to crocidolite asbestos. *Carcinogenesis* 1996; **17**: 2525–2527.

81. Fung H., Y. W. Kow, B. Van Houten and B. T. Mossman. Patterns of 8-hydroxydeoxyguanosine formation in DNA and indications of oxidative stress in rat and human pleural mesothelial cells after exposure to crocidolite asbestos. *Carcinogenesis* 1997; **18**: 825–832.

82. Ollikainen T., Linnainmaa K., and Kinnula V. L. DNA single strand breaks induced by asbestos fibres in human pleural mesothelial cells in vitro. *Environ Mol Mutagen* 1999; **33**: 153–160.

83. Levresse V., Renier A., Levy F., Broaddus V. C. and Jaurand M. DNA breakage in asbestos-treated normal and transformed (TSV40) rat pleural mesothelial cells. *Mutagenesis* 2000; **15**: 239–244.

84. Olofsson K. and J. Mark. Specificity of asbestos-induced chromosomal aberrations in short-term cultures of human mesothelial cells. *Cancer Genet Cytogenet* 1989; **41**: 33–40.

85. Jaurand M.-C., L. Kheuang, L. Magne and J. Bignon. Chromosomal changes induced by chrysotile fibres or benzo(3-4) pyrene in rat pleural mesothelial cells. *Mutat Res* 1986; **169**: 141–148.

86. Pelin K., A. Hirvonen, M. Taavitsainen and K. Linnainmaa. Cytogenetic response to asbestos fibres in cultured human primary mesothelial cells from 10 different donors. *Mutat Res* 1995; **334**: 225–233.

87. Pelin K., P. Kivipensas and K. Linnainmaa. Effects of asbestos and man-made vitreous fibres on cell division in cultured human mesothelial cells in comparison to rodent cells. *Environ Mol Mutagen* 1995; **25**: 118–125.

88. Yegles M., L. Saint-Etienne, A. Renier, Z. Janson and M.-C. Jaurand. Induction of metaphase and anaphase/telophase abnormalities by asbestos fibres in rat pleural mesothelial cells *in vitro. Am J Respir Cell Mol Biol* 1993; **9**: 186–191.

89. Lee W. C. and J. R. Testa. Somatic genetic alterations in human malignant mesothelioma. *Int J Oncol* 1999; **14**: 181–188.

90. Lechner J. F., J. Tesfaigzi and B. I. Gerwin. Oncogenes and tumor-suppressor genes in mesothelioma – a synopsis. *Environ Health Perspect* 1997; **105**: 1061–1067.

91. Bianchi A. B., S. Mitsunaga, J. Cheng, W. Klein, S. C. Jhanwar, B. Seizinger, N. Kley, A. Klein-Szanto and J. Testa. High frequency of inactivating mutations in the neurofibromatosis type 2 gene (NF2) in primary malignant mesothelioma. *Proc Natl Acad Sci U S A* 1995; **92**: 10854–10858.

92. Deguen B., L. Goutebroze, M. Giovannini, C. Boisson, R. Ven der Neut, M. C. Jaurand and G. Thomas. Heterogeneity of mesothelioma cell lines as defined by altered genomic structure and expression of the NF2 gene. *Int J Cancer* 1998; **77**: 554–560.

93. Sekido Y., H. I. Pass, B. S., D. J. Y. Mew, M. F. Christmas and A. F. Gazdar. Neurofibromatosis type 2 (NF2) gene is somatically mutated in mesothelioma but not in lung cancer. *Cancer Res* 1995; **55**: 1227–1231.

94. Gerwin B. I. Asbestos and the mesothelial cell: a molecular trail to mitogenic stimuli and suppressor gene suspects. *Am J Respir Cell Mol Biol* 1994; **11**: 507–508.

95. Narasimhan S. R., L. Yang, B. I. Gerwin and V. C. Broaddus. Resistance of pleural mesothelioma cell lines to apoptosis: relation to expression of Bcl-2 and Bax. *Am J Physiol Lung Cell Mol Physiol* 1998; **275**: L165–L171.

96. Broaddus, V. C., L. Yang, L. M. Scavo, J. D. Ernst and A. M. Boylan. Asbestos induces apoptosis of human and rabbit pleural mesothelial cells via reactive oxygen species. *J Clin Invest* 1996; **98**: 2050–2059.

97. Jimenez L. A., C. Zanella, H. Fung, Y. M. Janssen, P. Vacek, C. Charland, J. Goldberg and B. T. Mossman. Role of extracellular signal-regulated protein kinases in apoptosis by asbestos and H_2O_2. *Am J Physiol* 1997; **273**: L1029–L1035.

98. Goldberg J. L., C. L. Zanella, Y. M. W. Janssen, C. R. Timblin, L. A. Jimenez, P. Vacek, D. J. Taatjes and B. T. Mossman. Novel cell imaging techniques show induction of apoptosis and proliferation in mesothelial cells by asbestos. *Am J Respir Cell Mol Biol* 1997; **17**: 265–271.

99. Broaddus, V. C. Asbestos, the mesothelial cell and malignancy: a matter of life or death. *Am J Respir Cell Mol Biol* 1997; **17**: 657–659.

100. Marsella J. M., B. L. Liu, C. A. Vaslet and A. B. Kane. Susceptibility of p53-deficient mice to induction of mesothelioma by crocidolite asbestos fibres. *Environ Health Perspect* 1997; **105**: 1069–1072.

101. Levresse V., S. Moritz, A. Renier, L. Kheuang, F. Galateau-Salle, J. P. Mege, P. Piedbois, B. Salmons, W. Guenzburg and M. C. Jaurand. Effect of simian virus large T antigen expression on cell cycle control and apoptosis in rat pleural mesothelial cells exposed to DNA damaging agents. *Oncogene* 1998; **16**: 1041–1053.

102. Roggli V. L. and T. L. Benning. Asbestos bodies in pulmonary hilar lymph nodes. *Modern Pathol* 1990; **3**: 513–517.

103. Dodson R. F., M. G. Williams, C. J. Corn, A. Brollo and C. Bianchi. Asbestos content of lung tissue, lymph nodes, and pleural plaques from former shipyard workers. *Am Rev Respir Dis* 1990; **142**: 843–847.

104. Viallat J. R., F. Raybuad, M. Passarel and C. Boutin. Pleural migration of chrysotile fibres after intratracheal injection in rats. *Arch Environ Health* 1986; **41**: 282–286.

105. Choe N., S. Tanaka, W. Xia, D. R. Hemenway, V. L. Roggli and E. Kagan. Pleural macrophage recruitment and activation in asbestos-induced pleural injury. *Environ Health Perspect* 1997; **105** (Suppl 5): 1257–1260.

106. Broaddus, V. C., J. P. Wiener-Kronish, Y. Berthiaume and N. C. Staub. Removal of pleural liquid and protein by lymphatics in awake sheep. *J Appl Physiol* 1988; **64**: 384–390.

107. Fasske E. Pathogenesis of pulmonary fibrosis induced by chrysotile asbestos: longitudinal light and electron microscopic studies on the rat model. *Virchows Arch* 1986; **408**: 329–346.

108. Boutin, C., P. Dumortier, F. Rey, J. R. Viallat and P. DeVuyst. Black spots concentrate oncogenic asbestos fibres in the parietal pleura: thoracoscopic and mineralogic study. *Am J Respir Crit Care Med* 1996; **153**: 444–449.

109. Bryks, S. and F. D. Bertalanffy. Cytodynamic reactivity of the mesothelium. *Arch Environ Health* 1971; **23**: 469–472.

110. Adamson, I. Y. R., J. Bakowska, and D. H. Bowden. Mesothelial cell proliferation: a nonspecific response to lung injury associated with fibrosis. *Am J Respir. Cell Mol Biol* 1994; **10**: 253–258.

111. Adamson, I. Y. R., J. Bakowska, and D. H. Bowden. Mesothelial cell proliferation after instillation of long or short asbestos fibres into mouse lung. *Am J Pathol* 1993; **142**: 1209–1216.

112. Adamson, I. Y., H. Prieditis, and L. Young. Lung mesothelial cell and fibroblast responses to pleural and alveolar macrophage supernatants and to lavage fluids from crocidolite-exposed rats. *Am J Respir Cell Mol Biol* 1997; **16**: 650–656.

113. Kinnula V. L., K. O. Raivio, K. Linnainmaa, A. Ekman and M. Klockars. Neutrophil and asbestos fibre-induced cytotoxicity in cultured human mesothelial and bronchial epithelial cells. *Free Radic Biol Med* 1995; **18**: 391–399.

114. Hesterberg T. W., G. A. Hart, J. Chevalier, W. C. Miiler, R. D. Hamilton, J. Bauer and P. Thevenaz. The importance of fibre biopersistence and lung dose in determining the chronic inhalation effects of X607, RCF1, and chrysotile asbestos in rats. *Toxicol Appl Pharmacol* 1998; **153**: 68–82.

115. Marchi E., Liu W., Broaddus V.C. Mesothelial cell apoptosis is confirmed in vivo by morphological change in cytokeratin distribution. *Am J Physiol Lung Cell Mol Physiol* 2000; **278**: L528–535.

=16=

Novel Molecular, Epidemiological, and Therapeutic Issues in Mesothelioma: The Role of SV40

Michele Carbone, Amy Powers, Susan Fisher, Paola Rizzo, Robert Bright and Harvey I. Pass

The rise in mesothelioma cases that has occurred since 1950 has been associated with the widespread commercial use of asbestos. However, less than 10% of asbestos workers exposed to high levels of asbestos actually develop the disease, suggesting that additional factors may increase an individual's susceptibility to the carcinogenic effects of asbestos.[1] In addition, about 20% of mesotheliomas are not associated with asbestos exposure, suggesting that alternative factors may also cause mesothelioma. The occurrence of mesothelioma in children, although a rare event, also supports the possibility that mesothelioma is not solely caused by asbestos exposure.[2] Mesothelioma generally develops in adults at least 20 years after asbestos exposure. Thus, unless asbestos-related disease acts differently in children, cases of mesothelioma reported in children are not the result of asbestos exposure.

SV40

SV40 is a DNA tumour virus which was introduced into a significant portion of the human population between 1955 and 1963 through polio vaccines and adenovaccines contaminated with the virus.[3] By 1961, 80–90% of all US children under the age of 20 had received at least one polio vaccination potentially contaminated with SV40. In fact, during this nine-year distribution period, it is estimated that 98 million people – children *and* adults – may have been injected with an SV40-contaminated vaccine in the USA alone.[4] Although the vaccine substantially decreased the incidence of polio around the world, questions over its safety began to emerge. In 1960, Sweet and Hilleman demonstrated that SV40 contaminated both Salk and Sabin polio vaccines, which were prepared in the kidney cells of rhesus monkeys.[5] In 1962, Eddy reported that rhesus monkey cells infected with SV40 caused sarcoma when injected into hamsters,[6] and the intracranial injection of SV40 was found to cause ependymomas.[7] In parallel experiments in tissue culture, SV40 was shown to be capable of infecting and transforming hamster and other rodent, and human cells.[8]

While hamster and other rodent cells were found to be nonpermissive, meaning they could be transformed but could not support viral replication, it was determined that SV40 had different replication patterns in humans. Human cells were described as semi-permissive, as they could be both transformed and support low-level viral replication. The virus was proven capable of infecting humans when SV40-contaminated syncytial virus stocks given intranasally to volunteers caused SV40 infection.[9] In addition, in 1962, Shein and Enders found that SV40 could infect human cells in tissue culture, and that some of these cells became transformed.[10] Furthermore, in 1964, Jensen et al. determined that human cells transformed by SV40 and injected into human volunteers produced subcutaneous tumours.[11]

The ability of SV40 to transform cells and induce tumour formation is a function of the large tumour antigen (Tag), a 90 kDa protein produced by the virus that is found predominantly in the nuclei of SV40-infected and transformed cells.[8] Tag causes transformation by binding and inactivating the products of several tumour suppressor genes, including p53, pRb, p107, p130/Rb2, p300, and p400, which all prevent the cell from cycling. In uninfected cells, these tumour suppressor products must be inactivated by phosphorylation/dephosphorylation events to allow movement from G1 to S phase. Tag inactivates these proteins when binding to them, and thus allows the cell to cycle. In addition, Tag inactivates an essential checkpoint by inhibiting p53. p53 normally terminates mitosis in cells if DNA damage is detected. If the DNA is unable to be repaired, p53 then induces apoptosis. However, if p53 is complexed with and inactivated by Tag, the cell is able to continue to cycle even in the presence of DNA damage. Furthermore, Tag itself is able to cause DNA alterations, as it has been found to cause a number of chromosomal aberrations and aneuploidy. Aside from Tag, SV40 also produces a small t-antigen (tag), a protein found in the cytoplasm of infected and transformed cells. In addition to increasing the production of Tag, small t-antigen aids in inactivating p53 and stimulates mitosis in quiescent cells.[8]

Despite SV40's ability to transform both rodent and human cells, initial epidemiological studies concluded that the virus was not oncogenic in humans. However, only a few short-term studies were performed to determine if recipients of the contaminated polio vaccine developed a greater than average number of malignancies. In addition, only one long-term study investigated SV40's role in tumour incidence. In a longitudinal study, Mortimer et al. followed 1073 children inoculated with potentially contaminated polio vaccine for a period of 17–19 years.[12] No excess risk of mortality was observed in these children, as only one developed a malignancy. However, the authors cautioned that the 17–19 year follow-up may not have been sufficient to detect an increased risk of cancer in these children, as this time frame did not approach the 20–40 year latency period needed for other carcinogens to cause cancer. In addition, the small number of children used in the study would not allow accurate detection of an increased incidence of rare cancers. In a retrospective, cross-sectional study, Geissler, while in the German Federal Republic, compared cancer incidence in 885 783 people born between 1959 and 1961, 86% of whom were assumed to have been vaccinated with contaminated polio vaccines, to that of 891 321 people born between 1962 and 1964, the majority of whom were assumed to have been inoculated with SV40-free vaccines.[13] This study did not detect an overall difference in cancer incidence between the two groups. However, in the SV40-exposed cohort, many people were unlikely to have received contaminated polio vaccines, as not all lots were contaminated. The viral titer also differed among batches of the vaccine, so those who received contaminated polio vaccinations did not necessarily receive the same amounts of virus. Most importantly, 14% of those born in the SV40-exposed cohort were not vaccinated at all. Furthermore, in the presumed unexposed cohort, some of the individuals may have received contaminated vaccines, since distribution continued until 1963. Despite these limitations, the study concluded that the contaminated vaccines did not affect overall cancer rates in humans. However, it was not possible to exclude an increase in certain types of rare tumours that would not be detected through this study. Of interest, an increase of certain types of brain tumours was noted, and SV40 DNA was detected by Southern blotting hybridisation in 14 out of 53 brain tumours of different histology from the 'presumably' contaminated group (1959–1961), and SV40 large T antigen (Tag) expression in 18 out of 60 in the same group. Among people vaccinated after 1961, only one meningioma from a 6-year-old girl contained and expressed SV40.[13]

SV40 and hamsters

Despite reports that SV40-contaminated vaccines have not increased cancer incidence, there are recent studies that have associated SV40 with a variety of rare human and animal neoplasms. In a study done in our laboratory, 60% of hamsters injected intracardially with SV40 developed pleural mesotheliomas.[14] These results were surprising, since viruses had never been associated with mesotheliomas in mammals. Furthermore, when we injected SV40 into the pleural space, 100% of the animals developed mesothelioma in 3–6 months. SV40 injected into the femoral vein,[15] intracerebrally[7] or subcutaneously,[16] however, did not result in mesothelioma development. These findings suggest that SV40 reached the pericardium and/or pleura through the external surface of the needle during intracardial injection, and therefore that only a small amount of SV40 is needed to cause malignant mesothelioma.

SV40 and human tumours

The discovery that SV40 produced tumours in hamsters led to the PCR analysis of human mesotheliomas for the presence of SV40. Our group was the first to investigate whether there was any correlation between Polyomavirus and mesothelioma, and this was accomplished in two separate series of patients.[17,18] DNA was extracted from 48 frozen human mesothelioma specimens and 2 benign fibrous tumours of pleura (FTP) from patients undergoing resection of their tumours at the National Cancer Institute, Bethesda, Maryland. In 28 instances, the corresponding DNA was extracted from lung tissue not infiltrated with mesothelioma. To reduce the chance of PCR carry-over or contamination, DNA and PCR reactions were prepared in one building, while PCR amplifications, gel electrophoreses, and Southern blot hybridisations were performed in a separate building.

DNA was first assessed for PCR analysis by a control reaction designed to amplify the IgG gamma chain using primers AG1 and AG2 as described by Bergsagel.[19] Next, to amplify a 105 bp fragment of the SV40 early region that codes for Tag, we used the primers SV.for3 and SV.rev (Figure 16.1). Genomic DNA from the SV40-induced hamster mesothelioma tumour H9A was used as a positive control. When the PCR products were investigated by Southern blot, 29 of the 48 mesothelioma samples (60%) contained sequences of 105 bp that hybridised with a specific probe under high stringency (Figure 16.2). The 2 FTP as well as 27 of the 28 lungs did not hybridise.

To resolve ambiguities regarding the possible confusion with other papovaviruses, mesothelioma samples were analysed by direct DNA sequencing with the primers Pyv.for and Pyv.rev. These primers were previously described by Bergsagel *et al.* to identify SV40-like sequences in human ependymomas.[19] These primers amplify a 172 bp region of Tag containing the Rb-family binding domain common to several papovaviruses including SV40. The SV40 sequence, however, can be distinguished from the other papovaviruses because it lacks a 9 bp insert between positions 4516 and 4517. The sequences obtained from our three mesothelioma specimens lacked this 9 bp insert and were 95–97% homologous to SV40.

Frozen specimens from 14 mesothelioma samples were evaluated immunohistochemically, and 11 of these revealed Tag nuclear staining (Figure 16.3). The percentage of Tag positive tumour cells varied from 1% to 50%, and varied not only from specimen to specimen, but within a given specimen. Nine of these 11 Tag positive specimens contained SV40-like sequences. In two cases, viral sequences could not be detected despite the presence of Tag immunoreactivity. Since differing papovavirus Tags share antigenicity, the possibility that these specimens contained a different DNA virus has been considered. The other 3 Tag negative samples did not contain detectable SV40-like sequences.

To confirm the specificity of the immunohistochemical reaction, we attempted to immunoprecipitate Tag from 5 mesothelioma samples that contained SV40-like sequences and were positive for Tag staining. A band with a molecular weight of approximately 90 kDa that specifically reacted with a monoclonal anti-Tag antibody was immunoprecipi-

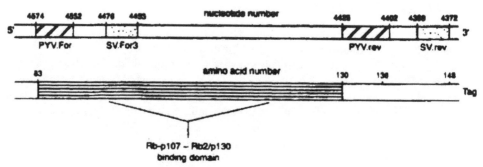

Figure 16.1. *Oligonucleotide primers used for PCR amplification of the RB-p107-RB2/130 binding domain of SV40 Tag.*

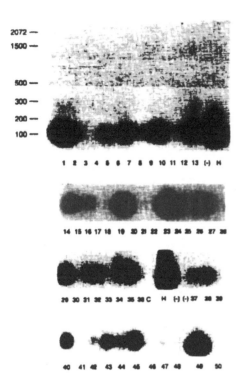

2072 —
1500 —
500 —
300 —
200 —
100 —

1 2 3 4 5 6 7 8 9 10 11 12 13 (-) H

14 15 16 17 18 19 20 21 22 23 24 25 26 27 28

29 30 31 32 33 34 35 36 C   H (-)(-) 37   38 39

40 41 42 43 44 45 46 47 48   49   50

Figure 16.2. Hybridisation of PCR amplified DNA from mesotheliomas to a probe specific for SV40 Tag sequences. Primers used were those described in Figure 16.1. H, SV40 induced hamster mesothelioma (positive control).

tated from all five mesotheliomas. Overall, of 16 different mesothelioma specimens evaluated for Tag-like expression, 13 (81%) were positive (Figure 16.4).

We have analysed an additional 42 mesotheliomas to determine: 1. whether our initial observations could be verified in a different set of mesothelioma tumours; and 2. the extent to which the SV40 genome is present in mesotheliomas.[20] Genomic DNA in this second series of tumours was extracted by a protocol of Butel to ensure that episomal DNA would be recovered. PCR primers were used to amplify two regions of the SV40 large T-antigen (Tag) *amino terminus* fragment containing the Rb pocket binding region, a 281 bp *carboxyl terminus* fragment, and a 310 bp fragment of the *enhancer promoter* region. Endonuclease digestions and Southern blotting were used to verify the expected product. Thirty of the 42 (71%) samples amplified Tag amino sequences, and specificity was verified by Southern hybridisation, and, as opposed to the first series of 48 mesotheliomas, 93% of the specimens hybridised with the specific probe.

Sixteen of 42 samples (38%) amplified the appropriate size fragment for the carboxyl terminus, and digestion with BsaB1 matched that of H9A while 22 of 42 samples (52%) amplified SV40 enhancer promoter sequences and FokI digestion matched that of the hamster control tumour. Sequence analysis of the enhancer promoter regions in 4 patients revealed 100% homology with the enhancer promoter region of wild-type SV40 strain 776.

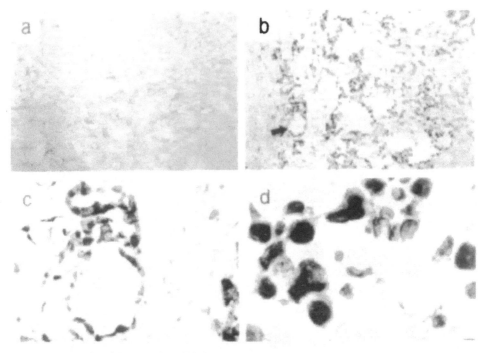

Figure 16.3. Histochemical reactivity of Tag in human malignant pleural meso-thelioma: (a) control, (b) staining with Tag monoclonal, × 20, (c) × 40, (d) × 63. Note intranuclear Tag staining and lack of staining of normal stroma.

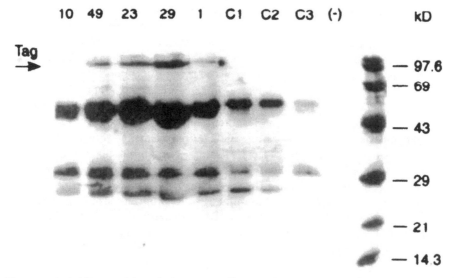

Figure 16.4. Western blot of 5 human malignant pleural mesothelioma tumor samples for Tag. C1 and C2, negative controls; (–), empty lane.

These results were soon independently confirmed by Cristaudo *et al.*, who found SV40 sequences in 72% of the mesothelioma specimens they tested,[21] and later, other labs also obtained similar results.[22-26]

These findings were the first to reveal an association of a DNA virus with *thoracic* malignancy, and, as such, have raised considerable controversy. The presence of SV40-like sequences and Tag expression in human mesotheliomas does not by itself establish a cause and effect relationship to the development of the tumour, but raises further issues regarding 'conventional wisdom' for the pathogenesis of mesothelioma and its relationship to asbestos. To investigate if SV40 played a causative role in mesothelioma development, we studied the ability of Tag to bind and inactivate p53 and other tumour suppressors in these tumours.[8] RNA *in situ* hybridisation, immunohistochemistry, and Western blot experiments indicated that Tag was able to bind, stabilise, and inactivate wild-type p53 in the mesotheliomas studied. In addition, De Luca *et al.*, in an analysis of mesothelioma samples, found that Tag was able to bind and inactivate the tumour suppressors pRB, p107, and pRB2/p130.[23] Thus, SV40 Tag found in mesothelioma samples targets and inactivates p53 and members of the retinoblastoma family, and this interaction may contribute to the development of mesothelioma, especially in people exposed to asbestos.[27]

In a recent collaboration with Kaija Linnainmaa at the Finnish Occupational Health Institute, we were unable to detect SV40 in Finnish mesothelioma specimens.[28] In light of our earlier finding that the presence of SV40 in human bone tumours differs depending on the geographic region from which the tumour specimen was obtained,[29] our inability to detect SV40 in the Finnish mesotheliomas suggests geographic differences for the presence of SV40 in human tumours. These differences may be related to the fact that the Finnish polio vaccines were not contaminated with SV40, or may be related to other presently unknown factors.

Epidemiology

Epidemiological studies investigating the incidence of specific types of cancer reported to contain SV40 DNA, such as mesothelioma, osteosarcoma, and ependymoma, are difficult to conduct due to the poor quality of existing data resources concerning cancer mortality. Available databases include the national mortality statistics, the Connecticut Tumor Registry, and the Surveillance, Epidemiology, and End Results Program (SEER). National mortality data provide population data about causes of death as reported on death certificates, but are not necessarily an accurate reflection of cancer incidence. The Connecticut Cancer Registry, established in 1935, includes incidence data and tumour histology from every cancer patient within the state. However, it is difficult to make general claims about cancer incidence using information from this registry, since SV40 exposure and cancer rates in the small, homogeneous state of Connecticut may not be representative of the entire USA. Trends related to rare tumours, such as mesothelioma, may also be imprecise, due to the small population considered. The SEER database provides the best representation of cancer incidence in the USA, since it provides tumour-specific information on all histologically proven malignancies occurring in selected geographic sites throughout the USA. The sample used represents approximately 12% of the USA population and is thought to represent the general characteristics of residents in the USA.[4]

Recently, in a retrospective cohort study done by Strickler *et al.*, data from the SEER program (1973–1993), the Connecticut Tumor Registry (1950–1969), and national mortality statistics (1947–1973) were used to compare specific cancer rates in SV40-exposed versus unexposed cohorts.[30] Strickler *et al.* compared three cohorts: 1. individuals likely to have been injected with SV40-contaminated polio vaccine as infants, born between 1956 and 1962; 2. individuals likely to have been injected with the contaminated vaccine as children, born between 1947 and 1952; and 3. individuals unlikely to have been vaccinated with contaminated vaccine, born between 1964 and 1969. It was concluded that after 30 years of follow-up, exposure to SV40-contaminated polio vaccine was not associated with a significant increase of ependymoma, osteosarcoma, or mesothelioma. In the case of mesothelioma, however, the study determined that children injected with potentially contaminated polio vaccines had an increased risk. However, the overall low number of mesotheliomas in children limited these analyses, which did not reach statistical significance. It was stated that the cohorts studied did not reach the age at which most mesotheliomas occur, resulting in imprecise estimates of risk. Because the number of mesotheliomas developing in children of the cohorts studied was not stated, we searched this number in the SEER database and found that there were just two cases of mesothelioma among the unexposed cohort as compared with 45 and 23 in the childhood and infancy exposed groups respectively. The higher rate of mesotheliomas in children vaccinated with SV40 could be related to SV40 or to the fact that older people are included in these cohorts. Thus, it is difficult to make conclusions using this data.

In conclusion, simply considering tumour incidence may lead to inaccurate findings concerning the relationship between SV40-contaminated vaccines and the incidence of certain human tumours. Furthermore, it is now known that different batches of vaccines contained different amounts of SV40. This complicates the interpretation of these analyses, because SV40 carcinogenesis, at least in hamsters, is dose-related (i.e., only people who received highly contaminated SV40 vaccines could be at higher risk for cancer). However, it is possible to state that the available SEER data indicate that SV40 exposure through the contaminated polio vaccines is unlikely to have caused cancer directly.

It would be highly unlikely, however, that SV40 'per se' caused cancer, because most, if not all, of the known human carcinogens require additional factors to cause cancer. SV40 may 'just' inhibit Rb and p53, in mesothelial cells, possibly rendering infected people more susceptible to asbestos carcinogenicity. The possibility that people infected with SV40 are at higher risk of developing mesothelioma if exposed to asbestos is intriguing. In spite of the fact that the risk of asbestos exposure was first noted in workers within the asbestos industry, a large proportion of cases now occur in workers in other occupations where exposure may be higher than that of the normal population, but the levels of exposure are much lower than those classically found in asbestos miners. The high proportion of carpenters, electricians and construction workers among current mesothelioma patients is probably a reflection of this. If SV40 and asbestos are co-carcinogens, people who are SV40 positive might be at a higher risk of developing mesothelioma when exposed to asbestos. Therefore, among workers at some risk of developing mesothelioma, it might be possible to detect those at higher risk and to develop some strategies that reduce their risk. The possibility that SV40 is a co-carcinogen with asbestos does not exclude that SV40 could also contribute directly to mesothelioma development in mesothelioma patients without asbestos exposure. Occasionally, multiple cases of mesotheliomas have been detected in the same family; it seems possible, and it would be of great interest to study, that SV40 contributed to the development of these mesotheliomas. If SV40 potentiates the carcinogenicity of asbestos, it may also play a role in the other tumour types that contain SV40 sequences – for example, choroid plexus tumours, ependymomas, and bone tumours.

The potential for mesothelioma therapy in the future

Although the role that SV40 plays in the development of human malignancies is under investigation, its presence in these human tumours raises the possibility of its use as a therapeutic target. The differential expression of SV40 Tag is fortunate, in that a viral-encoded tumour specific antigen (SV40 Tag) represents a foreign protein and an immunologic target for potential cancer vaccines. Investigators have already employed a murine SV40-tumour model to demonstrate the ability to protect animals against a lethal tumour challenge with syngeneic SV40 Tag positive tumour cells by vaccination with either recombinant, purified SV40 Tag protein[31] synthetic peptides corresponding to putative B cell epitopes on SV40 Tag[32] or plasmid DNA containing the gene for SV40 Tag.[33] Recently, a vaccine virus construct containing a safety modified SV40 Tag was developed, which when injected into mice elicited a cytotoxic T lymphocyte response against syngeneic SV40 Tag-expressing tumours.[34] Immunisation of these mice with a single dose of the vaccination resulted in protection against subsequent injection of a lethal mouse cancer expressing SV40 Tag. Administration of the vaccine with IL-2 produced a therapeutic effect against pre-administered Tag-containing tumour cells. These results indicate that vaccination with a modified Tag-expressing construct can provide a potent immunologic response in mice, which may allow for a similar therapy for human cancers associated with SV40.

These vaccination studies confirm the efficacy of inducing SV40 Tag specific protective tumour immunity *in vivo*, as well as the feasibility of targeting SV40 Tag for the immunotherapy of lethal tumours that express SV40 Tag. Evidence for the induction of SV40 Tag specific T cell responses has been demonstrated in this murine SV40 tumour model supporting the established importance of T cell induction for the specific immunologic destruction of tumour cells. Recent advances in the field of tumour immunology have demonstrated that human T cells can recognise and destroy human tumours, and that immunotherapy can be beneficial for some patients with advanced melanoma or kidney cancer. To facilitate the development of reagents and clinical protocols for T-cell-based immunotherapy of SV40-associated human malignancies (e.g., malignant pleural mesothelioma or osteosarcoma), it will be beneficial to characterise the anti-SV40 Tag cellular immune response and identify peptide epitopes on SV40

Tag recognized by cytotoxic T cells from the SV40 Balb/c tumour model for subsequent *in vivo* evaluation of T-cell transfer therapies and peptide-based vaccines. Finally, molecular approaches are being developed at the NCI to treat SV40-positive tumours.[35]

References

1. Carbone, M., Kratzke, R.A., and Testa J.R. The pathogenesis of mesothelioma. *Semin Oncol* (in press).
2. Cooper, S.P., Fraire, A.E., Buffler, P.A., Greenberg, S.D., and Lanston, C. Epidemiologic aspects of childhood mesothelioma. *Pathol Immunopathol Res* 1989; **8**: 276–286.
3. Carbone, M., SV40: From monkeys to humans. *Semin Cancer Biol* 2001; **11**: 1–3.
4. Klein, G., Powers, A., Croce, C. Association of SV40 with human tumours. *Oncogene* (in press).
5. Sweet, B.H. and Hilleman, R.M. The vacuolating virus SV40. *Proc Soc Exp Biol Med* 1960; **105**: 420–427.
6. Eddy, B.E., Borman, G.S., Berkeley, W.H., and Young, R.D. Tumors induced in hamsters by injection of rhesus monkey kidney cell extracts. *Proc Soc Exp Biol Med* 1961; **107**: 191–197.
7. Gerber, P. and Kirschsten, R.L. SV40 induced ependymomas in newborn hamster. I. Virus–tumor relationships. *Virology* 1962; **18**: 582–588.
8. Carbone, M., Rizzo, P., Grimley, P.M., Procopio, A., Mew, D.J., Shridhar, V., de Bartolomeis, A., Esposito, V., Giuliano, M.T., Steinberg, S.M., Levine, A.S., Giordano, A., and Pass, H.I. Simian virus-40 large-T antigen binds p53 in human mesotheliomas. *Nat Med* 1997; **3**: 908–912.
9. Morris, J.A., Johnson, K.M., Aulisio, C.G., Chanock, R.M., and Knight, V. Clinical and serologic responses in volunteers given vacuolating virus (SV40) by respiratory route. *Proc Soc Exp Biol Med* 1961; **108**: 56–59.
10. Shein, H.M. and Enders, J.F. Transformation induced by simian virus 40 in human renal cell cultures. Morphology and growth characteristics. *Proc Natl Acad Sci U S A* 1962; **48**: 1164–1169.
11. Jensen, F., Koprowski, H., Pagano, J.S., Ponten, J., and Ravdin, R.G. Autologous and homologous implantation of human cells transformed in vitro by SV40. *J Natl Cancer Inst* 1964; **32**: 917–925.
12. Mortimer, E.A., Lepow, M.L., Gold, E., Robbins, F.C., Burton, G.J., and Fraumeni, J.F. Long-term follow-up of persons inadvertently inoculated with SV40 as neonates. *N Engl J Med* 1981; **305**: 1517–1518.
13. Geissler, E. SV40 and human brain tumors. *Prog Med Virol* 1990; **37**: 211–222.
14. Cicala, C., Pompetti, F., and Carbone, M. SV40 induces mesotheliomas in hamsters. *Am J Pathol* 1993; **142**: 1524–1533.
15. Diamandopoulous, G.T. Leukemia, lymphoma and osteosarcoma induced in the Syrian golden hamster by simian virus 40. *Science* 1972; **176**: 73–75.
16. Eddy, B.E. Simian virus 40: an oncogenic virus. *Prog Exp Tumor Res* 1964; **4**: 1–26.
17. Carbone, M., Pass, H.I., Rizzo, P., Marinetti, M., Di Muzio, M., Mew, D.J.Y., Levine, A.S., and Procopio, A. Simian virus 40-like DNA sequences in human pleural mesothelioma. *Oncogene* 1994; **9**: 1781–1790.
18. Pass, H.I., Donington, J.S., Wu, P., Rizzo, P., Nishimura, M., Kennedy, R.C., and Carbone, M. Human mesotheliomas contain the simian virus 40 regulatory region and large tumor antigen DNA sequences. *J Thorac Cardiovasc Surg* 1998; **116**: 854–9.

19. Bergsagel, D.J., Finegold, M.J., Butel, J.S., Kupsky, W.J., and Garcea, R. DNA sequences similar to those of simian virus 40 in ependymomas and choroid plexus tumors of childhood. *N Engl J Med* 1992; **36**: 988–993.
20. Pass, H., Rizzo, P., Donington, J., Wu, P., and Carbone, M. Further validation of SV40-like DNA in human pleural mesotheliomas. *Dev Biol Stand* 1998; **94**: 143–145.
21. Cristaudo, A., Vivaldi, A., Sensales, G., Guglielmi, G., Ciancia, E., Elisei, R., and Ottenga, F. Molecular biology studies on mesothelioma tumor samples: preliminary data on H-ras, p21, and SV40. *J Environ Path Toxicol Oncol* 1995; **14**: 29–34.
22. Testa, J.R., Giordono, A. SV40 and cell cycle perturbations in malignant mesothelioma. *Semin Cancer Biol* 2001; **11**: 73–80.
23. De Luca, A., Baldi, A., Esposito, V., Howard, C.M., Bagella, L., Rizzo, P., Caputi, M., Pass, H.I., Giordano, G.G., Baldi, F., Carbone, M., and Giordano, A. The retinoblastoma gene family pRb/p105, p107, pRb2/p130 and simian virus-40 large T-antigen in human mesotheliomas. *Nat Med* 1997; **3**: 913–916.
24. Griffiths, D. and Weiss, R. Simian virus 40: a possible human polyomavirus workshop. National Institutes of Health, Bethesda, MD, 27–28 January 1997. **1**: 171–176. Washington, DC, SAG, Corp.
25. Galateau-Salle, F., Bidet, P., Iwatsubo, Y., Gennetay, E., Renier, A., Letourneux, M., Pairon, J.C., Moritz, S., Brochard, P., Jaurand, M.C., and Freymuth, F. SV40-like DNA sequences in pleural mesothelioma, bronchopulmonary carcinoma, and non-malignant pulmonary diseases. *J Pathol* 1998; **184**: 252–257.
26. Testa, J.R., Carbone, M., Hirvonen, A., Khalili, K., Krynska, B., Linnainmaa, K., Pooley, F.D., Rizzo, P., Rusch, V., and Xiao, G.H. A multi-institutional study confirms the presence and expression of simian virus 40 in human malignant mesotheliomas. *Cancer Res* 1998; **58**: 4505–4509.
27. Wiman, K. G. and Klein, G. An old acquaintance resurfaces in human mesothelioma. Nat Med 1997; **3**: 839–840.
28. Hirvonen, A., Mattson K., Karjalainen, A., Ollikainen, T., Tammilehto, L., Hovi, T., Vainio, H., Pass H.I., Di Resta, I., Carbone, M., and Linnainmaa, K. Simian virus 40 (SV40)-like DNA sequences not detectably in Finnish mesothelioma patients not exposed to SV40-contaminated polio vaccines. *Mol Carcinog* 1999; **26**: 93–99.
29. Carbone, M., Rizzo, P., Procopio, A., Giuliano, M., Pass, H.I., Gebhardt, M.C., Mangham, C., Hansen, M., Malkin, D.F., Bushart, G., Pompetti, F., Picci, P., Levine, A.S., Bergsagel, J.D., and Garcea, R.L. SV40-like sequences in human bone tumors. *Oncogene* 1996; **13**: 527–535.
30. Strickler, H.D., Rosenberg, P.S., Devesa, S.S., Hertel, J., Fraumeni, J.F., Jr., and Goedert, J.J. Contamination of poliovirus vaccines with simian virus 40 (1955–1963) and subsequent cancer rates. *JAMA* 1998; **279**: 292–295.
31. Shearer, M.H., Bright, R.K., Lanford, R.E., and Kennedy, R.C. Immunization of mice with baculovirus derived recombinant SV40 large tumor antigen induces protective immunity to a lethal challenge with SV40 transformed cells. *Clin Exp Immunol* 1993; **91**: 266–271.
32. Bright, R.K., Shearer, M.H., and Kennedy, R.C. Immunization of BALB/c mice with recombinant simian virus 40 large tumor antigen induces antibody dependent cell mediated cytotoxicity against simian virus 40 transformed cells: an antibody based mechanism for tumor immunity. *J Immunol* 1994; **153**: 2064–2071.
33. Bright, R.K., Shearer, M.H., Pass, H.I., and Kennedy, R.C. Immunotherapy of SV40 induced tumours in mice: a model for vaccine development. *Dev Biol Stand* 1998; **94**: 341–353.

34. Xie, Y. C., Hwang, C., Overwijk, W, Mule, J. J., and Sanda, M. G. Induction of tumor anti-gen-specific immunity in vivo by a novel vaccinia vector encoding safety modified simian virus 40 T antigen. *J Nat Cancer Inst* 1999; **91**: 169–175.
35. Schrump, D.S., and Waheed, I. Strategies to circumvent SV40 oncoprotein expression in malignant pleural mesotheliomas. *Semin Cancer Biol* 2001; **11**: 73–80.

=17=

The Molecular Pathogenesis of Mesothelioma

Blair R. Mclaren and Bruce W. S. Robinson

Significant advances have been made in the last 10 to 20 years in the understanding of how tumours arise and progress. The rapidly expanding field of molecular biology has been a major factor in these advances. Using the many new tools developed in this discipline we can now investigate changes at a genetic level looking at such things as growth factors, oncogenes and tumour suppressor genes. Already these approaches have opened up potential new therapeutic fields for the management of solid tumours including the use of monoclonal antibodies, gene therapy and antisense oligonucleotides.

Such advances are welcome for a tumour such as malignant mesothelioma (MM). Traditional therapeutic modalities such as surgery, radiotherapy and chemotherapy have been infrequently successful and demonstrate scant evidence of any prolongation of life. While continuing attempts to use these standard treatments optimally are important, it seems likely that the key to significant progress in the management of this tumour will be to improve our understanding of how the disease arises, and what features it possesses which enable it to maintain a growth advantage over normal cells.

The aim of this chapter therefore is to outline what is already known about the pathogenesis of MM. Other chapters have discussed the role of asbestos and other potentially important factors such as simian virus 40 (SV40) and while these will be briefly mentioned in this chapter, the focus will be on factors at a cellular level which may be important in the development of this uncommon tumour.

Asbestos – the dominant carcinogen

Following the original description of the association between asbestos exposure and MM in 1960 by Wagner (see Chapter 4),[1] it was rapidly accepted that this was the major causative factor in the development of MM. Although there has been some debate about the amount of exposure required to cause disease, it is also generally accepted that the duration and cumulative levels of asbestos exposure correlate with the risk of developing MM.[2]

Asbestos types and MM

Animal studies indicate that asbestos is a complete carcinogen, acting as both an initiator and promoter of carcinogenesis. There are two main types of asbestos, long, thin fibres (amphiboles) and leafy, sheet-like fibres (chrysotiles). In humans, it is generally believed that the amphibole forms of asbestos, particularly crocidolite, are the most carcinogenic forms.[3] Experimentally, both types of asbestos fibres have been found to be equally mutagenic to mesothelial cells, but in these studies chrysotile had generally been introduced intrapleurally. The shape of chrysotile fibres makes it difficult for them to penetrate the lung parenchyma deeply enough by inhalation *in vivo*, however. Most investigators attribute the MM that occurs with exposure to chrysotiles to contaminating amphiboles, such as tremolite.

Initial events

Animal studies in which asbestos fibres were injected into the peritoneum have shown initial macrophage activation[4] with resulting inflammation and cytokine production. In response to the release of cytokines such as TNF-α, the mesothelial cells proliferate and induce collagen synthesis.[5] This results in granulomatous lesions consisting of the asbestos fibres surrounded by a dense acellular collagen layer, a layer of mesenchymal cells and a surface layer of mesothelium.[6]

DNA and chromosomal damage

In vitro experiments have shown that the presence of asbestos fibres causes the production of reactive oxygen species, a scenario that would normally result in apoptosis.[7,8] The uptake of crocidolite by cells leads to the generation of iron-catalysed reactive oxygen metabolites and the presence of iron on the fibres appears to increase DNA damage. In early exposure it seems that activated macrophages release the majority of free radicals generated and only later do mesothelial cells contribute to production. These free radicals have direct toxic effects causing DNA point mutations, strand breaks and chromosomal breaks.[9] Asbestos fibres themselves may cause chromosomal spindle formation leading directly to karyotypic changes.

Asbestos and apoptosis

The avoidance of apoptosis may lead to survival of abnormal cells. It has been shown that while asbestos fibres induce apoptosis in mesothelial cells,[10] MM cells have a significantly higher resistance to asbestos cytotoxicity.[11] The combination of direct mitotic damage to cells by asbestos,[12] selection for apoptosis resistance and the increased proliferation associated with inflammation has led to speculation that the end result is an increased likelihood of cells with mutations surviving and proliferating, eventually leading to the development of mesothelioma. Asbestos also causes the upregulation of manganese superoxide dismutase, a superoxide radical scavenging agent[13] and AP-endonuclease, a DNA repair enzyme, in mesothelial cells.[14] While these are probably an attempted adaptive response to the toxic effects of asbestos fibres, apoptosis induced by asbestos has been shown to be inhibited by superoxide dismutase in the presence of catalase.[8] The high levels of these agents and of hydrogen peroxide scavenging antioxidant enzymes such as glutathione and glutathione-S-transferase (g-s-t) may be some of the reasons for the subsequent chemoresistance of MM.[15]

Other potential carcinogens

As has been discussed in another chapter, the recent discovery of SV40-like sequences in around 60% of human MM tissue samples[16] raises the possibility that this virus may act as a co-carcinogen in the development of mesothelioma. The T antigen (TAG) of SV40 in MM has been shown to retain the ability to inactivate the tumour suppressors p53[17] and the retinoblastoma protein (pRb).[18] While not all investigators have found SV40 sequences in MM tissue,[19] there have been several further studies which confirm Carbone's findings.[18,20,21] Further investigation of this area could well prove illuminating.

Around 25% of people with MM have no known history of contact with asbestos. A proportion of these cases has probably had occult exposure but it is likely that there is a subset of patients who have had no asbestos exposure. Other agents that have been proposed as carcinogens include thoracic radiotherapy,[22] intrapleural thorium dioxide[23] and other silicates including erionite and zeolite, but these are not all universally accepted.

Genetic predisposition

There have been reported clusters of MM within families, giving rise to speculation that there may be a genetic predisposition to the disease[24,25] The number of cases discussed in these publications is small, however, and the importance of an inherited tendency remains unproven. One study has shown that people who lack the g-s-t M1 gene are at increased risk of developing MM following asbestos exposure.[26] Members of the g-s-t family are involved in the repair of the free-radical induced lipid peroxidation that occurs with carcinogens such as asbestos. Such an association is therefore not unexpected. This group also found, however, that slow acetylators of *N*-acetyltransferase 2 (usually associated with the biotransformation of aromatic amines) were at increased risk of MM and those with both of these features had an additive risk.

Molecular changes in MM

The development of a cancer is now regarded as a process in which a series of multistep genetic changes eventually lead to the hallmarks of a malignancy – uncontrolled growth with autocrine/paracrine stimulation, tissue invasion and ability to metastasise. This complex process requires that the malignant cell provide its own stimuli for proliferation through oncogene activation and autocrine growth factor loops, to avoid cellular detection of DNA alterations by cell cycle regulators such as tumour suppressor genes and to enable tumour enlargement by stimulating angiogenesis. This process has best been described in the model proposed for colon cancer by Vogelstein *et al*,[27] but it is felt that it is likely to apply to most cancers.

The study of the pathogenesis of MM is made difficult by the long latency period between exposure to asbestos and development of the disease, which averages around 30–40 years. This prolonged latency period would seem to argue for a higher number of mutations being required for malignant development. While animal models have been developed which in many respects mimic the disease, these do not always reflect the situation in humans. Despite this reservation, a significant amount of valuable information has been gleaned from these studies. When discussing the findings below we will indicate which studies have been in animals and which in humans.

DNA array analysis

While this approach promises to yield much information in the future, only one preliminary study of 6500 overexpressed or underexpressed genes has been published, without clear-cut patterns emerging.[28] The relevant website is listed with the reference.

Chromosomal abnormalities

As was briefly discussed above, asbestos fibres have been found to be directly genotoxic. This may be due to interference with the mitotic spindle or through direct chromosomal adherence resulting in fragmentation. Free radical generation has also been shown to be important.

A wide variety of chromosomal abnormalities has been described in MM reflecting this effect and it would seem likely that those which are the most important to the development of MM would be most frequently noted. No specific abnormality has been found, however. The majority of MMs that have been cytogenetically examined show karyotypic changes with abnormalities involving both chromosome structure and number.[29] Losses of chromosomes are as common as gains.[30] The mean number of chromosomes has also been shown to correlate with survival.[31] Patients with more than 46 chromosomes had a median survival of 13 months in this study, as opposed to 26 months with less than 46 chromosomes and 31 months with a mean of 46 chromosomes.

Despite the heterogeneity of changes both between tumours and even within a single tumour, some studies show changes which appear to be non-random.[32] This group found 90% of abnormal karyotypes had chromosome 3 abnormalities, for instance, and they have also found frequent losses of 4, 9p and 22 with gains of 5, 7 and 20.[33] Of the many abnormalities described, some do appear to be more common and a number are of particular interest due to possible connections with other pathogenic factors postulated.

Alteration or loss of at least one locus of 1p[34,35] and particularly 1p22[36] has been frequently found in studies. Structural aberrations in 1p and loss of material in chromosomes 1 and 4 have been found to be related to a higher level of asbestos burden.[29]

Loss of heterozygosity in 3p has also been commonly reported[37] and localised to 3p21.[38] This region corresponds to the location of a known tumour suppressor gene.[39] Some 61% of MM were found to have allelic losses of various regions of chromosome 6q, often with more than one abnormal region in a tumour.[40] This group has postulated that such consistent losses may well be associated with a site for tumour suppressor genes.

The number of copies of the short arm of chromosome 7 was inversely correlated with survival in one study.[35] The loci for the epidermal growth factor (EGF) receptor and platelet derived growth factor (PDGF) A chain are both present on this chromosome (see below).

Other abnormalities of potential importance are deletions, both homozygous and hemizygous, of 9p21–22.[41] This region contains the gene for CDKN2, which codes for p16[INK4] (see below). Monosomy 22 has been described as the most consistent specific whole chromosome loss.[34] This alteration has been correlated with mutations in the neurofibromatosis type 2 (NF2) gene.[42] Chromosome 22 also contains the genetic locus for the PDGF B chain (see below). The importance of these will be further discussed in the following sections.

Of interest also were the findings of early chromosomal changes in a single patient who presented with a pleural effusion and 4 years later developed MM. Chromosomal examination at initial presentation showed changes to chromosomes 1, 4, 21 and 22. Abnormalities to these chromosomes may therefore be earlier steps in the development of MM.[43]

Oncogenic expression in MM

Proto-oncogenes are naturally occurring genetic sequences which are usually associated with the regulation of proliferation of a cell. When such sequences become 'switched on' in the absence of required signals, they are then known as oncogenes. Such a change can occur as a result of point mutations, translocations or amplification and they usually act in a dominant fashion.

As yet there have been no specific consistent oncogenic abnormalities found in MM. Two genes have been shown to have oncogenic potential with the v-*src* gene causing MM in chickens[44] and the EJ-*ras* gene having the ability to cause malignant transformation of mesothelial cells following transfection.[45] There is no evidence that these oncogenes are important in human MM.

Induction of the proto-oncogenes c-*fos* and c-*jun* has been demonstrated in rat mesothelial cells exposed to asbestos,[46] but the levels of c-*fos* were found to be similar in neoplastic and non-neoplastic mesothelium.[47] Otherwise wild-type K-*ras* has been found in 20 MM cell lines,[48] no H-*ras* mutations were found in primary MM specimens by Cristaudo *et al.*[49] and c-*myc* was not amplified in murine MM cell lines.[50]

Tumour suppressor genes

While oncogenes are usually associated with a gain of function in terms of cellular activity, it is the loss of function of tumour suppressor genes which is associated with an increase in malignant potential. Tumour suppressor genes are generally involved in negative regulation of the cell cycle and in the maintenance of genomic integrity. Tumour suppressor genes usually act in a recessive fashion and hence a loss of function generally requires the loss or mutation of both alleles. In some uncommon conditions (e.g., Li-Fraumeni cancer syndrome) there may be an inherited loss of one allele and a propensity to early development of malignancies when the other arm is spontaneously lost or mutated. A significant number of cancers are associated with the spontaneous loss of both alleles during the gradual development of the malignant phenotype.

In MM a number of tumour suppressor genes have been investigated with a view to determining their significance in the pathogenesis of this disease. The role of the most well known tumour suppressor gene, p53, has been studied by a number of groups by various methods. As perhaps would be expected, a murine mesothelial cell line with a point mutation in p53 was more susceptible to DNA damage by crocidolite asbestos.[51] Mutations in the p53 gene have been found in 76% of murine MM cell lines,[52] but in human cell lines, 18 of 20 lines examined expressed wild-type p53.[48] No mutations of p53 were found in tumour paraffin sections by PCR in two different studies.[53,54]

Immunohistochemical (IHC) studies show evidence of overexpression of p53 protein in a proportion of MM, however. Wild-type p53 is usually not detectable by IHC as the protein is only normally present in low levels. Mutant type p53 protein has a prolonged half-life and if overexpressed is readily detected. A number of studies have found MM to frequently express p53 by IHC. These have included positive findings in 44%,[55] 70%[56] and 85.7%[57] of tumours examined. One study in 1992 used three different antibodies for p53 and concluded that while 25% of cells had positive nuclear staining, none reacted to an antibody against mutant p53 type protein.[58] The current evidence would seem to indicate that wild-type p53 is present in most human MM and so the reason for the common finding of overexpression of p53 protein remains unclear.

There are other means of bypassing the p53 control point. One of these that may be applicable in MM has already been mentioned – the large TAG of SV40 present in MM tumours has been shown to retain its ability to bind to and inactivate p53.[17] Another group looked for the presence of mouse double-minute 2 (MDM2), a protein that can inhibit the function of both p53 and pRb. No amplification of the gene was seen in 18 MM cell lines,[59] but 6 of 15 tumours examined have been shown to exhibit positive staining for MDM2.[60]

pRb is another important tumour suppressor, the loss of which can be associated with malignant progression. The level of expression of pRb has been found to be normal in human MM cell lines[61,62] and in primary tumours by IHC.[62] A single study questions whether such expressed pRb is abnormal in that they found all mesotheliomas examined to stain with a polyclonal antiserum but no immunoreactivity was seen to an antibody specific for the epitopes between exon 21–27.[63] As with p53, SV40 TAG in MM specimens has also been found to still be capable of blocking pRb.[8]

Another control point associated with pRb is p16[INK4]. This is the product of the CDKN2 gene and normally inhibits phosphorylation of pRb. The loss of this gene would therefore be associated with uncontrolled progress through this part of the cell cycle. Chromosome 9, the site of the CDKN2 gene, is frequently abnormal in MM (see above). A number of studies have consistently found abnormalities with this pathway. Prins et al.[64] found homozygous deletions of the locus for CDKN2A on chromosome 9, but not for CDKN2B in all of 12 examined cell lines. These results confirmed those of Cheng et al.[65] who had found 85% of cell lines to contain deletions but only 22% of primary tumours. Codeletions of p15 and p16 CDK4 genes have also been found in 72% of primary tumours in a third study.[66] IHC analysis for p16[INK4] determined that all of 15 cell lines and 12 primary tumours had abnormal expression of this protein.[62] This group went on to show that transfection of the CDKN2 gene into two MM cell lines inhibited their growth, a finding recently confirmed by a second study.[67] This tumour suppressor appears to be a significant factor in the development of MM.

The NF2 gene is another tumour suppressor which has been frequently reported as abnormal in MM. Sekido *et al.* found mutations of this gene in 41% of cell lines[68] and Bianci *et al.* described abnormalities in 53% of cell lines and 75% of corresponding primary tumours.[69] Analysis of 7 cell lines (of 18 examined) with NF2 gene alterations showed decreased NF2 transcript in these lines and also in an additional 4 lines with apparently normal NF2 genes.[70] All of these 11 lines had undetectable NF2 protein. The presence of NF2 is one situation where an animal model may not correlate with human disease as no mutations of NF2 were found in rats with MM.[71]

The Wilms' tumour (WT1) gene is expressed in normal mesothelium during embryogenesis and is thought to play a role in the transition of mesenchymal tissues to epithelial cells. WT1 protein is of particular interest in MM with one of its functions being to control the transcription of the genes which encode for PDGF-A,[72] insulin-like growth factor (IGF)-II,[73] transforming growth factor (TGF) beta 1[74] and the IGF-I receptor.[75] Each of these has been described as being a possible autocrine growth factor in MM (see below) and the deletion of the WT1 gene could contribute to overproduction.

WT1 has been found to be present in the majority of MM cell lines and primary tumours.[39,76] Although the level of expression has been found to be variable, no inverse correlation was seen between WT1 levels and those of IGF II or PDGF-A.[77] Mutational analysis of tumours found only single deletions in 2 of 42 tumours, neither of which altered function, and no correlation was found between WT1 immunostaining and EGF receptor or IGF I receptor levels.[78,79] It appears likely that WT1 lesions are not directly involved in the pathogenesis of MM.

Growth factors

A large number of growth factors that could potentially act as autocrine or paracrine stimulators of MM proliferation have been described. The most convincing arguments in favour of a role for these are those which demonstrate not only the presence of the specific factor and its receptor but also decreased proliferation where the pathway is blocked. These criteria have now been fulfilled for several factors.

The best described are probably the platelet derived growth factors. Elevation of mRNA for both PDGF A- and B-chain was found in MM cell lines in comparison with normal mesothelial cells as early as 1987.[80] Since then, cell lines have been shown to express predominantly the PDGF β-receptor mRNA and protein.[81,82] This result has been confirmed by IHC in human tumours where PDGF and PDGF β-receptors were seen.[83] This group also found PDGF α-receptors in MM cell lines. The use of a hammerhead ribozyme directed against PDGFβ mRNA decreased MM cell growth.[84] The transfection and subsequent overexpression of PDGF A-chain has been shown to cause malignant transformation of a human mesothelial cell line.[85] In murine and human cell lines, antisense oligonucleotides to PDGF A, but not PDGF B, inhibited *in vitro* cell growth.[86,87] This group postulated that the effects of PDGF A in MM may be less well recognised due to an action on an internal autocrine loop that could only be detected using antisense approaches.

TGF-β has been shown to be produced by both murine and human MM.[80,88] It is known to stimulate the growth of normal mesenchymal cells[89] and Gerwin's group did not find TGF-β mRNA expression to be higher in MM cell lines than in normal human mesothelial cells. All three major isoforms appear to be expressed in MM, but particularly TGF-β1 and TGF-β2, and both latent and active forms have been found.[88]

Antisense mRNA against TGF-β has reduced tumorigenicity of murine MM when transfection was undertaken before tumour inoculation.[88] This study also found that inhibition of TGF-β was associated with increased numbers of tumour-infiltrating leukocytes with increased expression of functional surface molecules on the T lymphocytes. This indicates that this factor may be involved in the immune suppression associated with MM. It has also been shown that antisense oligonucleotides (ASON) to TGF-β decreased the growth of MM not only *in vitro* but also when encapsulated in liposomes and injected intratumorally.[90] ASON to TGF-β1 and TGF-β2 both inhibited *in vitro* tumour growth but the effect was not enhanced when both isotypes were combined. This growth factor could therefore be central to many aspects of tumour development as it has angiogenic properties and is immunosuppressive as well as being a potential autocrine factor.

The receptor for EGF has been found to be expressed by human MM cell lines.[91,92] Morocz *et al.* examined four MM cell lines, however, and while the EGF receptor was ubiquitously expressed, none secreted EGF.[93] Two of the cell lines secreted TGF-α (which can interact with the EGF receptor) but only one cell line showed decreased DNA synthesis when TGF-α and EGF receptor antibodies were used.

IGF I, its receptor and IGF-binding protein 3 have been shown to be present in MM cell lines but not at higher levels than in normal mesothelial cells.[94] The use of IGF I receptor antisense transcripts has resulted in decreased growth of hamster MM.[95-97]

There has also been some recent interest in hepatocyte growth factor/scatter factor (HGF) and its receptor c-*met*. IHC analysis in human MM specimens has found immunoreactivity for both HGF and c-met to be common.[98,99] In 11 human MM cell lines, only 3 produced HGF but all 11 expressed the c-met receptor and recombinant HGF increased motility and was mitogenic in all cells. Harvey *et al.* found that epithelioid MM cell lines did not produce HGF while fibroblast-like and mixed-morphology cells did.[100] Of two cell lines extensively examined in this study, only one proliferated with HGF but cell motility was increased in both. Further investigation of this pathway is required.

A number of cytokines are also commonly produced by MM but there is no evidence at this time that these are involved in the proliferation of the cells. Interleukin-6 (IL-6) has been frequently found to be secreted by both human and murine MM cell lines[101,102] and in the latter study the use of anti-IL-6 antibodies decreased symptoms, particularly cachexia, in tumour-bearing mice. The growth of the tumour was not inhibited, suggesting that this was not acting as an autocrine factor. High levels of IL-6 in the pleural fluid of patients with MM have also been found[103] and there was a significant correlation between pleural fluid levels and the degree of thrombocytosis.[104] It appears most likely that IL-6 is associated with paraneoplastic symptoms of MM but not with the growth of the tumour.

Other cytokines described in association with MM cell lines but not apparently involved in the growth of the tumour are M-CSF, G-CSF and GM-CSF.[101,105]

Apoptosis, angiogenesis and immortalisation

In the last 10 years a significant amount of attention has been directed at the role of angiogenesis as a key factor in the growth of tumours and at the avoidance of apoptosis by malignant cells. At this time little research has been done with regard to either of these processes in MM.

It is now accepted that the ability to promote angiogenesis is essential if a tumour is to enlarge to a size more than a few millimetres across. The degree of angiogenesis has been examined as a possible prognostic feature in MM and tumours with the highest intratumoral microvascular density were associated with shorter survival times.[78,79] HGF and its receptor c-met have been found to be present in a large proportion of MM as discussed in the section on growth factors. Their presence has also been correlated with higher microvessel density[99] with HGF being a known inducer of angiogenesis. This area could be one of great interest in the future.

A number of the growth factors that have been described in the previous section are known to be associated with angiogenesis. TGF-β, PDGF, and IGF-I have all been shown to have a role in blood vessel growth. Whether this is one of the roles of each of these factors in the progression of MM has yet to be determined.

The avoidance of apoptosis is essential if a malignant cell population is to escape normal cellular controls and may also be important in subsequent resistance to chemotherapy. It has been postulated that apoptosis resistance may be central to MM development.[11] Many cancers achieve this by having mutations of p53 but as has been discussed, this does not appear to be the case in many MM. Alterations in other steps of this pathway then become critical for the survival of the cell. The apoptosis blocking protein bcl-2 has been looked for by IHC in two studies and is infrequently overexpressed in MM. IHC immunoreactivity was only found in 8% of tumours by Segers *et al.*[106] and in no tumours examined by Chilosi *et al.*[107] Only one of three apoptosis-resistant cell lines examined expressed Bcl-2 in a further study and with immunoblotting only 3 of 14 additional cell lysates showed expression.[108] All of these lines expressed the proapoptotic protein Bax with a low ratio of Bcl-2 to Bax. This combination would generally be associated with cellular sensitivity to apoptosis. As this group has postulated, other mechanisms to prevent apoptosis must therefore be operating. They speculated on Bax mutations or antagonists, and abnormalities to other Bcl-2 members such as Bad, Bak, Bcl-xl or Mcl-1.

The lifespan of replicating cells is controlled by gradual shortening of telomeres. The majority of malignancies have been shown to express telomerases that prevent this shortening and allow cell immortalisation. Of MM examined, 91% were telomerase positive using a non-isotopic dilution assay of the telomeric repeat amplification protocol, whereas none of six normal mesothelial cell cultures showed activity.[109]

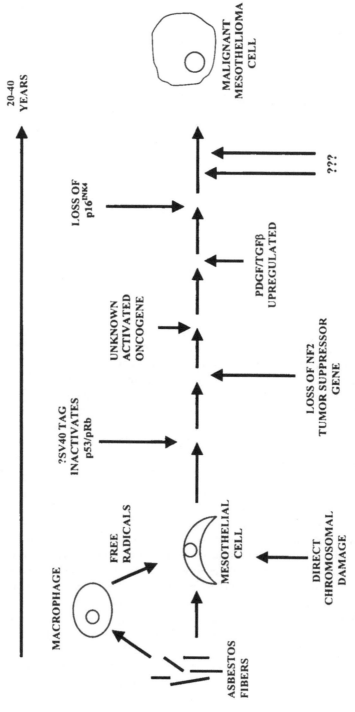

Figure 17.1. Possible mechanisms for the pathogenesis of malignant mesothelioma (after Vogelstein[27]).

Summary

Despite progress in the management of many cancers in the past 30 years, the outlook for patients with MM remains depressingly bleak. Investigation of the pathogenesis of this tumour and particularly the molecular basis is a new area of research that has the potential to give us insights into novel methods of treatment.

It seems likely from the current evidence that the development of MM follows a similar pathway to that of many other malignancies, the best described of which is colorectal cancer. The carcinogen, asbestos, is unable to be removed by the mesothelium. Its continued presence generates free radical production, initially from macrophages but subsequently directly from mesothelial cells. These, in conjunction with the direct genotoxic effects of asbestos, cause cellular DNA damage. The presence of potential cofactors such as SV40 may decrease the detection of such damage by inactivating p53 or pRb. The accumulation of certain DNA abnormalities, such as loss of the tumour suppressor genes for NF2 and p16^{INK4}, and the activation of as yet undetermined oncogenes allow the uncontrolled proliferation of these cells. This is supported by the autocrine production of growth factors such as PDGF and TGF-β. These and other factors also cause immune suppression and angiogenesis, further enhancing the ability of the tumour to proliferate. The end result of this process is malignant transformation (see Figure 17.1).

While it is clear that many gaps still remain to be filled in this scenario, this should not disguise the fact that significant progress has been made. Although such findings are individually interesting, they also give us potential windows for new management strategies. The use of gene therapy, antisense oligonucleotides, and monoclonal antibodies directed against autocrine receptors offers therapeutic possibilities against abnormalities already described. Each of these techniques is discussed in other chapters of this book. Further investigations of the pathogenesis of this tumour can only increase the possibility of improving the outlook for those who are unfortunate enough to suffer from this dire disease.

Acknowledgement

B.R.M. is supported by a grant from the National Health and Medical Research Council of Australia.

References

1. Wagner, J.C., Sleggs, C.A., Marchand, P. Diffuse pleural mesothelioma and asbestos exposure in the North Western Cape Province. *Br J Ind Med* 1960; **17**: 260–271.
2. Hansen, J., Deklerk, N.H., Musk, A.W., Hobbs, M.S.T. Environmental exposure to crocidolite and mesothelioma – exposure-response relationships. *Am J Respir Crit Care Med* 1998; **157**: 69–75.
3. McDonald, J.C., McDonald, A.D. The epidemiology of mesothelioma in historical context [Review]. *Eur Respir J* 1996; **9**: 1932–1942.

4. Branchaud, R.M., Garant, L.J., Kane, A.B. Pathogenesis of mesothelial reactions to asbestos fibres. Monocyte recruitment and macrophage activation. *Pathobiology* 1993; **61**: 154–163.

5. Owens, M.W., Grimes, S.R. Pleural mesothelial cell response to inflammation: tumor necrosis factor-induced mitogenesis and collagen synthesis. *Am J Physiol* 1993; **265**: L382–388.

6. Davis, J.M. Ultrastructure of human mesotheliomas. *J Natl Cancer Inst* 1974; **52**: 1715–1725.

7. Mossman, B.T., Marsh, J.P. Evidence supporting a role for active oxygen species in asbestos-induced toxicity and lung disease. *Environ Health Perspec* 1989; **81**: 91–94.

8. Broaddus, V.C., Yang, L., Scavo, L.M., Ernst, J.D., Boylan, A.M. Crocidolite asbestos induces apoptosis of pleural mesothelial cells – role of reactive oxygen species and poly(adp-ribosyl) polymerase. *Environ Health Perspec* 1997; **105**: 1147–1152.

9. Walker, C., Everitt, J., Barrett, J.C. Possible cellular and molecular mechanisms for asbestos carcinogenicity. *Am J Ind Med* 1992; **21**: 253–273.

10. Broaddus, V.C., Yang, L., Scavo, L.M., Ernst, J.D., Boylan, A.M. Asbestos induces apoptosis of human and rabbit pleural mesothelial cells via reactive oxygen species. *J Clin Invest* 1996; **98**: 2050–2059.

11. Gabrielson, E.W., Van der Meeren, A., Reddel, R.R., Reddel, H., Gerwin, B.I., Harris, C.C. Human mesothelioma cells and asbestos-exposed mesothelial cells are selectively resistant to amosite toxicity: a possible mechanism for tumor promotion by asbestos. *Carcinogenesis* 1992; **13**: 1359–1363.

12. Yegles, M., Saint-Etienne, L., Renier, A., Janson, X., Jaurand, M.C. Induction of metaphase and anaphase/telophase abnormalities by asbestos fibers in rat pleural mesothelial cells in vitro. *Am J Respir Cell Mol Biol* 1993; **9**: 186–191.

13. Kinnula, V.L., Pietarinenruntti, P., Raivio, K., *et al.* Manganese superoxide dismutase in human pleural mesothelioma cell lines. *Free Radic Biol Med* 1996; **21**: 527–532.

14. Fung, H., Kow, Y.W., Vanhouten, B., *et al.* Asbestos increases mammalian ap-endonuclease gene expression, protein levels, and enzyme activity in mesothelial cells. *Cancer Res* 1998; **58**: 189–194.

15. Kinnula, K., Linnainmaa, K., Raivio, K.O., Kinnula, V.L. Endogenous antioxidant enzymes and glutathione S-transferase in protection of mesothelioma cells against hydrogen peroxide and epirubicin toxicity. *Br J Cancer* 1998; **77**: 1097–1102.

16. Carbone, M., Pass, H.I., Rizzo, P., *et al.* Simian virus 40-like DNA sequences in human pleural mesothelioma. *Oncogene* 1994; **9**: 1781–1790.

17. Carbone, M., Rizzo, P., Grimley, P.M., *et al.* Simian virus-40 large-T antigen binds P53 in human mesotheliomas. *Nat Med* 1997; **3**: 908–912.

18. De Luca, A., Baldi, A., Esposito, V., *et al.* The retinoblastoma gene family pRb/p105, p107, pRb2/p130 and simian virus-40 large T-antigen in human mesotheliomas. *Nat Med* 1997; **3**: 913–916.

19. Strickler, H.D., Goedert, J.J., Fleming, M., *et al.* Simian virus 40 and pleural mesothelioma in humans. *Cancer Epidemiol Biomarkers Prev* 1996; **5**: 473–475.

20. McLaren BR, Haenel T, Stevenson S, Mukherjee S, Robinson BWS, Lake RA. SV40 like sequences in cell lines and tumour biopsies from Australian malignant mesothelioma. *Aust N Z J Med* 2000; **30**: 450–456.

21. Pepper, C., Jasani, B., Navabi, H., Wynford-Thomas, D., Gibbs, A.R. Simian virus 40 large T antigen (SV40LTAg) primer specific DNA amplification in human pleural mesothelioma tissue. *Thorax* 1996; **51**: 1074–1076.

22. Hofmann, J., Mintzer, D., Warhol, M.J. Malignant mesothelioma following radiation therapy. *Am J Med* 1994; **97**: 379–382.
23. Andersson, M., Wallin, H., Jonsson, M., *et al.* Lung carcinoma and malignant mesothelioma in patients exposed to Thorotrast: incidence, histology and p53 status. *Int J Cancer* 1995; **63**: 330–336.
24. Martensson, G., Larsson, S., Zettergren, L. Malignant mesothelioma in two pairs of siblings: is there a hereditary predisposing factor? *Eur J Respir Dis* 1984; **65**: 179–184.
25. Risberg, B., Nickels, J., Wagermark, J. Familial clustering of malignant mesothelioma. *Cancer* 1980; **45**: 2422–2427.
26. Hirvonen, A., Pelin, K., Tammilehto, L., Karjalainen, A., Mattson, K., Linnainmaa, K. Inherited GSTM1 and NAT2 defects as concurrent risk modifiers in asbestos-related human malignant mesothelioma. *Cancer Res* 1995; **55**: 2981–2983.
27. Vogelstein, B., Fearon, E.R., Hamilton, S.R., *et al.* Genetic alterations during colorectal-tumor development. *N Engl J Med* 1988; **319**: 525–532.
28. Rihn H, Mohr S, McDowell S, Binet S, Loubinoux J, Galateu F, Keith G, Leikauf G. Differential gene expression in mesothelioma. *FEBS Lett* 2000; **480**: 95–100.
    General site: http://www.inrs.fr/dossiers/amiante/genemesoen.htm
    http://www.inrs.fr/dossiers/amiante/gene.txt
29. Knuutila, S., Tiainen, M., Tammilehto, L., *et al.* Cytogenetics of human malignant mesotheliomas. *Eur Respir Rev* 1993; **3**: 25–28.
30. Bjorkqvist, A.M., Tammilehto, L., Nordling, S., *et al.* Comparison of DNA copy number changes in malignant mesothelioma, adenocarcinoma and large-cell anaplastic carcinoma of the lung. *Br J Cancer* 1998; **77**: 260–269.
31. Tiainen, M., Rautonen, J., Pyrhonen, S., Tammilehto, L., Mattson, K., Knuutila, S. Chromosome number correlates with survival in patients with malignant pleural mesothelioma. *Cancer Genet Cytogenet* 1992; **62**: 21–24.
32. Hagemeijer, A., Franken-Postma, E., Versnel, M. Cytogenetic studies of forty malignant mesotheliomas. *Eur Respir Rev* 1993; **3**: 64–67.
33. Hagemeijer, A., Versnel, M.A, Van Drunen, E., *et al.* Cytogenetic analysis of malignant mesothelioma. *Cancer Genet Cytogenet* 1990; **47**: 1–28.
34. Flejter, W.L., Li, F.P., Antman, K.H., Testa, J.R. Recurring loss involving chromosomes 1, 3, and 22 in malignant mesothelioma: possible sites of tumor suppressor genes. *Genes Chromosomes Cancer* 1989; **1**: 148–154.
35. Tiainen, M., Tammilehto, L., Rautonen, J., Tuomi, T., Mattson, K., Knuutila, S. Chromosomal abnormalities and their correlations with asbestos exposure and survival in patients with mesothelioma. *Br J Cancer* 1989; **60**: 618–626.
36. Lee, W.C., Balsara, B., Liu, Z., Jhanwar, S.C., Testa, J.R. Loss of heterozygosity analysis defines a critical region in chromosome 1p22 commonly deleted in human malignant mesothelioma. *Cancer Res* 1996; **56**: 4297–4301.
37. Zeiger, M.A., Gnarra, J.R., Zbar, B., Linehan, W.M., Pass, H.I. Loss of heterozygosity on the short arm of chromosome 3 in mesothelioma cell lines and solid tumors. *Genes Chromosomes Cancer* 1994; **11**: 15–20.
38. Pitterle, D.M., Jolicoeur, E.M., Bepler, G. Hot spots for molecular genetic alterations in lung cancer. *In Vivo* 1998; **12**: 643–58.
39. Walker, C., Rutten, F., Yuan, X.Q, Pass, H., Mew, D.M., Everitt, J. Wilms tumor suppressor gene expression in rat and human mesothelioma. *Cancer Res* 1994; **54**: 3101–3106.
40. Bell, D.W., Jhanwar, S.C., Testa, J.R. Multiple regions of allelic loss from chromosome arm 6q in malignant mesothelioma. *Cancer Res* 1997; **57**: 4057–4062.

41. Cheng, J.Q., Jhanwar, S.C., Lu, Y.Y., Testa, J.R. Homozygous deletions within 9p21-P22 identify a small critical region of chromosomal loss in human malignant mesotheliomas. *Cancer Res* 1993; **53**: 4761–4763.

42. Huncharek, M. Genetic factors in the aetiology of malignant mesothelioma. *Eur J Cancer* 1995; **31A**: 1741–1747.

43. Hansteen, I.L., Hil, B., Lien, J.T., Skaug, V., Haugen, A. Karyotypic changes in the preclinical and subsequent stages of malignant mesothelioma: a case report. *Cancer Genet Cytogenet* 1993; **70**: 94–98.

44. England, J.M., Panella, M.J., Ewert, D.L., Halpern, M.S. Induction of a diffuse mesothelioma in chickens by intraperitoneal inoculation of v-*src* DNA. *Virology* 1991; **182**: 423–429.

45. Reddel, R.R, Malan-Shibley, L., Gerwin, B.I., Metcalf, R.A., Harris, C.C. Tumorigenicity of human mesothelial cell line transfected with EJ-*ras* oncogene. *J Natl Cancer Inst* 1989; **81**: 945–948.

46. Heintz, N.H, Janssen, Y.M., Mossman, B.T. Persistent induction of c-*fos* and c-*jun* expression by asbestos. *Proc Natl Acad Sci U S A* 1993; **90**: 3299–3303.

47. Ramael, M., Vandenbossche, J., Buysse, C., Deblier, I., Segers, K., Vanmarck, E. Immunoreactivity for c-*fos* and c-*myc* protein with the monoclonal antibodies 14eio and 6e10 in malignant mesothelioma and nonneoplastic mesothelium of the pleura. *Histol Histopathol* 1995; **10**: 639–643.

48. Metcalf, R.A., Welsh, J.A., Bennett, W.P., *et al.* p53 and Kirsten-*ras* mutations in human mesothelioma cell lines. *Cancer Res* 1992; **52**: 2610–2615.

49. Cristaudo, A., Vivaldi, A., Sensales, G., *et al.* Molecular biology studies on mesothelioma tumor samples: preliminary data on H-*ras*, p21, and SV40. *J Environ Pathol, Toxicol Oncol* 1995; **14**: 29–34.

50. Moyer, V.D., Cistulli, C.A., Vaslet, C.A., Kane, A.B. Oxygen radicals and asbestos carcinogenesis. *Environ Health Perspect* 1994; **102**: 131–136.

51. Marsella, J.M., Liu, B.L., Vaslet, C.A., Kane, A.B. Susceptibility of p53-deficient mice to induction of mesothelioma by crocidolite asbestos fibers. *Environ Health Perspect* 1997; **105**: 1069–1072.

52. Cora, E.M., Kane, A.B. Alterations in a tumour suppressor gene, p53, in mouse mesotheliomas induced by crocidolite asbestos. *Eur Respir Rev* 1993; **3**: 148–150.

53. Mor, O., Yaron, P., Huszar, M., *et al.* Absence of P53 mutations in malignant mesotheliomas. *Am J Respir Cell Mol Biol* 1997; **16**: 9–13.

54. Kitamura, F., Araki, S., Tanigawa, T., Miura, H., Akabane, H., Iwasaki, R. Assessment of mutations of Ha- and Ki-ras oncogenes and the p53 suppressor gene in seven malignant mesothelioma patients exposed to asbestos – PCR-SSCP and sequencing analyses of paraffin-embedded primary tumors. *Ind Health* 1998; **36**: 52–56.

55. Mayall, F.G., Goddard, H., Gibbs, A.R. The frequency of p53 immunostaining in asbestos-associated mesotheliomas and non-asbestos-associated mesotheliomas. *Histopathology* 1993; **22**: 383–386.

56. Kafiri, G., Thomas, D.M., Shepherd, N.A., Krausz, T., Lane, D.P., Hall, P.A. p53 expression is common in malignant mesothelioma. *Histopathology* 1992; **21**: 331–334.

57. Esposito, V., Baldi, A., Deluca, A., *et al.* P53 immunostaining in differential diagnosis of pleural mesothelial proliferations. *Anticancer Res* 1997; **17**: 733–736.

58. Ramael, M., Lemmens, G., Eerdekens, C., *et al.* Immunoreactivity for p53 protein in malignant mesothelioma and non-neoplastic mesothelium. *J Pathol* 1992; **168**: 371–375.

59. Ungar, S., Vandemeeren, A., Tammilehto, L., Linnainmaa, K., Mattson, K., Gerwin, B.I. High levels of mdm2 are not correlated with the presence of wild-type p53 in human malignant mesothelioma cell lines. *Br J Cancer* 1996; **74**: 1534–1540.

60. Segers, K., Backhovens, H., Singh, S.K., *et al.* Immunoreactivity for p53 and mdm2 and the detection of p53 mutations in human malignant mesothelioma. *Virchows Arch* 1995; **427**: 431–436.

61. Van de Meeren, A., Seddon, M.B., Kispert, J., Harris, C.C., Gerwin, B.I. Lack of expression of the retinoblastoma gene is not frequently involved in the genesis of human mesothelioma. *Eur Respir Rev* 1993; **3**: 177–179.

62. Kratzke, R.A, Otterson, G.A., Lincoln, C.E., *et al.* Immunohistochemical analysis of the P16(Ink4) cyclin-dependent kinase inhibitor in malignant mesothelioma. *J Natl Cancer Inst* 1995; **87**: 1870–1875.

63. Ramael, M., Segers, K., Vanmarck, E. Differential immunohistochemical staining for retinoblastoma protein with the antibodies-C15 and 1f8 in malignant mesothelioma. *Pathol, Res Pract* 1994; **190**: 138–141.

64. Prins, J.B., Williamson, K.A., Kamp, M.M.K., *et al.* The gene for the cyclin-dependent-kinase-4 inhibitor, Cdkn2a, is preferentially deleted in malignant mesothelioma. *Int J Cancer* 1998; **75**: 649–653.

65. Cheng, J.Q., Jhanwar, S.C., Klein, W.M., *et al.* p16 alterations and deletion mapping of 9p21–p22 in malignant mesothelioma. *Cancer Res* 1994; **54**: 5547–5551.

66. Xiao, S., Li, D.Z., Vijg, J., Sugarbaker, D.J., Corson, J.M., Fletcher, J.A. Codeletion of P15 and P16 in primary malignant mesothelioma. *Oncogene* 1995; **11**: 511–515.

67. Frizelle, S.P., Grim, J., Zhou, J., *et al.* Re-expression of P16(Ink4a) in mesothelioma cells results in cell cycle arrest, cell death, tumor suppression and tumor regression. *Oncogene* 1998; **16**: 3087–3095.

68. Sekido, Y., Pass, H.I., Bader, S., *et al.* Neurofibromatosis type 2 (NF2) gene is somatically mutated in mesothelioma but not in lung cancer. *Cancer Res* 1995; **55**: 1227–1231.

69. Bianchi, A.B., Mitsunaga, S.I., Cheng, J.Q., *et al.* High frequency of inactivating mutations in the neurofibromatosis type 2 gene (NF2) in primary malignant mesotheliomas. *Proc Natl Acad Sci U S A* 1995; **92**: 10854–10858.

70. Deguen, B., Goutebroze, L., Giovannini, M., *et al.* Heterogeneity of mesothelioma cell lines as defined by altered genomic structure and expression of the Nf2 gene. *Int J Cancer* 1998; **77**: 554–560.

71. Kleymenova, E.V., Bianchi, A.A., Kley, N., Pylev, L.N., Walker, C.L. Characterization of the rat neurofibromatosis 2 gene and its involvement in asbestos-induced mesothelioma. *Mol Carcinog* 1997; **18**: 54–60.

72. Wang, Z.Y., Madden, S.L., Deuel, T.F., Rauscher, F.J.D. The Wilms' tumor gene product, WT1, represses transcription of the platelet-derived growth factor A-chain gene. *J Biol Chem* 1992; **267**: 2199–2002.

73. Drummond, I.A., Madden, S.L., Rohwer-Nutter, P., Bell, G.I., Sukhatme, V.P., Rauscher, F.J.D. Repression of the insulin-like growth factor II gene by the Wilms tumor suppressor WT1. *Science* 1992; **257**: 674–678.

74. Dey, B.R., Sukhatme, V.P., Roberts, A.B., Sporn, M.B., Rauscher, F. Jr, Kim, S.J. Repression of the transforming growth factor-beta 1 gene by the Wilms' tumor suppressor WT1 gene product. *Mol Endocrinol* 1994; **8**: 595–602.

75. Werner, H., Re, G.G., Drummond, I.A., *et al.* Increased expression of the insulin-like growth factor I receptor gene, IGF1R, in Wilms tumor is correlated with modulation of IGF1R promoter activity by the WT1 Wilms tumor gene product. *Proc Natl Acad Sci U S A* 1993; **90**: 5828–5832.

76. Amin, K.M., Litzky, L.A., Smythe, W.R., *et al.* Wilms tumor 1 susceptibility (Wt1) gene products are selectively expressed in malignant mesothelioma. *Am J Pathol* 1995; **146**: 344–356.

77. Langerak, A.W., Williamson, K.A., Miyagawa, K., Hagemeijer, A., Versnel, M.A., Hastie, N.D. Expression of the Wilms tumor gene Wti in human malignant mesothelioma cell lines and relationship to platelet-derived growth factor A and insulin-like growth factor 2 expression. *Genes Chromosomes Cancer* 1995; **12**: 87–96.

78. Kumarsingh, S., Segers, K., Rodeck, U., *et al.* Wt1 mutation in malignant mesothelioma and Wt1 immunoreactivity in relation to P53 and growth factor receptor expression, cell-type transition, and prognosis. *J Pathol* 1997; **181**: 67–74.

79. Kumarsingh, S., Vermeulen, P.B., Weyler, J., *et al.* Evaluation of tumour angiogenesis as a prognostic marker in malignant mesothelioma. *J Pathol* 1997; **182**: 211–216.

80. Gerwin, B.I., Lechner, J.F., Reddel, R.R, *et al.* Comparison of production of transforming growth factor-beta and platelet-derived growth factor by normal human mesothelial cells and mesothelioma cell lines. *Cancer Res* 1987; **47**: 6180–6184.

81. Versnel, M.A., Claesson-Welsh, L., Hammacher, A., *et al.* Human malignant mesothelioma cell lines express PDGF beta-receptors whereas cultured normal mesothelial cells express predominantly PDGF alpha-receptors. *Oncogene* 1991; **6**: 2005–2011.

82. Prins, J.B., Langerak, A.W., Dirks, R.P.H., *et al.* Identification of regulatory sequences in the promoter of the PDGF β-chain gene in malignant mesothelioma cell lines. *Biochim Biophys Acta* 1996; **1317**: 223–232.

83. Langerak, A.W., Delaa,t P., Vanderlindenvanbeurden, C.A.J., *et al.* Expression of platelet-derived growth factor (PDGF) and PDGF receptors in human malignant mesothelioma in vitro and in vivo. *J Pathol* 1996; **178**: 151–160.

84. Dorai, T., Kobayashi, H., Holland, J.F., Ohnuma, T. Modulation of platelet-derived growth factor-beta mRNA expression and cell growth in a human mesothelioma cell line by a hammerhead ribozyme. *Mol Pharmacol* 1994; **46**: 437–444.

85. Van der Meeren, A., Seddon, M.B., Betsholtz, C.A., Lechner, J.F., Gerwin, B.I. Tumorigenic conversion of human mesothelial cells as a consequence of platelet-derived growth factor-A chain overexpression. *Am J Respir Cell Mol Biol* 1993; **8**: 214–221.

86. Garlepp, M.J., Christmas, T.I., Manning, L.S., *et al.* The role of platelet-derived growth factor in the growth of human malignant mesothelioma. *Eur Respir Rev* 1993; **3**: 189–191.

87. Garlepp, M.J., Christmas, T.I., Mutsaers, S.E., Manning, L.S., Davis, M.R, Robinson, B.W.S. Platelet-derived growth factor as an autocrine factor in murine malignant mesothelioma. *Eur Respir Rev* 1993; **3**: 192–194.

88. Fitzpatrick, D.R., Bielefeldt-Ohmann, H., Himbeck, R.P., Jarnicki, A.G., Marzo, A.L., Robinson, B.W. Transforming growth factor-beta: antisense RNA-mediated inhibition affects anchorage-independent growth, tumorigenicity and tumor-infiltrating T-cells in malignant mesothelioma. *Growth Factors* 1994; **11**: 29–44.

89. Moses, H.L., Yang, E.Y., Pietenpol, J.A. TGF-beta stimulation and inhibition of cell proliferation: new mechanistic insights. *Cell* 1990; **63**: 245–247.

90. Marzo, A.L., Fitzpatrick, D.R., Robinson, B.W.S., Scott, B. Antisense oligonucleotides specific for transforming growth factor beta-2 inhibit the growth of malignant mesothelioma both in vitro and in vivo. *Cancer Res* 1997; **57**: 3200–3207.

91. Dazzi, H., Hasleton, P.S., Thatcher, N., Wilkes, S., Swindell, R., Chatterjee, A.K. Malignant pleural mesothelioma and epidermal growth factor receptor (EGF-R). Relationship of EGF-R with histology and survival using fixed paraffin embedded tissue and the F4, monoclonal antibody. *Br J Cancer* 1990; **61**: 924–926.

92. Ramael, M., Segers, K., Buysse, C., Van den Bossche, J., Van Marck, E. Immunohistochemical distribution patterns of epidermal growth factor receptor in malignant mesothelioma and non-neoplastic mesothelium. *Virchows Arch – A, Pathol Anat Histopathol* 1991; **419**: 171–175.

93. Morocz, I.A., Schmitter, D., Lauber, B., Stahel, R.A. Autocrine stimulation of a human lung mesothelioma cell line is mediated through the transforming growth factor alpha epidermal growth factor receptor mitogenic pathway. *Br J Cancer* 1994; **70**: 850–856.

94. Lee, T.C., Zhang, Y.H., Aston, C., *et al.* Normal human mesothelial cells and mesothelioma cell lines express insulin-like growth factor-I and associated molecules. *Cancer Res* 1993; **53**: 2858–2864.

95. Pass, H.I., Mew, D.J.Y. In vitro and in vivo studies of mesothelioma. *J Cell Biochem* 1996: 142–151.

96. Pass, H.I., Mew, D.J.Y., Carbone M, *et al.* Inhibition of hamster mesothelioma tumorigenesis by an antisense expression plasmid to the insulin-like growth factor-1 receptor. *Cancer Res* 1996; **56**: 4044–4048.

97. Pass, H.I., Kennedy, R.C., Carbone, M. Evidence for and implications of SV40-like sequences in human mesotheliomas. *Important Adv Oncol* 1996: 89–108.

98. Harvey, P., Warn, A., Newman, P., Perry, L.J., Ball, R.Y, Warn, R.M. Immunoreactivity for hepatocyte growth factor/scatter factor and its receptor, met, in human lung carcinomas and malignant mesotheliomas. *J Pathol* 1996; **180**: 389–394.

99. Tolnay, E., Kuhnen, C., Wiethege, T., Konig, J.E., Voss, B., Muller, K.M. Hepatocyte growth factor scatter factor and its receptor c-met are overexpressed and associated with an increased microvessel density in malignant pleural mesothelioma. *J Cancer Res Clin Oncol* 1998; **124**: 291–296.

100. Harvey, P., Warn, A., Dobbin, S., *et al.* Expression of Hgf/Sf in mesothelioma cell lines and its effects on cell motility, proliferation and morphology. *Br J Cancer* 1998; **77**: 1052–1059.

101. Schmitter, D., Lauber, B., Fagg, B., Stahel, R.A. Hematopoietic growth factors secreted by seven human pleural mesothelioma cell lines: interleukin-6 production as a common feature. *Int J Cancer* 1992; **51**: 296–301.

102. Bielefeldt-Ohmann, H., Marzo, A.L., Himbeck, R.P., Jarnicki, A.G., Robinson, B.W., Fitzpatrick, D.R. Interleukin-6 involvement in mesothelioma pathobiology: inhibition by interferon alpha immunotherapy. *Cancer Immunol Immunother* 1995; **40**: 241–250.

103. Monti, G., Jaurand, M.C., Monnet, I., *et al.* Intrapleural production of interleukin 6 during mesothelioma and its modulation by gamma-interferon treatment. *Cancer Res* 1994; **54**: 4419–4423.

104. Nakano, T., Chahinian, A.P., Shinjo, M., *et al.* Interleukin 6 and its relationship to clinical parameters in patients with malignant pleural mesothelioma. *Br J Cancer* 1998; **77**: 907–912.

105. Demetri, G.D., Zenzie, B.W., Rheinwald, J.G., Griffin, J.D. Expression of colony-stimulating factor genes by normal human mesothelial cells and human malignant mesothelioma cells lines in vitro. *Blood* 1989; **74**: 940–946.

106. Segers, K., Ramael, M., Singh, S.K., *et al.* Immunoreactivity for bcl-2 protein in malignant mesothelioma and non-neoplastic mesothelium. *Virchows Arch* 1994; **424**: 631–634.

107. Chilosi, M., Facchettti, F., Dei Tos, A.P., *et al.* bcl-2 expression in pleural and extrapleural solitary fibrous tumours. *J Pathol* 1997; **181**: 362–367.

108. Narasimhan, S.R., Yang, L., Gerwin, B.I., Broaddus, V.C. Resistance of pleural mesothelioma cell lines to apoptosis – relation to expression of Bcl-2 and Bax. *Am J Physiol – Lung Cell Mol Physiol* 1998; **19**: L165–L171.

109. Dhaene, K., Hubner, R., Kumarsingh, S., Weyn, B., Vanmarck, E. Telomerase activity in human pleural mesothelioma. *Thorax* 1998; **53**: 915–918.

=18=
Immunotherapy of Malignant Mesothelioma

Sutapa Mukherjee and Bruce W. S. Robinson

Given the poor response of malignant mesothelioma to conventional treatment modalities, such as surgery, radiotherapy and chemotherapy, an ideal approach to the treatment of mesothelioma would be to enlist the host immune system to become active against tumour and eradicate it. This forms the basis of immunotherapy for any cancer and in animal models of this disease there is evidence to support the use of immunologically active molecules (e.g., cytokines) to facilitate an anti-tumoral response in malignant mesothelioma. Numerous cytokines have been studied, including interleukin-2 (IL-2), interferons alpha (IFN-α), beta (IFN-β) and gamma (IFN-γ) as well as granulocyte macrophage–colony stimulating factor (GM-CSF) and more recently tumour necrosis factor (TNF). Other cytokines that may show promise include the co-stimulatory molecule B7-1 and interleukin-12. Many of these agents have been studied extensively in the animal model and this has led to human trials being performed with modest results. In this chapter we will review the rationale of immunotherapy; what is known about the general immune response to tumours and to malignant mesothelioma; and the animal and human immunotherapy studies which have been performed. We will also discuss the difficulties involved in delivery of cytokines to patients and the toxicities which limit their use therapeutically. Finally we will discuss the future of immunotherapy in malignant mesothelioma with respect to its use in combination with other therapies, such as gene therapy, chemotherapy and surgery.

General overview of the immune response against tumours

Immunotherapy uses unique host defences to initiate and effect tumour regression. This is different from radiation therapy and chemotherapy, which are directly cytotoxic to cancer cells and kill a fixed percentage of tumour cells rather than a fixed number of cancer cells. Interestingly, complete responses to several cycles of chemotherapy may not be possible unless there was an effective host immune response generated against the tumour when the tumour burden had been reduced to a level to allow the immune response to occur.

The immune response against all tumours can be broadly classified into a humoral (antibody) response and a cell-mediated (effector) response that is more effective in its ability to destroy malignant cells. T lymphocytes are the critical mediators of tumour immunity. These are derived from marrow stem cells and initially migrate to the thymus where they mature and migrate to all lymphatic organs and lymph node regions. They circulate from these areas and after stimulation by the presence of antigens or in response to various cytokines they are capable of migration to specific areas, including within the tumour environment, and these T lymphocytes are called tumour infiltrating lymphocytes (TILs). Cytotoxic T lymphocytes (CD8+) are able to lyse tumour cells when they have been activated. These cytotoxic T cells must recognise as foreign tumour antigens presented by MHC Class I molecules on the surface of tumour cells to perform the function of cell-specific killing. In human malignant mesothelioma the extent of lymphocytic infiltration is variable and depends on the individual tumour.[1,2] The lack of TILs within malignant mesothelioma tumours suggests a lack of tumour antigen expression and/or recognition by the host or the production of other factors, such as the secretion of immunosuppressive cytokines to limit the overall immunogenicity of the tumour.[3]

The monocyte is also involved in the immune response against tumours and is derived from myeloid precursors. These cells are present in the peripheral circulation but larger numbers are found in the lung, liver and spleen, where they are called macrophages. Macrophages are important in presenting tumour antigens to T-cells but also in non-specific killing after activation by lymphokines released from T-cells. Macrophages are able to release soluble mediators that lead to an improved immune response by activation of T cells. In both human and mouse malignant mesothelioma there is a significant macrophage infiltration of the tumours. These macrophages are predominantly Class II negative and are therefore unactivated and are unlikely to be capable of generating an effective anti-tumour response in their present state. However, it seems plausible that under appropriate conditions these macrophages could become activated and participate in an anti-tumour response.

Humoral immunity is also important and antibodies may bind to tumour cells and lead to disruption of tumour cell membranes. The antibodies may also bind to macrophages, neutrophils or natural killer (NK) cells, allowing these effector cells to remain in close proximity to the tumour cells. In a recent study of malignant mesothelioma patients a significant proportion (28%) were found to have an immune response against their tumour.[4] In this study, patients' sera reacted with a number of human malignant mesothelioma cells lines, as determined by Western blot analysis. When sera were analysed sequentially it was found that the titre increased with disease progression. This work will, it is hoped, lead to the subsequent identification of a number of potential tumour-associated antigens for malignant mesothelioma which can be used in future vaccination and immunotherapy strategies.

NK cells are other important cells involved in the immune response against tumours. NK cells can lyse a number of human tumour cell lines in the absence of previous exposure to tumour antigens. Importantly, IFN-α can lead to increased NK cell activity against tumours. In mesothelioma, NK cell resistance exists because fresh and cultured human malignant mesothelioma cells are not susceptible to NK cell lysis.[5]

Lymphokine activated killer (LAK) cells are also important in the immune response against tumours. These cells are generated when IL-2 binds to NK cells and induces them to proliferate and activates them to kill a wider range of tumour lines. Both human and murine malignant mesothelioma cell lines are susceptible to non-MHC restricted lysis by LAK cells *in vitro*.[5, 6]

The five basic requirements for the induction of an anti-tumour immune response are shown in Figure 18.1. In summary, these five steps are as follows:

1. *Tumour antigen expression*: No tumour will be rejected by a host immune response if it is not antigenic, i.e. if it is not recognised by the host immune response as a target. Tumour antigens are of two types: 'neo'-antigens and 'self'-antigens. Neo-antigens are antigens to which the host is not tolerant, such as oncogenic viruses (human papillomavirus in cervical carcinoma, hepatitis B virus in hepatoma, Epstein-Barr virus in lymphoma and nasopharyngeal carcinoma, etc.) or mutated proteins which induce the formation of neo-antigens, e.g., some *ras* mutations. Self-antigens represent normal body proteins to which the host has only partial tolerance. These are either differentiation antigens (e.g., tyrosinase), onco-fetal or self-antigens (e.g., MAGE) or over-expressed proteins (e.g., p53 protein). Few such antigens have been identified in mesothelioma, although we have recently described topoisomerase-2-beta as a potential mesothelioma tumour antigen since the majority of patients

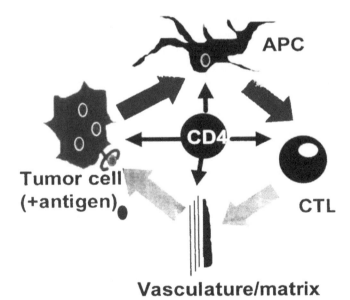

Figure 18.1. *Diagram illustrating the main components of an anti-tumour immune response. (See text for details.)*

with mesothelioma have evidence of serological reactivity against this protein.[7] Other patients do exhibit anti-mesothelioma immune reactivity but in many cases this is patient-specific, i.e. 'private', reactivity.

2. *Tumour antigen presentation*: Tumour antigens that remain sequestered in tumour sites are unable to induce an anti-tumour immune response. They must travel to the draining lymph node and be cross-presented by dendritic cells to the host T cell repertoire before any immune response can be generated. Therefore, the role of the lymph nodes draining any tumour is crucial. In animal models, mesothelioma antigens are efficiently cross-presented in lymph nodes draining the tumour, and therefore it is unlikely that sequestration of mesothelioma antigens is occurring.[8] Thus immunotherapy studies in mesothelioma will need to focus on the induction of an appropriate immune response to these presented antigens, rather than focusing on the induction of cross-presentation of such antigens, as the latter is already occurring, apparently efficiently.

3. *Induction of an appropriate T cell effector response*: Immune responses to any antigen vary according to the nature of the antigen, the dose and context in which it is presented. It is considered that tumours such as mesothelioma induce weak or tolerogenic responses to the antigens that are presented and evidence from mouse mesothelioma models suggest that this is occurring in mesothelioma. Anti-tumour T cell responses are usually weak or, if they are induced, fail to eradicate tumours. Immunotherapeutic approaches therefore aim to induce an appropriate 'immune response' (i.e., one which induces high-level cytotoxic T cell responses with early and persistent CD-4 'helper' responses, the latter being required at both the induction arm and the effector arm of the anti-tumour response).[9]

4. *Traffic to the tumour site*: Cytotoxic T cells with anti-tumour specificity can be generated from a number of animal models of mesothelioma but in some cases the tumour still grows; i.e., the circulating anti-mesothelioma T cells fail to traffic to the tumour. Evidence from these models suggests that if the T cells can be brought into contact with the tumour cells then tumour eradication may occur. No method has yet been successfully devised to ensure that tumour-specific T cells effectively traffic to the tumour site. This is particularly important in mesothelioma as it is impossible to be certain exactly where the tumour deposits are and the host immune system must be relied upon to detect and eradicate occult tumour deposits.

5. *Local tolerance mechanisms must be overcome*: All tumours exhibit some form of self-protection. This may include the production of immunosuppressive molecules, such as transforming growth factor-beta (TGF-β), the expression of molecules which disable damaging T cells (e.g., FasL expression), downregulation of immune recognition molecules (e.g., MHC class I, TAP) and altered 'killability', e.g., modified expression of TNF receptor family molecules. Successful immunotherapy requires that these defenses must be overcome. For example, mesothelioma produces large amounts of TGF-β, which, when blocked, allows T-cell infiltration to occur.[3]

Types of immunotherapy

The most clinically relevant types of immunotherapy are listed below.

1. *Passive:* This involves treatment with monoclonal antibodies that may be given alone or attached to isotopes or chemotherapeutic agents; or

2. *Active*: This involves specific or non-specific stimulation of the host immune system. Specific stimulation involves the use of vaccines comprised of tumour cells or fragments of tumour cells which can stimulate cytotoxic T cells with or without other cells such as DCs. Non-specific stimulation involves macrophages and/or NK cells using adjuvants. The most commonly used adjuvant in humans has been Bacille Calmette-Guérin (BCG), which is an extract of mycobacteria. Cytotomodulatory therapy aims to increase the number of tumour-associated or MHC antigens on the surface of tumour cells to enable immune effector cells to recognise tumour cells and ultimately eliminate them. Examples in this category include IFN-γ and TNF-α. IFN-α upregulates MHC antigen expression but also has other other properties (see below).

The transfer of cells such as NK cells, macrophages, and cytolytic T cells, can either have anti-tumour activity themselves or can modify and stimulate the patient's own immune response.

Immunology of mesothelioma

Evidence exists that mesothelioma cells are susceptible to immune mechanisms. Mesothelioma cells can be killed directly by lymphocyte effector mechanisms. In both human and murine-derived mesothelioma cell lines, LAK cells and certain gamma-delta T lymphocytes are able to cause non-MHC restricted lysis *in vitro*[5,10] As mentioned previously, NK cells are unable to cause lysis of the tumour cells. The ability of these cells to kill mesothelioma cells is not changed when the cells are exposed to IFN-γ or IFN-α.[10] These studies support the concept that there is potential for mesothelioma to be eradicated by immunological means. It is therefore important to develop immunotherapy strategies that exploit the weaknesses of the mesothelioma tumour and this knowledge comes from the animal studies as well as *in vitro* human studies. The ability of tumour cells to promote an immune response or to act as targets for antigen-specific immune effector cells is determined by the cell surface antigens and the soluble factors released by those cells. In human and murine mesothelioma cell lines it has been shown that large amounts of MHC class-1 molecules exist on the cell surface and that this expression can be up-regulated by treatment with IFN-α or IFN-γ.[10,11] However, mesothelioma cell lines express little or no class-II MHC molecules although IFN-γ can upregulate class-II expression in some cell lines. This is significant because although mesothelioma cells have abundant class-I MHC molecules that are important in activation of cytotoxic (CD8+) T cells these cells are poorly able to activate CD4+ positive T cells. This may be one of the ways the tumour is able to escape immune recognition by the host.[12]

Human immunotherapy studies

Most of the human immunotherapy studies of malignant mesothelioma have focused on single agents. However, it seems unlikely that single therapy interventions will be successful because the tumour has several mechanisms to evade immune recognition and certainly so far single treatments have shown only modest responses. Combination therapy combining surgery, irradiation and/or chemotherapy with immunotherapy and gene therapy may have more success. A review of the the various biological and immunological agents that have been used in malignant mesothelioma follows.

BCG in malignant mesothelioma

One of the earliest immunotherapy studies of malignant mesothelioma was performed using BCG.[13] Regular injections of BCG were given intradermally in 30 patients and although no improvement in survival was found, a reduction in tumour-related symptoms was seen in those with minimal or modest disease. There was, however, little or not response seen in those patients who had massive disease. Since this study no further patient studies of BCG have been performed.

Interleukin-2 (IL-2) in malignant mesothelioma

Several clinical studies have shown objective anti-tumoral responses after intrapleural administration of IL-2 for the treatment of malignant pleural mesothelioma and metastatic malignant pleurisy.[14-16] Intrapleural therapy allows high and prolonged intrapleural concentration of cytokines with low circulating levels to cause systemic toxicity. Intrapleural IL-2 at doses ranging from $4-14 \times 10^6$ units with activated autologous LAK cells was administered to 5 patients with mesothelioma intrapleurally on the same side as the tumour.[13] Severe local side effects occurred including empyema, non-cardiogenic pulmonary oedema, encephalopathy, skin rash and abnormal blood biochemistry, effects which limit its clinical use.

Astoul *et al.* have used intrapleural infusions of IL-2 and have determined the maximum tolerated dose of recombinant IL-2 to be 24×10^6 IU/m^2/day.[14,17] This has been followed by a Phase 2 study where intrapleural IL-2 at a dose of 21×10^6 IU/m^2/day was administered continuously for 5 days to 22 patients with malignant pleural mesothelioma.[18] Sixteen of these patients had stage 2 disease (involvement of the mediastinal pleura as well as involvement of the costal or diaphragmatic and visceral pleura.) There were 11 partial responses and 1 complete response. Complete response was defined as the disappearance of macroscopic and microscopic disease and partial response was defined as a greater than 50% reduction in tumour size or as the disappearance of macroscopic disease but persistence of positive cytology or biopsy. The overall median survival time was 18 months, with the median survival time of responders being 28 months compared to non-responders at 8 months ($P<0.01$). The 24 and 36 month survival rates for responders were 58% and 41% respectively. The major side effects were fever, weight gain due to fluid retention and empyema. One of the advantages of this study is that all patients (except 2) underwent a second thoracoscopy to evaluate the macroscopic evidence of response. This study suggests that patients with limited disease (Stage 1 or 2) may benefit from IL-2 therapy although local intrapleural reactions limit the efficiency of this therapy.

Twelve of the 22 patients who achieved objective responses had mesotheliomas of the epithelial histological type, suggesting that histological type may play an important role in the response to IL-2. Further studies are needed to determine the dosing schedule of IL-2, in particular for further cycles of treatment, as in this study only 1 cycle was administered, as well as the optimal treatment schedule when IL-2 is combined with chemotherapy or surgery.

In a study by Nano *et al.*,[19] 6 patients received 1 500 000 IU units of recombinant IL-2 every 8 hours for 5 days as an infusion into the pleural cavity, followed by systemic therapy with 4×10^6 IU of IL-2 administered every day for 5 days per week for 6 weeks. In this study activation of the immune system, as shown by an increase in lymphocytes, monocytes and eosinophils, was observed. The therapy did not lead to significant changes in disease progression. However, in one patient necrosis at the tumoral site was observed after loco-regional recombinant IL-2 administration. Further studies are required to document the effects on the immune system that develop after intracavitary and systemic IL-2 treatment.

IL-2 has been combined with epirubicin in the treatment of malignant mesothelioma.[20] This study was a multi-centre phase 2 study by the Italian Group on Rare Tumours and 21 patients were studied. Treatment included intravenous administration of epirubicin on day 1 and IL-2 at a dose of 9×10^6 units subcutaneously from day 8 to 12 and from day 15 to 19. Cycles were repeated every 3 weeks, up to 6 times, if there was no evidence of progressive disease. There was an overall response rate of 5% with a median progression free and overall survival of 5 and 10 months respectively. There was significant toxicity and this led to treatment cessation in several patients. Therefore the use of IL-2 with other chemotherapy agents needs to be investigated; however, it appears that toxicity will be a major problem. Importantly, it is unclear how patients will tolerate long-term repeated doses of IL-2.

Gene therapy using immunomodulatory agents

This is described in Chapter 12.

Use of IFN-α as a single agent in humans

IFN-α can interfere with cellular growth signals and also upregulate MHC class-I antigens. A trial of 25 patients with malignant mesothelioma was undertaken using recombinant human IFN-α2a (Roferon A).[21] This study administered 3–18 x 10^6 units of recombinant IFN-α2a subcutaneously daily for 12 weeks. Twenty patients completed the 3 months of treatment and 5 of these progressed; 3 patients demonstrated responses with 2 partial responders and 1 complete responder. One patient exhibited a delayed partial response with complete regression over the next 18 months. Therefore recombinant human IFN-α has only modest effects when given subcutaneously.

Combined therapy of IFN-α with chemotherapeutic agents has been studied and has the advantage of the potential synergism that has been demonstrated previously.[22-25] The mechanism is possibly due to altered drug metabolism and promotion of apoptosis of

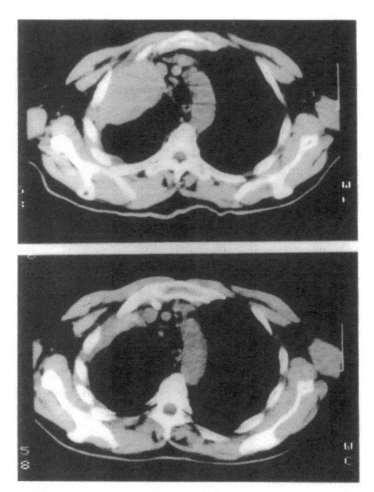

Figure 18.2. IFN-α-induced mesothelioma regression. This patient had a histologically confirmed mesothelioma with a large, solid intrathoracic mass (upper panel). After 3 months of therapy with SC recombinant IFN-α2a there was clear evidence of near-total regression (lower panel).

chemotherapy-damaged cells. Twenty-five patients received IFN-α2a at a dose of 9×10^6 units subcutaneously daily combined with doxorubicin 25 mg/m² intravenously weekly for 12 weeks.[26] A partial response was seen in 4 subjects and 11 remained stable while 6 progressed. Four patients were withdrawn from the study within the first month because of toxicity. Dose modification due to toxicity was required in all patients, with the most common side effects being lethargy, weight loss, leukopenia and vomiting. This study shows that the addition of doxorubicin did not improve the response to IFN-α alone.

Other trials have combined adjuvant immunochemotherapy in the form of cisplatinum, tamoxifen,[27-29] cisplatinum, and mitomycin C, with IFN-α2a.[30,31] Soulie *et al.*

and Purohit *et al.*[31] looked at the combination of weekly cisplatinum/IFN-α2a in mesothelioma. All these studies show partial response rates of between 10% and 35%, but it is difficult to determine the effect of IFN-α on these chemotherapeutic regimens.

IFN-γ in human malignant mesothelioma

IFN-γ has a limited effect on malignant mesothelioma cell lines *in vivo*.[32-34] However, Boutin[35] has shown that IFN-γ used intrapleurally in patients with early stage disease may be useful. Twenty-two patients were treated with IFN-γ 40×10^6 units infused intrapleurally twice weekly for 2 months. Response was determined using serial CT scans and follow-up thoracoscopy. The overall response rate was 56%. This is an encouraging study, but given that most patients with malignant mesothelioma do not present with early stage 1 disease few patients are suitable for this treatment. The effect of cyto-reductive surgery combined with IFN-γ given intrapleurally at the time of surgery has not been studied, and this would be an important study to undertake.

IFN-β in malignant mesothelioma

A phase 2 trial conducted by the South West Oncology Group (SWOG) failed to show any benefit from IFN-β therapy in malignant mesothelioma.[36]

GM-CSF in malignant mesothelioma

GM-CSF activates mature white blood cell effector function and augments antigen presentation.[37] It is able to enhance anti-tumour activity by increasing phagocytic activity of granulocytes and to stimulate antigen presentation by cells such as macrophages and dendritic cells.[38] A study was undertaken of 14 patients who received 2.5–10 mg/kg/day of recombinant human GM-CSF (Molgramostin) intralesionally for 6 weeks using a portable pump.[39,40] One patient developed histologically confirmed necrosis of the tumour surrounding the distal catheter, and one developed lymphocytic infiltrate within the tumour and had a partial response as seen on CT scan (50% tumour shrinkage). Ten patients progressed and 3 were unresponsive to the treatment. There were significant problems with catheter-related infections, blocked catheters, catheter dislodgement, sterile pus at the insertion site and local discomfort related to the positioning of the catheter. This study highlights the technical difficulties in the administration of cytokines intralesionally. Intralesional catheter insertion is difficult and time-consuming and there is an ongoing need to maintain sterility and avoid catheter dislodgement. Some studies have tried to overcome these technical difficulties[41] and future studies should focus on how to administer intrapleural substances effectively whilst minimising side effects.

Animal models

Numerous models have been established in animals to enable better understanding of the biology of malignant mesothelioma.[11,42] The murine malignant mesothelioma cells are diagnostically similar to human MM tumours.[10,11] Upon subcutaneous injection

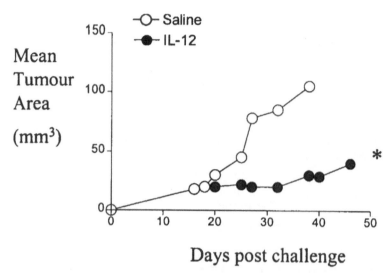

Figure 18.3. *Intratumoral administration of recombinant IL-12 inhibits tumour growth. Balb/c mice were inoculated subcutaneously with 10⁶ AB1 murine malignant mesothelioma cells. Starting on day 16, mice were given intratumoral injection of 0.5 mg of recombinant IL-12 (n=13) or saline (n=10) three times per week for 2 weeks. Data are presented as means, and represent one of three experiments. *Animals treated with recombinant IL-12 had significantly inhibited tumour growth (p<0.0001).*

into mice solid tumours form and grow rapidly. There is minimal evidence of lymphocytic infiltration and the most prominent infiltrating leukocyte is the macrophage, which makes up 50% of the tumour mass. These macrophages are predominantly class II negative and are of the unactivated phenotype, a fact which suggests that they are unlikely to contribute to the initiation of an effective anti-tumour response.

These murine malignant mesothelioma cell lines have been transfected with a number of immunologically relevant molecules including the costimulatory molecules B7-1 and B7-2, plus the cytokines IL-2, IL-4, IL-12, GM-CSF and others.[43-46] Experiments in the animal model indicate that whilst the tumour itself is generally unable to induce an effective anti-tumour response it is susceptible to eradication by the immune system when agents such as these are available. The transduction of B7-1 can lead to the induction of cytotoxic T cells (CD8+) which can recognise and destroy both the transfectant and the parental cell line.[44] Malignant mesothelioma transfected with the IL-12 gene is unable to grow in syngeneic mice.[46,47] This is an immune mediated response as the tumorigenicity of the transfected line is unaffected in immune deficient mice. It has been shown that CD4+ and CD8+ T cells are required and can be seen to infiltrate the site of tumour inoculation before tumour is completely eradicated. IL-12 is a cytokine that is associated with the differentiation of T-cell-mediated cytolytic responses and when it is given systemically in mice with established tumour, IL-12 can cause delay of tumour growth and in some cases eradicate the tumour.

However, in the animal model it has been shown that the cytokine needs to be present continuously and cessation of treatment leads to continued growth of the tumour.

Future directions

There is some modest evidence that immunotherapy for malignant mesothelioma is possible; however we need to develop better regimes to deliver the cytokines to the local tumour environment which do not cause significant side effects. It is also important to perform other studies in conjunction with other therapeutic modalities such as chemotherapy, gene therapy and cytoreductive surgical debulking to see whether combination therapy will be more successful. We also need to determine the optimal method to deliver cytokines (i.e. continuously or intermittently). There is some evidence to suggest that continuous cytokine delivery via intratumoral or intracavitary catheters is more effective. The animal models suggest that other agents such as IL-12 are likely to be important and may hold promise.

References

1. Corson, J.M. Pathology of malignant mesothelioma. *In*: A. J. Antman K, editor. *Asbestos-related malignancy*. Orlando: Grune and Stratton, 1987; 176–200.
2. Henderson, D.W., K.B., Shilkin, D., Whitaker. The pathology of malignant mesothelioma, including immunohistochemistry and ultrastructure. *In* DW Henderson, KB Shilkin, SLP Langlois and D Whitaker, editors. *Malignant mesothelioma*. New York: Hemisphere, 1992; 69–139.
3. Marzo, A. L., D. R. Fitzpatrick, B. W. Robinson, B. Scott. Antisense oligonucleotides specific for transforming growth factor beta2 inhibit the growth of malignant mesothelioma both in vitro and in vivo. *Cancer Res* 1997; **57**: 3200–3207.
4. Robinson, C., B. W. Robinson, R. A. Lake. Sera from patients with malignant mesothelioma can contain autoantibodies. *Lung Cancer* 1998; **20**:175–184.
5. Manning, L. S., R. V. Bowman, S. B. Darby, B. W. Robinson. Lysis of human malignant mesothelioma cells by natural killer (NK) and lymphokine-activated killer (LAK) cells. *Am Rev Respir Dis* 1989; **139**: 1369–1374.
6. Mavaddat, N., B. W. Robinson, A. H. Rose, L. S. Manning, M. J. Garlepp. An analysis of the relationship between gamma delta T cell receptor V gene usage and non-major histocompatibility complex-restricted cytotoxicity. *Immunol Cell Biol* 1993; **71**: 27–37.
7. Robinson, C., M. Callow, S. Stevenson, B. Scott, B. W. S. Robinson, R. A. Lake. Serologic responses in patients with malignant mesothelioma: evidence for both public and private specificities. *Am J Respir Cell Mol Biol* 2000; **22**: 550–556.
8. Marzo, A. L., R. A. Lake, M. Callow, B. W. S. Robinson, B. M. Scott, D. Lo, L. Sherman. Tumor antigens are constitutively presented in the draining lymph nodes. *J Immunol* 1999; **162**: 5838–5845.
9. Marzo, A. L., B. F. Kinnear, R. A. Lake, J. J. Frelinger, E. J. Collins, B. W. S. Robinson, B. Scott. Tumor-specific CD4+ T cells have a major 'post-licensing' role in CTL mediated anti-tumor immunity. *J Immunol* 2000; **165**: 6047–6055.
10. Christmas, T. I., L. S. Manning, M. R. Davis, B. W. Robinson, M. J. Garlepp. HLA antigen expression and malignant mesothelioma. *Am J Respir Cell Mol Biol* 1991; **5**: 213–220.

11. Davis, M.R., L.S. Manning, D. Whitaker, M.J. Garlepp, and B. W. Robinson. Establishment of a murine model of malignant mesothelioma. *Int J Cancer* 1992; **52**: 881–886.

12. Upham, J. W., M. J. Garlepp, A. W. Musk, and B. W. Robinson. Malignant mesothelioma: new insights into tumour biology and immunology as a basis for new treatment approaches. *Thorax* 1995; **50**: 887–893.

13. Webster, I., J. W. Cochrane, and K. R. Burkhardt. Immunotherapy with BCG vaccine in 30 cases of mesothelioma. *S Afr Med J* 1982; **61**: 277–278.

14. Astoul, P., J. R. Viallat, J. C. Laurent, M. Brandely, and C. Boutin. Intrapleural recombinant IL-2 in passive immunotherapy for malignant pleural effusion. *Chest* 1993; **103**: 209–213.

15. Viallat, J. R., C. Boutin, F. Rey, P. Astoul, P. Farisse, and M. Brandely. Intrapleural immunotherapy with escalating doses of interleukin-2 in metastatic pleural effusions. *Cancer* 1993; **71**: 4067–4071.

16. Robinson, B. W. S., L. S. Manning, R. V. Bowman, T. I. Christmas, A. W. Musk, M. R. Davis, *et al.* The scientific basis for the immunotherapy of human malignant mesothelioma. *Eur Respir Rev* 1993; **3**: 195–198.

17. Astoul, P., P. Bertault-Peres, A. Durand, J. Catalin, F. Vignal, and C. Boutin. Pharmacokinetics of intrapleural recombinant interleukin-2 in immunotherapy for malignant pleural effusion. *Cancer* 1994; **73**: 308–313.

18. Astoul, P., D. Picat-Joosen, J. Viallet, and C. Boutin. Intrapleural administration of interleukin-2 for the treatment of patients with malignant pleural mesothelioma. *Cancer* 1998; **83**: 2099–2104.

19. Nano, R., E. Capelli, M. Civallero, G. Terzuolo, E. Volpini, C. Nascimbene, and P. Cremaschi. Effects of interleukin-2 for the treatment of malignant mesothelioma. *Oncol Res* 1998; **5**: 489–492.

20. Bretti, S., A. Berruti, L. Dogliotti, B. Castagneto, R. Bertulli, P. Spadaro, G. Toscano, P. Astorre, C. Verusio, R. Lionetto, P. Bruzzi, and A. Santoro. Combined epirubicin and interleukin-2 regimen in the treatment of malignant mesothelioma: a multicenter phase II study of the Italian Group on Rare Tumours. *Tumori* 1998; **84**: 558–561.

21. Christmas, T. I., L. S. Manning, M. J. Garlepp, A. W. Musk, and B. W. Robinson. Effect of interferon-alpha 2a on malignant mesothelioma. *J Interferon Res* 1993; **13**: 9–12.

22. Wadler, S., R. Wersto, V. Weinberg, D. Thompson, and E. L. Schwartz. Interaction of fluorouracil and interferon in human colon cancer cell lines: cytotoxic and cytokinetic effects. *Cancer Res* 1990; **50**: 5735–5739.

23. Wadler, S., and E. L. Schwartz. Antineoplastic activity of the combination of interferon and cytotoxic agents against experimental and human malignancies: a review. *Cancer Res* 1990; **50**: 3473–3486.

24. Wadler, S., M. Goldman, A. Lyver, and P. H. Wiernik. Phase I trial of 5-fluorouracil and recombinant alpha 2a-interferon in patients with advanced colorectal carcinoma. *Cancer Res* 1990; **50**: 2056–2059.

25. Wadler, S., and P. H. Wiernik. Clinical update on the role of fluorouracil and recombinant interferon alfa-2a in the treatment of colorectal carcinoma. *Semin Oncol* 1990; **17(1 Suppl 1)**: 16–21; Discussion 38–41.

26. Upham, J. W., A. W. Musk, G. van Hazel, M. Byrne, and B. W. Robinson. Interferon alpha and doxorubicin in malignant mesothelioma: a phase II study. *Aust N Z J Med* 1993; **23**: 683–6837.

27. Pass, H. W., B. K. Temeck, K. Kranda, S. M. Steinberg, and H. I. Pass. A phase II trial investigating primary immunochemotherapy for malignant pleural mesothelioma and the

feasibility of adjuvant immunochemotherapy after maximal cytoreduction. *Ann Surg Oncol* 1995; **2**: 214–220.

28. Ardizzoni, A., M. C. Pennucci, B. Castagneto, G. L. Mariani, A. Cinquegrana, D. Magri, A. Verna, F. Salvati, and R. Rosso. Recombinant interferon alpha-2b in the treatment of diffuse malignant pleural mesothelioma. *Am J Clin Oncol* 1994; **17**: 80–82.

29. Tansan, S., S. Emri, T. Selcuk, Y. Koc, P. Hesketh, T. Heeren, R. P. McCaffrey, and Y. I. Baris. Treatment of malignant pleural mesothelioma with cisplatin, mitomycin C and alpha interferon. *Oncology* 51994; **1**: 348–351.

30. Soulie, P., P. Ruffie, L. Trandafir, I. Monnet, A. Tardivon, P. Terrier, E. Cvitkovic, T. Le Chevalier, and J. P. Armand. Combined systemic chemoimmunotherapy in advanced diffuse malignant mesothelioma. Report of a phase I-II study of weekly cisplatin/interferon alfa-2a. *J Clin Oncol* 1996; **14**: 878–885.

31. Purohit, A., L. Moreau, A. Dietemann, R. Seibert, G. Pauli, J. M. Wihlm, and E. Quoix. Weekly systemic combination of cisplatin and interferon alpha 2a in diffuse malignant pleural mesothelioma. *Lung Cancer* 1998; **22**: 119–125.

32. Phan-Bich, L., A. Buard, J. F. Petit, L. Zeng, J. P. Tenu, P. Chretien, I. Monnet, C. Boutin, J. Bignon, G. Lemaire, and M. C. Jaurand. Differential responsiveness of human and rat mesothelioma cell lines to recombinant interferon-gamma. *Am J Respir Cell Mol Biol* 1997; **16**: 178–186.

33. Monti, G., M. C. Jaurand, I. Monnet, P. Chretien, L. Saint-Etienne, L. Zeng, A. Portier, P. Devillier, P. Galanaud, J. Bignon, *et al*. Intrapleural production of interleukin 6 during mesothelioma and its modulation by gamma-interferon treatment. *Cancer Res* 1994; **54**: 4419–4423.

34. Zeng, L., A. Buard, I. Monnet, C. Boutin, J. Fleury, L. Saint-Etienne, P. Brochard, J. Bignon, and M. C. Jaurand. In vitro effects of recombinant human interferon gamma on human mesothelioma cell lines. *Int J Cancer* 1993; **55**: 515–520.

35. Boutin, C., J. R. Viallat, N. Van Zandwijk, J. T. Douillard, J. C. Paillard, J. C. Guerin, P. Mignot, J. Migueres, F. Varlet, A. Jehan, *et al*. Activity of intrapleural recombinant gamma-interferon in malignant mesothelioma. *Cancer* 1991; **67**: 2033–2037.

36. Von Hoff, D. D., B. Metch, J. G. Lucas, S. P. Balcerzak, S. M. Grunberg, and S. E. Rivkin. Phase II evaluation of recombinant interferon-beta (IFN-beta ser) in patients with diffuse mesothelioma: a Southwest Oncology Group study. *J Interferon Res* 1990; **10**: 531–534.

37. Metcalf, D. Haemopoietic growth factors 1. *Lancet* 1989; **1**: 825–827.

38. Morrissey, P. J., L. Bressler, L. S. Park, A. Alpert, and S. Gillis. Granulocyte-macrophage colony-stimulating factor augments the primary antibody response by enhancing the function of antigen-presenting cells. *J Immunol* 1987; **139**: 1113–1119.

39. Davidson, J. A., A. W. Musk, B. R. Wood, S. Morey, M. Ilton, L. L. Yu, P. Drury, K. Shilkin, and B. W. Robinson. Intralesional cytokine therapy in cancer: a pilot study of GM-CSF infusion in mesothelioma. *J Immunother* 1998; **21**: 389–398.

40. Robinson, B., S. Mukherjee, A. Davidson, S. Morey, A. Musk, I. Ramshaw, D. Smith, R. Lake, T. Haenel, M. Garlepp, J. Marley, C. Leong, I. Caminschi, and B. Scott. Cytokine gene therapy or infusion as treatment for solid human cancer. *J Immunother* 1998; **21**: 211–217.

41. Driesen, P., C. Boutin, J. R. Viallat, P. H. Astoul, J. P. Vialette, and J. Pasquier. Implantable access system for prolonged intrapleural immunotherapy. *Eur Respir J* 1994; **7**: 1889–1892.

42. Cora, E. M., and A. B. Kane. Alterations in a tumour suppressor gene, p53, in mouse mesotheliomas induced by crocidolite asbestos. *Eur Respir Rev* 1993; **3**: 148–150.

43. Leong, C. C., B. W. Robinson, and M. J. Garlepp. Generation of an antitumour immune response to a murine mesothelioma cell line by the transfection of allogeneic MHC genes. *Int J Cancer* 1994; **59**: 212–216.
44. Leong, C. C., J. V. Marley, S. Loh, N. Milech, B. W. Robinson, and M. J. Garlepp. Transfection of the gene for B7-1 but not B7-2 can induce immunity to murine malignant mesothelioma. *Int J Cancer* 1997; **71**: 476–482.
45. Leong, C. C., J. V. Marley, S. Loh, B. W. Robinson, and M. J. Garlepp. The induction of immune responses to murine malignant mesothelioma by IL-2 gene transfer. *Immunol Cell Biol* 1997; **75**: 356–359.
46. Caminschi, I., E. Venetsanakos, C. C. Leong, M. J. Garlepp, B. Scott, and B. W. Robinson. Interleukin-12 induces an effective antitumour response in malignant mesothelioma. *Am J Respir Cell Mol Biol* 1998; **19**: 738–746.
47. Caminschi, I., E. Venetsanakos, C. C. Leong, M. J. Garlepp, B. W. Robinson, and B. Scott. Cytokine gene therapy of mesothelioma. Immune and antitumour effects of transfected interleukin-12. *Am J Respir Cell Mol Biol* 1999; **21**: 347–356.

$=19=$

Epidemiology of Mesothelioma

Nicholas H. de Klerk and A. William Musk

Background

Put simply, the epidemiology of a disease is a summary of who gets the disease, where when and why they get it, and what happens once they have it. Such a summary is therefore usually specified by some age and time trends; sex and geographical differences in the principal disease measures (incidence, mortality, prevalence); and the natural history of the disease, including efficacy of treatments, aetiology, and possibly, avenues for prevention. There is little scope for controversy in this description unless of course the definition of the disease itself or aspects of its enumeration are open to variable interpretation. A good example of such a disease is asthma, which has recently merited yet another whole book on its epidemiology.[1]

The association between exposure to asbestos in its various forms and malignant mesothelioma (hereafter referred to just as mesothelioma) is so strong that the epidemiology of mesothelioma can be almost completely described in terms of the 'epidemiology' of exposure to asbestos, that is, using the above definition, a summary of who has been exposed to asbestos, what type of asbestos they were exposed to, where when and how they were exposed, and what happened to them afterwards. Indeed, some authors have preferred to describe the epidemiology of both together, and certainly the epidemiology of mesothelioma has been summarised previously on many occasions. Because of this we have aimed to summarise only briefly the generally accepted aspects of these 'epidemiologies' and to concentrate on more recent or perhaps controversial points. Interested readers wanting more basic descriptions and more numerical data are advised to look in these other reports.[2-7]

History

Most cases of mesothelioma arise after exposure to asbestos, especially the amphibole varieties, and the disease occurs long (10–50 years) after first exposure.

Major controversy arose after the Second World War about the definition of 'meso-thelioma' and, more recently, the definition of the term 'asbestos'. There have also been aspects of the disease that are unrelated to asbestos and these are discussed further below.

It is still not entirely clear why it was only after Wagner *et al.*'s seminal 1960 paper[8] that mesothelioma was accepted as a disease in its own right, together with its association with asbestos, when endothelioma of the pleura had been a recognised consequence of asbestos exposure for many years previously.[9]

One explanation is the influential declaration by Willis[10] (p 77) that there was no such entity:

> While the possibility of the occurrence of primary neoplasms of coelomic membranes cannot be denied, the great majority of cases so reported are certainly only examples of serosal disease secondary to undiscovered primary tumours in neighbouring viscera. The truth of this statement will be apparent from the following brief review.

He then went on to dismiss the various reports (usually of endothelioma of the pleura) in the literature as being in such a category.

Another explanation is deliberate obfuscation by 'scientists' working for the asbes-tos companies. Credence may be given to this theory by the revelations from Castleman's investigations into the history of asbestos company sponsored research from the 1930s onwards, where suppression of important findings and deliberate fraud[11] ranked alongside similar immoral behaviour by tobacco corporations.[12] Even 5 years after the Wagner paper a representative of Cape Industries was implying that, since no mesotheliomas had been recorded in South Africa after Wagner's departure and that numerous cases were then occurring in Britain coinciding with his arrival there, the diagnosis was largely a personal aberration.[13] A similar argument could be made that the erionite found in Karain did not cause any mesothelioma there until Baris and his colleagues arrived in the 1970s,[14] or that the – recently discontinued – export of crocidolite from South Africa to destinations un-known has not and will not cause mesothelioma there,[15] simply because there may be inadequate health statistics recorded in those destinations.

Descriptive epidemiology

Worldwide rates

Even though people with mesothelioma have a very short life expectancy,[16] mesothelioma mortality rates usually underestimate incidence rates, probably because of difficulties with diagnosis as well as the general drawbacks of death certification.[17] Highest rates are in those countries that have made the most use of crocidolite and amosite asbestos, in par-ticular in the shipbuilding industry. Mortality rates from the WHO mortality database for 1993 (Figs 19.1 and 19.2) are in almost exactly the same order as they were in 1988.[18]

Age and sex

Incidence increases with age and, in subjects with the same exposure, either occupa-tional, environmental or none at all, is the same in both sexes. The sex-related differ-ences are accounted for by exposure differences.

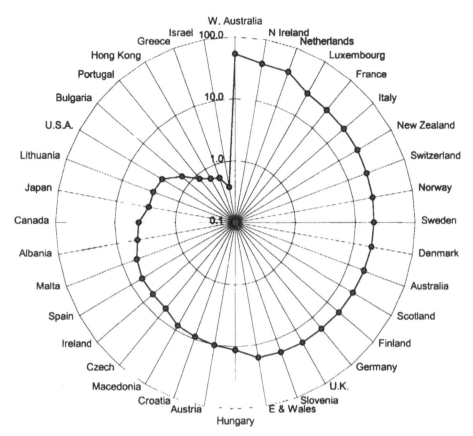

Figure 19.1. *Mortality rates (deaths per million population, all ages) for males, 1993, WHO reported data.*

Primary site: pleural or peritoneal

Nothing has been elucidated epidemiologically about the difference between the two main primary sites of mesothelioma. In populations where asbestos exposure has been documented and sufficient follow-up has occurred, the distribution of the latent period between exposure and onset of disease has been similar but survival is slightly shorter for peritoneal mesothelioma (an average of 6 months compared with 9 months). In general, however, apart from some exceptional populations, peritoneal mesothelioma is rarer than pleural mesothelioma and is almost unheard of in non-occupationally exposed populations where the overall incidence is low.

Calendar time

Mortality rates from mesothelioma appear to have ceased their dramatic increase in the developed world, and in places such as the USA and Western Australia they

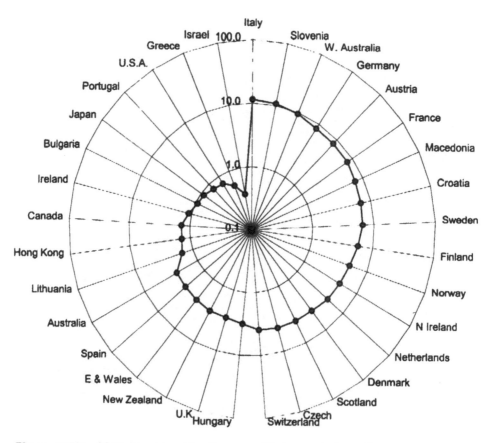

Figure 19.2. *Mortality rates (deaths per million population, all ages) for females, 1993, WHO reported data.*

are now actually declining. The effects of the decline in production and use of crocidolite particularly seems to be having beneficial effects. It is now over 33 years since the Wittenoom mine closed in 1966 and use of crocidolite has been declining since then.

Future rates

Several well-reasoned analyses have demonstrated the probable increase in mesothelioma rates, particularly in Europe, as a result of the continued use of amphibole asbestos in industry into the 1970s.

Rates in less well developed economies that were recipients of the continued export of South African crocidolite and amosite can be expected to rise.[15]

Aetiology

Asbestos

A recent extensive investigation has developed reliable exposure–response relationships for mesothelioma, separately for the 3 major fibre types: crocidolite, amosite and chrysotile. Very approximately, the study found that crocidolite was 10 times worse than amosite, which was in turn 10 times worse than chrysotile.[5]

Exposure–response relationships

These have been fully discussed elsewhere.[2,4,5,19 21] It is generally accepted that the incidence of mesothelioma increases with the 3rd to 4th power of time from first exposure to asbestos (or from birth if unexposed or if exposed uniformly throughout life) and increases approximately linearly with intensity of exposure, or:

$$I = K \times F \times T^p$$

where I = incidence (rate), T = time after first exposure, F = fibres/mL and p is between 3 and 4. The shape of the curve is similar for all asbestos types but K varies, being highest for crocidolite, then amosite and then chrysotile.

The amphibole hypothesis

There is ample evidence that crocidolite is the most mesotheliomagenic form of asbestos. The 'ordering' of the different types in terms of their capacity to cause mesothelioma is generally agreed on, but the implications perhaps are not (see, e.g., Wagner *et al.*[22]).

Arguments that chrysotile in its pure form does not cause mesothelioma and therefore can be safely used for certain products for which other substitutes perform worse are more theoretical than practical: firstly because it is almost never found in its pure form but is contaminated by tremolite (or even 'Balangeroite') and secondly because of its association with lung cancer. Hodgson also summarised the information relating to lung cancer, concluding that for the same amount of exposure (in fibres/mL years) the excess lung cancer due to chrysotile was 2–10% of that due to amosite or crocidolite.[5]

Types of exposure to asbestos

Inherent occupational exposure

The majority of cases of mesothelioma arise in people with direct exposure to asbestos incurred as a necessary part of their job. That is, the workers have mined or milled asbestos, worked on its manufacture into various products, or used the manufactured products in their work. Most of these types of exposure have been well described previously (e.g., de Klerk and Armstrong[2]).

Bystander occupational exposure

Some of the types of 'casual' exposure could have been foreseen. The Annual Report of the Chief Inspector of Factories for the year 1949 (HMSO) stated:[23]

> Several Inspectors refer to the unsatisfactory practice of packing raw asbestos fibre into unlined hessian or jute bags (frequently it is shipped at the country of origin and delivered to a factory in this manner) which renders workers handling them liable to considerable exposure to dust and fibre. The Regulations prohibit the use of such sacks or bags for transport of the material within the factory – for which purpose only containers constructed of impermeable material in good repair are permitted.

The Regulations referred to are the Code of Regulations for Asbestos, in force in the UK since 1931. Many of the cases of mesothelioma, certainly those arising in workers on the State Ships and in lumpers on the Point Sampson and Fremantle wharves in Western Australia, would have been avoided if the crocidolite from Wittenoom had been packed in impermeable material. Most of the cases arising among Aborigines in the Wittenoom area in Western Australia received their exposure via the leaky hessian bags, resulting in their having one of the highest population-based mesothelioma rates in the world.[24] Bags that had been used at Wittenoom were used at the chrysotile mine in Baryulgil, New South Wales, and were thought to be responsible for the cases of mesothelioma arising among workers there.[25]

Childhood exposure

Only the cohort study of former Wittenoom residents has been able to examine the question of whether childhood exposure to crocidolite confers greater risk of mesothelioma than that caused by exposure occurring later in life. Recent analyses indicated that no such increased risk was evident;[26] that is, the effects of duration, intensity and time since exposure were the same in adults and children.

Environmental exposure

A distinction is usually made between domestic/household exposure from living with an asbestos worker, and environmental exposure, from nearby asbestos works or natural occurrences of asbestos. There have been numerous descriptions of cases arising in people without occupational exposure and these and their implications have been discussed extensively elsewhere.[3,27] Rates in unexposed people in Western Australia have ceased increasing (Fig. 19.3), as have rates in females (Fig. 19.4). Previous increases could have been taken to be a reflection of an increase in general environmental levels, an issue which is moot.

Lung burden studies

Fibres clear from the lungs at different rates, chrysotile certainly clears much faster than the others due to its solubility and its propensity to break into smaller fibrils,

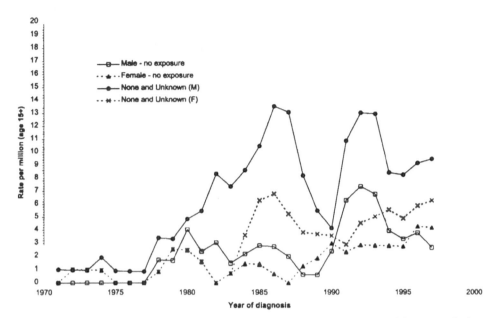

Figure 19.3. *Western Australian mesothelioma rates (cases per million population aged 15+), subjects with no known exposure to asbestos or unknown exposure status, 3-year moving averages, 1971–98.*

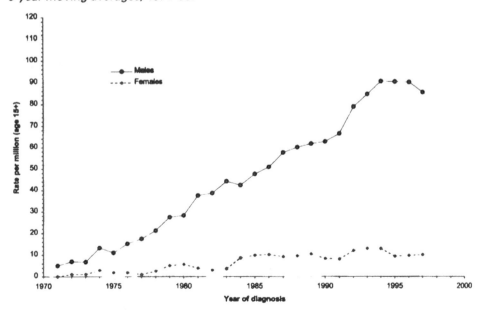

Figure 19.4. *Western Australian mesothelioma rates (cases per million population aged 15+), all cases, 3-year moving averages, 1971–98.*

making the value of lung burden studies of chrysotile questionable. Crocidolite appears to clear at about 9% per year or with a half-life of about 7 years.[28]

Erionite

The rate of mesothelioma after exposure to erionite is much higher than that for crocidolite. This difference in humans is also mirrored in inhalation experiments with rats, and although, in many respects, rat experiments may be somewhat misleading (see Berry[20] for a good discussion), the difference between the effect of crocidolite and erionite inhalation on rat mesothelioma mortality was striking.[29] The form of the exposure–response relationship derived from the Turkish studies of erionite is the same as for crocidolite, except that the increase in rate with 3–4th power of time from first exposure equates to an increase with 3–4th power of age, as it is also in people who are unexposed.[3]

Other causes

This has been reviewed elsewhere: radiation, in particular the use of Thorotrast, and chest injuries seem to be the only other established causes.[30]

Other fibres

Workers in other fibre industries have been under extensive scrutiny for many years because of the likelihood of disease due to the common size and shape and possibly durability of the fibres to which the workers are exposed and *in vitro* and *in vivo* evidence of their similar carcinogenic potential. No cases of mesothelioma have arisen in these industries that have not been linked to actual asbestos exposure.

SV-40

DNA sequences from simian virus 40 (SV-40) have been found in several series of mesothelial tumours worldwide. Similar sequences have not been found in surrounding tissue. The significance of this finding for the epidemiology of mesothelioma has not been established.[31] It is not known what the prevalence of SV-40 infection (previously thought to be harmless to humans) is in any populations. This lack of knowledge of the epidemiology of SV-40 in human populations hampers progress on this potentially interesting finding. Because numerous batches of polio vaccine in the 1950s were found to be infected with this virus, it has been suggested that this may be a 'cofactor' with asbestos in causing mesothelioma. Investigations so far have not been large enough (either in population size or length of follow-up) to rule out the possibility of increased rates of mesothelioma in recipients of the infected vaccine compared with recipients of uninfected vaccine.

Lack of association with smoking

Mesothelioma is one of the very few cancers that is not affected in any way by inhalation of tobacco smoke.

Familial associations

There have been several reports of clusters of cases of mesothelioma arising within families. It has not been possible to determine whether these have not been caused by common domestic, environmental or occupational asbestos exposure; however, it seems likely that genetic effects are implicated.

Migrants

Migrant studies, as well as studies of distinct ethnic groups, may further investigation of the possibility of differences in susceptibility due to different genetic backgrounds. For example, it has been suggested that Italian migrants who worked at Wittenoom have higher rates of mesothelioma than similarly exposed Australian workers.[33] The evidence is far from conclusive because precise exposures are unknown and it has been suggested that the Italians may have been given the more dusty work at Wittenoom, even within the recorded job titles.[32]

Precursors/predictors

The presence of pleural plaques on x-ray, while an indicator of past exposure to asbestos, is not a predictor of mesothelioma, if the level of exposure is taken into account.[33] Studies that have claimed the contrary have not been able adequately to control for asbestos exposure.

Prevention

The best prevention of mesothelioma is prevention of exposure to asbestos. Only one prevention trial has demonstrated the efficacy of any protective agent in people already exposed to substantial amounts of asbestos. While only a comparatively small study, administration of daily retinol (25 000 IU/day) was associated with much lower rates of mesothelioma in former Wittenoom workers than workers who took daily beta-carotene, or those who were not randomised into the study at all. [4,35] This study is continuing in modified form.

Treatment and survival

The average survival time after presentation with mesothelioma is about 9 months. Patients presenting with breathlessness survive longer than patients presenting with pain, presumably because the latter have solid tumour present rather than only malignant pleural effusion. Patients with peritoneal mesothelioma survive less long (median survival about 6 months) than patients with pleural tumours, probably for the same reason.

Various treatments have been tried, including chemotherapy, radiation and surgery. These are discussed at length elsewhere in this volume. Some of these may lead to temporary improvement in quality of life, and also an apparent increase in survival; however, groups of patients for whom increased survival has been described after various treatments are generally specially selected for treatment and are likely to have survived longer anyway. No treatments have yet been described that would justify Phase 3 trials.

References

1. Pearce, N., Beasley, R., Burgess, C., Crane, J. Asthma epidemiology: principles and methods. New York: Oxford University Press, 1998.
2. de Klerk, N.H., Armstrong, B.K. The epidemiology of asbestos and mesothelioma. In: Henderson, D.W., Shilkin, K.B., Langlois, S.L.P., Whitaker, D., eds. *Malignant Mesothelioma.* New York: Hemisphere, 1992; 223–250.
3. de Klerk, N.H. Environmental mesothelioma. In: Bignon J, Jaurand MC, eds. *Mesothelial Cell and Mesothelioma.* New York: Marcel Dekker, 1994; 19–36.
4. Health Effects Institute – Asbestos Research. *Asbestos in Public Buildings: A Literature Review and Synthesis of Current Knowledge.* Cambridge: HEI-AR, 1991.
5. Hodgson, J.T., Darnton, A. A review of the quantitative risks of mesothelioma and lung cancer in relation to asbestos exposure. *Ann Occup Hyg* 2000; **44**: 565–601.
6. McDonald, J.C., McDonald, A.D. The epidemiology of mesothelioma in historical context. *Eur Respir J* 1996; **9**: 1932–1942.
7. Western Australian Advisory Committee on Hazardous Substances. Asbestos cement products. Perth: Health Department of WA, 1990.
8. Wagner, J.C., Sleggs, C.A., Marchand, P. Diffuse pleural mesothelioma and asbestos exposure in The North Western Cape Province. *Br J Ind Med* 1960; **17**: 260–271.
9. Perry, K.M.A. Diseases of the lung resulting from occupational dusts other than silica. *Thorax* 1947; **2**: 91–113.
10. Willis, R.A. *The Spread of Tumours in the Human Body.* London: Churchill, 1934.
11. Lilienfeld, D.E. The silence: the asbestos industry and early occupational cancer research – a case study. *Am J Public Health* 1991; **81**: 791–800.
12. Glantz, S.A., Barnes, D.E., Bero, L., Hanauer, P., Slade, J. Looking through a keyhole at the tobacco industry – the Brown and Williamson documents. *JAMA* 1995; **274**: 219–224.
13. Gaze, R. Discussion of: Owen WG. Mesothelial tumors and exposure to asbestos dust. *Ann N Y Acad Sci* 1965; **132**: 674–684.
14. Baris, Y.I., Sahin, A.A., Ozesmi, M., *et al.* An outbreak of pleural mesothelioma and chronic fibrosing pleurisy in the village of Karain/Uerguep in Anatolia. *Thorax* 1978; **33**: 181–192.
15. Harington, J.S., McGlashan, N.D. South African asbestos: production, exports, and destinations, 1959–1993. *Am J Ind Med* 1998; **33**: 21–26.
16. Musk, A.W., Woodward, S.D. Conventional treatment and its effect on survival of malignant pleural mesothelioma in Western Australia. *Aust N Z J Med* 1982; **12**: 229–232.
17. Lilienfeld, D.E., Gunderson, P.D. The 'missing cases' of pleural malignant mesothelioma in Minnesota, 1979–81: preliminary report. *Public Health Reports* 1986; **101**: 395–399.
18. Williams, V.M., de Klerk, N.H., Musk, A.W., Whitake, D., Filion, P.R., Shilkin, K.B., Wolanski, K. Measurement of lung tissue content of asbestos: an example from Western Australia. In: Peters GA, Peters BJ, eds. *Sourcebook on Asbestos Diseases.* Charlottesville: Lexis Law Publishing, 1997; 17–46.
19. Peto, J. The hygiene standard for chrysotile asbestos. *Lancet* 1978; i: 484–489.
20. Berry, G. Models for mesothelioma incidence following exposure to fibers in terms of timing and duration of exposure and the biopersistence of the fibers. *Inhalation Toxicol* 1999; **11**: 111–130.

21. Berry, G. Prediction of mesothelioma, lung cancer and asbestosis in former Wittenoom asbestos workers. *Br J Ind Med* 1991; **48**: 793–802.
22. Wagner, J.C., Stayner, L.T., Dankovic, D.A., *et al.* Asbestos-related cancer and the amphibole hypothesis [Letters to the Editor] *Am J Public Health* 1997; **87**: 687–691.
23. Chief Inspector of Factories. Annual Report. London: HMSO, 1949.
24. Musk, A.W., de Klerk, N.H., Eccles, J.L., Hansen, J., Shilkin, K.B. Malignant mesothelioma in Pilbara Aborigines. *Aust J Public Health* 1995; **19**: 520–522.
25. House of Representatives Standing Committee on Aboriginal Affairs. *The Effects of Asbestos Mining on the Baryulgil Community.* Canberra: Australian Government Publishing Service, 1984.
26. Hansen, J., de Klerk, N.H., Musk, A.W., Hobbs, M.S.T. Environmental exposure to crocidolite and mesothelioma: exposure-response relationships. *Am J Respir Crit Care Med* 1998; **157**: 69–75.
27. Hillerdal, G. Mesothelioma: cases associated with non-occupational and low dose exposures. *Occup Environ Med* 1999; **56**: 505–513.
28. de Klerk, N.H., Musk, A.W., Williams, V.M., Filion, P.R., Whitaker, D., Shilkin, K.B. Comparison of measures of exposure to asbestos in former crocidolite workers from Wittenoom Gorge, W. Australia. *Am J Ind Med* 1996; **30**: 579–587.
29. Wagner, J.C., Skidmore, J.W., Hill, R.J., Griffiths, D.M. Erionite exposure and mesothelioma in rats. *Br J Cancer* 1985; **51**: 727–730.
30. Comin, C.E., de Klerk, N.H., Henderson, D.W. Malignant mesothelioma. *Ultrastruct Pathol* 1997; **21**: 315–320.
31. Butel, J.S., Lednicky, J.A. Cell and molecular biology of simian virus 40: implications for human infections and disease. *J Nat Cancer Inst* 1999; **91**: 119–134.
32. Merler, E., Ercolanelli, M., Cappelletto, F., de Klerk, N.H., Lund, H.G., Musk, A.W. On 1126 Italian migrants to Australia who worked at the crocidolite mine of Wittenoom Gorge between 1946 and 1966. In: Grieco A, Iavicoli S, Berlinguer G (eds), *Proceedings of the 1st International Conference of Occupational and Environmental Prevention*, Rome, 1998.
33. de Klerk, N.H., Musk, A.W., Armstrong, B.K., Hobbs, M.S.T. Non-malignant pleuro-pulmonary disease and the development of malignant mesothelioma in Western Australian crocidolite workers. *Proceedings of the 9th International Symposium on Epidemiology in Occupational Health.* US Dept of Health and Human Services. 1994; 161–166.
34. Musk, A.W., de Klerk, N.H., Ambrosini, G.L., Eccles, J.L., Hansen, J., Olsen, N., Watts, V.L., Lund, H.G., Pang, S.C., Beilby, J., Hobbs, M.S.T. Vitamin A and cancer prevention. I. Observations in workers previously exposed to asbestos at Wittenoom, Western Australia. *Int J Cancer* 1998; **75**: 355–361.
35. de Klerk, N.H., Musk, A.W., Ambrosini, G.L., Eccles, J.L., Hansen, J., Olsen, N., Watts, V.L., Lund, H.G., Pang, S., Beilby, J., Hobbs, M.S.T. Vitamin A and cancer prevention. II. Comparison of the effects of retinol and beta-carotene. *Int J Cancer* 1998; **75**: 362–367.

=20=

Mesothelioma in Japan

Takashi Nakano

Malignant mesothelioma is an insidious neoplasm which has a strong aetiological relationship with asbestos exposure. The incidence is still rising worldwide, but is expected to start dropping in industrialised countries because of recent prohibitions on the use of asbestos. Mesothelioma, and its relationship with asbestos and other aetiological factors in Japan, are discussed in this chapter.

Incidence

Malignant mesothelioma has been a relatively rare neoplasm, which was not separately listed in the Ministry of Health and Welfare's document 'Vital Statistics in Japan'. It was difficult to determine statistically the incidence of malignant mesothelioma in Japan because of this listing problem. In 1995, the 10th Revision of the *International Classification of Diseases* (ICD-10) was adopted in Japan for classifying the causes of death. In this document, mesothelioma is listed as a separate cause of death for use on death certificates. The annual numbers of deaths from mesothelioma in 1995, 1996, 1997 and 1998 were 500, 576, 597 and 570, respectively, and its proportional mortality rate was 0.19–0.22% (Fig. 20.1). The male:female ratio is approximately 3:1. The age distribution in 1995–98 was monophasic, peaking in the 65–69-year-old age group (Fig. 20.1). This rate of 500–600 cases per year seems to be a fairly small number, compared to that in other industrialised countries. About 2000 new cases of malignant mesothelioma are recorded in the United States each year.[1] According to 'Vital Statistics in Japan', which used the 9th Revision of ICD, the annual number of deaths from malignant neoplasms of pleura and pleural mesothelioma was about 100 in the early 1980s, and 250 in the late 1980s.[2] The number of cases of malignant mesothelioma is small, although mortality data in 'Vital Statistics' suggest that the incidence of mesothelioma is increasing in Japan. Specialised registry-based incidence and mortality data for mesothelioma in the whole of Japan are not available. The use of death certificate data to investigate the incidence of mesothelioma has led to inaccuracies because of uncertain diagnoses, due to lack of

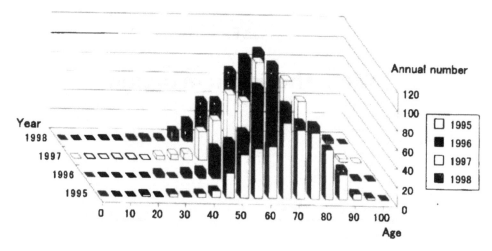

Figure 20.1. Number of deaths from malignant mesothelioma by age and year in Japan, 1995–98.

necropsy and/or lack of definite histological data. In the *Annual of the Pathological Autopsy Cases in Japan*, published by the Japanese Pathological Society, 222 cases with histologically confirmed malignant mesothelioma were recorded between 1974 and 1980, a frequency of 0.114% of all autopsy cases.[3] One-third of the cases of mesothelioma were of pleural origin. The reason for the low incidence of malignant mesothelioma is found in the history of the asbestos industry in Japan, as described below.

Aetiology

Asbestos and mesothelioma in Japan

A very small amount of asbestos, mainly chrysotile, is produced in Japan; therefore, the amount of asbestos imported is nearly equal to the total used. In the history of the Japanese asbestos industry, 30 000–40 000 tons was imported per year before World War II. Thereafter, imports of asbestos ceased between 1942 and 1948 because of the economic blockade of Japan during World War II and the complete destruction of industry as a result of the war. The latent period between initial exposure to asbestos and the onset of malignant mesothelioma is extremely long, nearly 40 years. The Australian Mesothelioma Surveillance Programme of 1979–85 has demonstrated that more than three-quarters of the 450 exposed cases were first exposed to asbestos during the time of its extensive use between 1930 and 1959.[4] The very low level of asbestos use in the period during and after the war (about 10 years) could account for the low incidence of mesothelioma in Japan today (Fig. 20.2), because of the long latent period associated with mesothelioma. The recovery of Japanese industry has been accelerating since the Korean War (1950–53), and the import

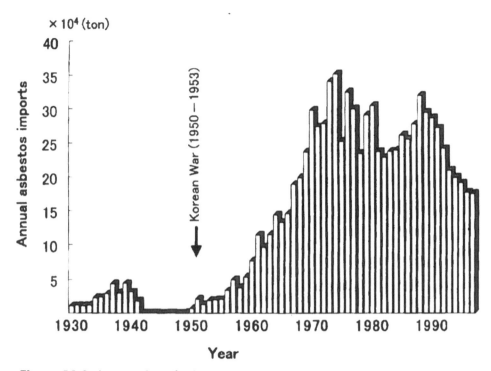

Figure 20.2. *Importation of asbestos into Japan, 1930–97.*

of asbestos vastly increased in the late 1960s. In contrast to the situation in Japan, the production and use of asbestos in the United States and other industrialised countries increased rapidly during and soon after World War II. In Japan, more than 300 000 tons of asbestos were imported between 1973 and 1977. Compared to the United States,[5] Great Britain,[6] and other industrialised countries, there is a time-lag of about 20 years in the increase in use of asbestos. After asbestos spraying was prohibited in 1974, asbestos consumption began to decrease in Japan. But, from the mid-1980s, an economic policy to increase domestic consumption so that Japan's trade surplus would decrease, markedly increased demand for building construction. The import of asbestos, therefore, rose again to 320 000 tons in 1988, but recently dropped again to 176 000 tons in 1997, because of the serious recession in the Japanese economy (Fig. 20.2). Japan is one of the greatest consumers of chrysotile asbestos and one of the largest producers of asbestos-containing products.[7,8] The highest incidences of mesothelioma are in those countries where there is or was a large production of crocidolite.[9,10] In Japan, however, only very small amounts of chrysotile and anthophyllite were produced. Considering the long latent period of about 40 years and the more than 300 000 tons of asbestos used between 1973 and 1977 in Japan, the incidence of malignant mesothelioma can be expected to increase dramatically hereafter, maybe from 2010.

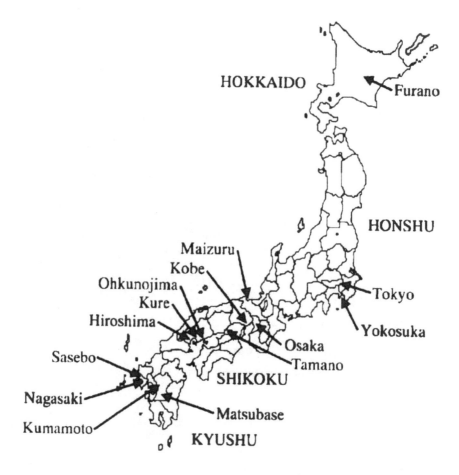

Figure 20.3. Map of Japan to show the locations of the naval shipyards (Yokosuka, Kure, Maizuru, Sasebo), private shipbuilding industries (Kobe, Osaka, Tamano), former asbestos mines (Matsubase, Furano), the former mustard-gas-weapons factory (Ohkunojima Island), Hiroshima and Nagasaki.

Geographical distribution of mesothelioma

The aetiological relationship between malignant mesothelioma and exposure to asbestos is well established.[11] Shipbuilding facilities are also clearly associated with significant increases in mortality as a result of pleural mesothelioma.[5,12] In Japan, there also tend to be clusters of cases of mesothelioma in areas where there are shipbuilding facilities.[13] The naval shipyards of the former Imperial Japanese Navy were located in Yokosuka (Kanagawa prefecture), Kure (Hiroshima prefecture), Sasebo (Nagasaki prefecture) and Maizuru (Kyoto prefecture) (Fig. 20.3). After World War II, the Maritime Self-Defence Forces used these shipyards. Private shipbuilding industries were located in Kobe (Hyogo prefecture), Osaka (Osaka prefecture) and Tamano (Okayama prefecture). Population-based epidemiological studies on asbestos-linked mesothelioma have been insufficient in Japan. Recently, a historical cohort mortality study of the workers at a United States Navy refitting shipyard in Yokosuka, Japan, was carried out.[14] However, the sample size was small and there was only one death from malignant pleural mesothelioma, of a boiler repairer, during the study period, to give a standardized mortality ratio of 55.56. Almost all the asbestos used in industry is imported, because of the very small amount of local chrysotile production.[15] Asbestos mines were located in the Matsubase district on Kyushu island and the Furano district on Hokkaido island (Fig. 20.3). In Matsubase, only small amounts of asbestos ore were mined initially from 1883, but the blockade of Japan during World War II compelled Japanese industries to obtain asbestos domestically. Therefore, several small-scale asbestos mines (chrysotile and anthophillite) were opened and factories operated actively.[16] Most of the asbestos was of poor quality, and only small amounts of high-quality fibres were moved to the asbestos factories in Osaka, Kobe and Tokyo. There was a high prevalence of pleural plaque in the residents in Matsubase who were more than 20 years old, but no cases of malignant mesothelioma were confirmed.[17] Fibre analysis of the lungs of 50 residents obtained at surgical resection or autopsy showed that the residents of Matsubase had significantly higher numbers of anthophyllite fibres in their lungs than the residents of regions where plaque occurred at the normal plaque frequency,[18] and that the fibres were quite long (mean length=25.1 μm) and thick (mean diameter=0.84 μm). These findings agree with Finnish studies.[19,20] Epidemiological studies in the Furano district on Hokkaido island have not yet been performed.

Radiation and other aetiological factors for mesothelioma

In approximately 20% of male and in most female mesothelioma patients, no history of asbestos exposure can be elicited.[1,21] Other aetiological factors are rare: the non-asbestos mineral fiber zeolite;[22] the virus SV-40;[23] and chronic inflammation as a result of tuberculosis, chemicals or radiation exposure.[24] Mesothelioma rarely develops as a second malignant neoplasm in the pleura within prior radiotherapy fields. In a cumulative review of 35 cases of post-irradiation malignant mesothelioma, the mean latent period between the radiation exposure and the development of mesothelioma was 19.5 years.[25] In 1945, during World War II, atomic bombs were dropped on Nagasaki and Hiroshima, where there were naval shipyards (Fig. 20.2). There is one case report of malignant pleural mesothelioma following exposure to atomic bomb radiation in Nagasaki.[26] This patient also had a history of asbestos exposure as a shipbuilder for a period of two years. According to the Atomic-Bomb Disasters database at Nagasaki University, 40 atomic bomb survivors died from primary malignant tumours of the pleura between 1970 and 1994, while 1217 survivors died from lung cancer.[26] It has been indicated that the morbidity rate of atomic bomb survivors with malignant mesothelioma is approximately 1/30 of that of atomic bomb survivors with lung cancer.[26] In preliminary experimental models, asbestos reacted synergistically with radiation to induce mesothelioma in rats.[27,28] The radiation-associated relative risk of a second primary cancer in patients whose first primary cancer was treated using radiotherapy has been compared with the radiation-associated relative risk estimates from the Japanese atomic bomb survivor cancer incidence data.[29] The relative risks in comparable (age at exposure, time since exposure, sex matched) subsets from the Japanese data are significantly greater than those in the majority of second primary cancer studies. There was no case report in English of malignant mesothelioma in atomic bomb survivors in Hiroshima. It is unfortunate that so little has been published in English in well-known journals. In the Japanese literature, however, a study of autopsied cases of malignant mesothelioma in Hiroshima district for 1959–85 shows a marked increase in malignant mesothelioma.[30] Age-adjusted mortality rates for mesothelioma from cancer registry data of 1982–86 were 0.8 per million in Hiroshima district and 2.5 per million in Nagasaki district, standardised to the world population.[2] Mesothelioma is sometimes difficult to diagnose, and a definite diagnosis requires well-trained clinicians and pathologists, so the true incidence may have been underestimated

Several chemicals, such as N-methyl-N-nitrosourea, sterigmatocystin (aflatoxin-B), and 3-methylcholanthrene, have been suggested as inducers of mesotheliomas in animal studies. In Japan, a factory manufacturing mustard gas (2,2'-dichlorodiethyl sulphide) weapons for the former Imperial Japanese Army was located on Ohkunojima island in the Hiroshima prefecture from 1929 until 1945 (Fig. 20.3). The workers in the gas factory suffered from respiratory illness. Autopsies were performed on 172 former workers, from 1952 to 1986, and showed that 54 (31.4%) had a malignant tumour in the respiratory tract, one of which was a malignant tumour of the pleura.[30]

The use of asbestos worldwide declined in the 1990s to approximately 50% of the peak in 1973. In most developed countries, asbestos is strictly banned, although Japan has not banned its use completely. Japan still imports a significant amount of chrysotile asbestos, and produces many asbestos-containing products under the controlled-use policy sponsored by the Japan Asbestos Association. There are on-going discussions of its risk on the incidence of malignant mesothelioma.

References

1. Chahinian, A.P., Rusch, V.W. Malignant mesothelioma. In: Holland, J.F., Bast, R.C., Morton, D.L., Frei, E., Kufe, D.W., Weichselbaum, R.R. eds. *Cancer medicine*. 4th edition. Baltimore: Williams & Wilkins, 1997; pp.1807–1826.
2. Morinaga, K., Fujimoto, I., Sakatani, M. *et al*. Epidemiology of asbestos-related diseases in Japan. In: Gibbs, G.W., Dunnigan, J., Kido, M., Higashi, T. eds. *Health risks from exposure to mineral fibers: an international perspective*. Ontario: Captus University Publications, 1993; pp. 247–253.
3. Baba, K. Indications of an increase of occupational pleural mesothelioma in Japan. *Sangyo Ika Daigaku Zasshi* 1983; **5**: 3–15.
4. Ferguson, D.A., Berry, G., Jelihovsky, T. *et al*. The Australian mesothelioma surveillance program 1979–1985. *Med J Aust* 1987; **147**: 166–172.
5. Enterline, P.E., Henderson, V.L. Geographic patterns for pleural mesothelioma deaths in the United States, 1968–81. *J Natl Cancer Inst* 1987; **79**: 31–37.
6. Peto, J., Hodgson, J.T., Matthews, F.E., *et al*. Continuing increase in mesothelioma mortality in Britain. *Lancet* 1995; **345**: 535–539.

7. Levy, B.S., Seplow, A. Asbestos-related hazards in developing countries. *Environ Res* 1992; **59**: 167–174.
8. Lemen, R.A., Bingham, E. A case study in avoiding a deadly legacy in developing countries. *Toxicol Ind Health* 1994: **10**: 59–87.
9. de Klerk, N., Armstrong, B. The epidemiology of asbestos and mesothelioma. In: Henderson, D.W., Shilkin, K.B., Langlois, S.P., Whitaker, D. eds. *Malignant mesothelioma*. New York : Hemisphere Publishing Corp., 1992; pp. 223–250.
10. Musk, A.W., de Klerk, N.H., Eccles, J.L. *et al*. Historical perspectives in occupational medicine. Wittenoom, Western Australia: a modern industrial disaster. *Am J Ind Med* 1992; **21**: 735–747.
11. McDonald, J.C., McDonald, A.D. Epidemiology of mesothelioma from estimated incidence. *Prev Med* 1977 **6**: 426–442.
12. Andersson, M., Olsen, J.H. Trend and distribution of mesothelioma in Denmark. *Br J Cancer* 1985; **51**: 699–705.
13. Kishimoto, T., Okada, K., Sato, T. *et al*. Evaluation of the pleural malignant mesothelioma patients with the relation of asbestos exposure. *Environ Res* 1989; **48**: 42-48.
14. Kurumatani, N., Natori, Y., Mizutani, R. *et al*. A historical cohort mortality study of workers exposed to asbestos in a refitting shipyard. *Ind Health* 1999; **37**: 9–17.
15. Morinaga, K., Kohyama, N., Yokoyama, K. *et al*. Asbestos fiber content in the lungs of mesothelioma in Osaka, Japan. In: Bignon J, Peto J, Saracci R, eds. Non-occupational exposure to mineral fibers. No. 90, Lyon: IARC Scientific Publications, 1989; pp. 438–443.
16. Hiraoka, T. Endemic pleural plaques in the town of Kyushu island of Japan. In: Gibbs GW, ed. Health risks from exposure to mineral fibers. Ontario: Captus University Publications, 1993; pp. 242–246.
17. Hiraoka, T., Ohkura, M., Morinaga, K. *et al*. Anthophyllite exposure and endemic pleural plaques in Kumamoto, Japan. *Scand J Work Environ Health* 1998; **24**: 392–397.
18. Murai, Y., Kitagawa, M., Hiraoka, T. Fiber analysis in lungs of residents of a Japanese town with endemic pleural plaques. *Arch Environ Health* 1997; **52**: 263–269.
19. Huuskonen, M.S. Asbestosis in Finland. Clinical and immunological findings and mortality among asbestosis patients. University of Helsinki: Academic Dissertation, 1979.
20. Kiviluoto, R. Pleural calcification as a roentgenologic sign of non-occupational endemic anthophyllite-asbestosis. *Acta Radiol* 1960; **194**(suppl): 1–65.
21. McDonald, J.C. Health implications of environmental exposure to asbestos. *Environ Health Perspect* 1985; **62**: 319.
22. Baris, Y.I., Saracci, R., Simonato, L. *et al*. Malignant mesothelioma and radiological chest abnormalities in two villages in central Turkey. An epidemiological and environmental investigation. *Lancet* 1981; **1**: 984.
23. Carbone, M., Pass, H.I., Rizzo, P. *et al*. Simian virus 40-like DNA sequences in human pleural mesothelioma. *Oncogene* 1994; **9**: 1781–1790.
24. Peterson, J.T., Greenberg, S.D., Buffler, P.A. Non-asbestos-related malignant mesothelioma. A review. *Cancer* 1984; **54**: 951–960.
25. Cavazza, A., Travis, L.B., Travis, W.D. *et al*. Post-irradiation malignant mesothelioma. *Cancer* 1996; **77**: 1379–1385.
26. Mizuki, M., Yukishige, K., Abe, Y., Tsuda, T. A case of malignant pleural mesothelioma following exposure to atomic radiation in Nagasaki. *Respirology* 1997; **2**: 201–205.
27. Lafuma, J., Hirsch, A., Monchaux, G. *et al*. Mesothelioma induced by intrapleural injection of different types of fibers in rats: Synergistic effect of other carcinogens. In: Wagner JC, ed. *Biological effects of mineral fibers*. No. 30, Lyon: IARC Scientific Publications, 1980; pp. 311–322.

28. Warren, S., Brown, C.E., Chute, R.N., *et al*. Mesothelioma relative to asbestos, radiation, and methylcholanthrene. *Arch Pathol Lab Med* 1981; **105**: 305–312.

29. Little, M.P., Muirhead, C.R., Haylock, R.G., *et al*. Relative risks of radiation-associated cancer: comparison of second cancer in therapeutically irradiated populations with the Japanese atomic bomb survivors. *Radiat Environ Biophys* 1999; **38**: 267–283.

30. Tokuoka, S., Inai, K. Lung cancer and related environmental factors. *Yakugaku Zasshi* 1988; **108**:1013–1022 [in Japanese].

Index

T - #0208 - 071024 - C0 - 246/174/20 - PB - 9780367396374 - Gloss Lamination